Dedicated to the memory of

Dr. Edward I. Curtiss

1938-2006

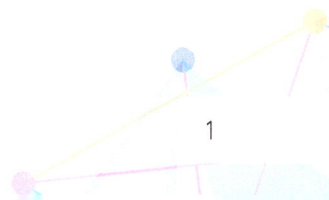

EKG PRIMER – YOUR GUIDE TO THE CARDIOLOGY ROTATION

ISBN-13: 978-0692490808 - ISBN-10: 0692490809

http://www.EKGPrimer.com

1st Edition

Printed in the United States of America by CreatSpace. Amazon.com Publishing Company

Disclaimer

The authors and the publisher of this book have taken care to use sources believed to be reliable to provide information that is accurate and compatible with standards generally accepted at the time of publication. The authors, editors, and publisher are not responsible for errors or omissions or for any consequences from application of the information in this book and make no warranty, expressed or implied, with respect to the completeness, or accuracy of the contents of the publication. Application of the information in a particular situation remains the professional responsibility of the practitioner. Medical science is continually advancing and our knowledge base continues to expand.

The authors, editors, and publisher have exerted every effort to ensure that the drug selection and dosage set forth in this text is in accordance with current recommendations and practice at the time of publication. However, in view of ongoing research, changes in government regulations, and the constant flow of information relating to drug therapy and drug reactions, the reader is urged to check the package insert for each drug for any change in indications and dosage and for added warnings and precautions. We recommend that the reader always consult current research and specific institutional policies before making clinical decisions. The authors have no responsibility for the persistence or accuracy of URLs for external or third-party Internet websites referred to in this publication and do not guarantee that any content on such websites is, or will remain, accurate or appropriate.

ISBN 978-0-692-49080-8

9 780692 490808 >

ABOUT THE AUTHORS

Samir F. Saba, MD, FACC, FHRS

Samir Saba (BE 1989, MD 1993) received his Bachelor's degree in Electrical Engineering in 1985 from the American University of Beirut and his Medical degree in 1993 from the same institution. He then finished his training in Internal Medicine (1993-1996), in Cardiolovascular Diseases (1996-1999), and in Cardiac Electrophysiology (1999-2000) all at the Tufts University – New England Medical Center in Boston, Massachusetts, prior to joining the faculty of the University of Pittsburgh Medical Center as an Assistant Professor of Medicine in the field of Cardiac Electrophysiology. Starting in 2005, Dr. Saba was appointed chief of the Cardiac Electrophysiology section and director of the cardiac electrophysiology laboratories at the University of Pittsburgh Medical Center. He was promoted to Associate Professor of Medicine and of Clinical and Translational Science in 2009. He was granted tenure by the University of Pittsburgh in August 2014 and promoted to Associate Chief of Cardiology for clinical affairs in 2015. He is currently a fellow of the American College of Cardiology and of the Heart Rhythm Society.

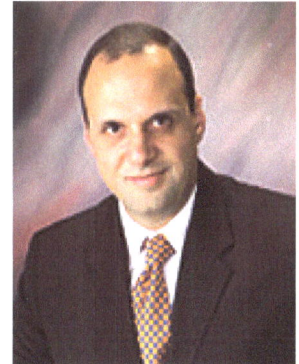

Mian Bilal Alam, MD

Mian Bilal Alam received his medical degree in 2005 from Ayub Medical College -Peshawar University, Pakistan. He then finished his Internal Medicine training from Temple University – Conemaugh Medical Center in Johnstown, Pennsylvania. He is currently working in the department of critical care medicine as a clinical Assistant Professor of Medicine at the University of Pittsburgh Medical Center.

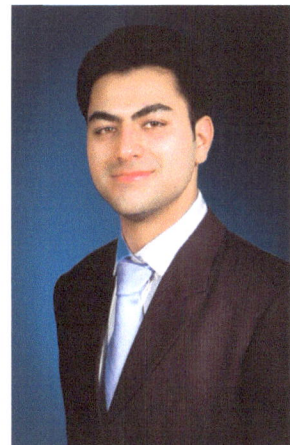

DEDICATIONS

TO MY WIFE, LAYLA AND CHILDREN NICOLAS, THOMAS, AND KARINA, WITH LOVE FOREVER.

SAMIR SABA

TO MY LOVING PARENTS, M. ALAM AND DR. SHAHEEN ALAM, MY WIFE, ZARA AND CHILDREN LUJAIN, HASSAN AND UMER.

BILAL ALAM

ACKNOWLEDGEMENTS

- Dr. Brahma N. Sharma. MD, FACC. Associate Professor of Medicine. University of Pittsburgh Medical Center

- Dr. Joon Sup Lee. MD, FACC. Chief, Division of Cardiology. Associate Professor of Medicine. University of Pittsburgh Medical Center

- Dr. Lydia S Davis MD, FACC. Clinical Assistant Professor of Medicine. University of Pittsburgh Medical Center

- Dr. Martha A. Pullins DO, FACC

- Dr. Saleem Ahmed. MD, FACC Clinical Assistant Professor of Medicine. Director Intervention Cardiology UPMC (Passavant)

- Dr. Sandeep Jain, MD, FACC. Associate Professor of Medicine. University of Pittsburgh Medical Center

- Dr. Shasank Rijal. MD, Hospital Medicine, University of Pittsburgh Medical Center

- Judy Galiano, Coordinator, Central Heart Station, University of Pittsburgh Medical Center

- Kathleen Zell, RN, MSN. Executive Director, Heart & Vascular Services. University of Pittsburgh Medical Center

- Dr. Asif Nawaz Khan, MD and Dr. Mehwish Asad, MD

Special thanks to Open-Source EKG resources

- Lifeinthefastlane.com (LIFL) and FOAM (Free Open Access Meducation). Support #FOAMed project. Some of the content (text and images) used in this book were reproduced with permission from LIFL.

- ECG University of Utah School of Medicine http://ecg.utah.edu/

- Wikidoc Wikidoc.org/index.php/The_electrocardiogram

- OpenStax College. Openstaxcollege.org/books

- ECGPedia.org

- ECGGuru.org

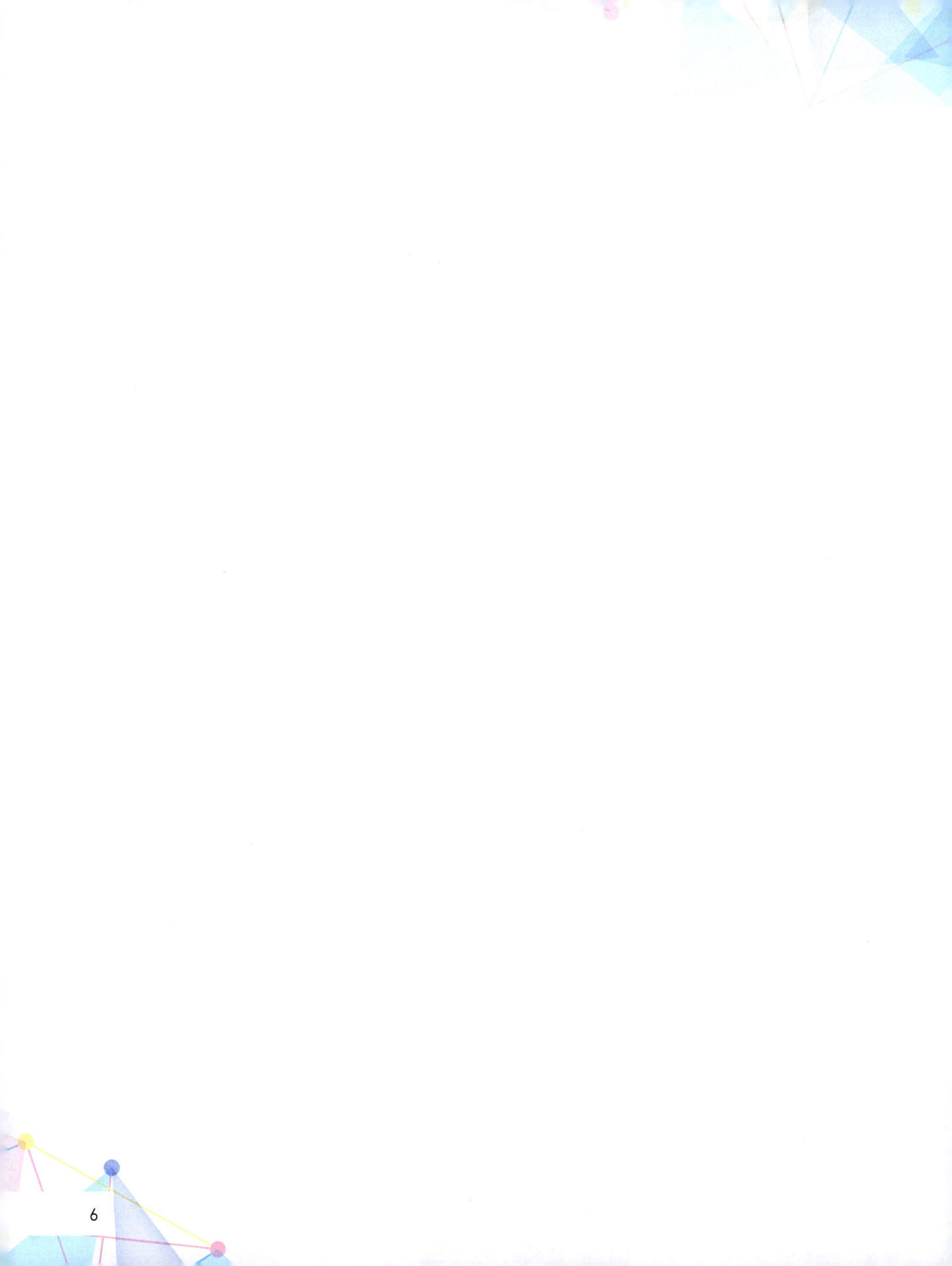

PREFACE

Although the surface electrocardiogram (abbreviated as ECG or EKG) was invented by the Dutch physician and physiologist Willem Einthoven in 1903—earning him the Nobel Prize in Medicine in 1924—it continues to be today, more than a century later, an essential tool used by clinicians for the detection and diagnosis of numerous cardiac conditions such as ischemia, arrhythmias, or congenital heart abnormalities, as well as for the immediate management of critically ill patients, such as those presenting to the emergency department with acute myocardial infarction. In addition, the EKG has also proven to be useful in detecting numerous non-cardiac conditions, such as drug toxicities, electrolyte abnormalities, or infectious illnesses like Lyme disease, to name just a few. From its original form as a simple resting measure of cardiac electrical activity projected onto 12 vectors or leads, the EKG morphed over the years into other forms better adapted to the ambulatory needs of monitoring. These other forms include Holter and event monitors, electrocardiographic stress test machines, and implantable EKG recorders, which can be triggered to store events either manually or automatically. Now there are even tools that allow patients to record a single-lead EKG tracing on their own iPhone through a battery pack that can be connected to the smartphone and held with both hands, each touching one of two built-in electrodes. This evolution of technology has resulted in a significant improvement in the diagnostic capability of EKG tracings, adapting to the varying needs of patients who present with diverging symptoms including chest pain, palpitations, dizziness, shortness of breath, syncope, and many others.

Because of its high importance in the clinical management of many patients across vast areas of medical and surgical specialties, it is not too surprising that the medical community has invested, over many decades, a lot of time, effort, and resources into training physicians, nurses, and other allied professionals on how to obtain, troubleshoot, and interpret EKGs. In fact, acquiring proficiency in EKG reading is a primary focus of medical training in general, particularly cardiology training. It is part of medical school *curricula* and of board examinations in cardiovascular diseases, but also in internal medicine and anesthesia. Equally important is the fact that student, residents, and even fellows are often put on the spot by a more senior physician asking them to interpret an interesting EKG or identify its main finding. Knowing how to read EKGs can turn this common but uncomfortable situation into an opportunity to impress and shine.

Like most tasks in life, learning how to read EKGs requires practice. Of course it involves acquiring a very basic understanding of the physics and physiology of EKG recordings, but it mostly hinges on being exposed to a lot of EKGs, both normal and abnormal. With time and practice, the process eventually becomes automatic, allowing the expert reader to rely more on pattern recognition to spot abnormalities and make a diagnosis rather than on a step-by-step, systematic reading (rate, then rhythm, then axis, etc.) the way we all started.

With of all these considerations in mind, we embarked on the journey of writing this book about a year ago, compiling relevant EKGs that cover most topics of interest (arrhythmias, conduction abnormalities, electrolyte imbalances, etc.), providing a clinical vignette for each case, a succinct interpretation of the findings, a mechanistic explanation of these findings, and often offering insight into possible treatment options. From the outset and throughout the process of putting together this book, we kept in mind the needs and desires of our potential readers, who include medical students, residents in internal medicine or anesthesia, general cardiology and electrophysiology fellows, as well as registered nurses, EKG technicians, and other allied professional, such as nurse practitioners and physician assistants. For all these groups, we wanted to provide an easy tool to help them learn and fine tune their skills in EKG interpretation. By providing them this book, with over hundred high-quality EKG tracings compiled over many years, we wanted to expose them to some of the most common EKG findings that they will undoubtedly encounter throughout their professional careers, thus preparing them to promptly recognize the condition and nail the correct diagnosis. Throughout this book, cases are grouped by categories (e.g, atrioventricular block or myocardial infarction) and each one will consist of an EKG, a clinical vignette, a diagnosis, and an explanation of the findings, and even a management plan. Book and manuscript references are cited at the end of each case. Often a case in this book will reference another when similar or related concepts are tested and discussed.

This project would have not been possible without contributions from many key individuals that we here recognize. Many thanks to Kitty Zell, Director of Operations within the Heart and Vascular Institute (HVI) at the University of Pittsburgh Medical Center (UPMC), who helped us navigate our institutional regulatory process in order to obtain the permissions necessary to publish this book. Also, a big thank you to Dr. Joon Lee MD, Chief of Cardiology and Co-Director of the UPMC HVI, for his support and encouragement for this project, as always. To Drs. Sandeep Jain, Brahma Sharma, Ahmed Saleem, Lydia Davis, and Martha Pullins, cardiologists at UPMC, who—in record time—did the thankless job of proofreading the book for accuracy of interpretation and clinical information: a big thank you. Finally, our acknowledgement and appreciation go to the late Dr. Ed Curtis to whose memory we dedicate this book: he was a superb cardiologist and clinician who taught EKG readings to many generations of medical students and trainees in cardiology, and to whose EKG library we owe many of the tracings that we include in this book.

Our ultimate goal with this book is to give current and future health professionals a tool that will provide them with the knowhow and confidence to hold an EKG tracing in their hands, troubleshoot it, read it, and move on to delivering high-quality care to patients. Academic life in medicine stands on three essential pillars: (1) We strive to improve patient outcomes through sound clinical care; (2) We advance knowledge through innovative research; and (3) We perpetuate knowledge through tireless and consistent teaching and training. This book is our small contribution to this third and most important pillar of academic medicine.

Samir Saba, MD, FACC, FHRS
Associate Professor of Medicine
Associate Professor in Clinical and Translational Science
Associate Chief of Cardiology, Clinical Affairs
Director, Cardiac Electrophysiology
University of Pittsburgh Medical Center
200 Lothrop Street, PUH B535
Pittsburgh, PA 15213
sabas@upmc.edu
Phone: (412) 647 6272
Fax: (412) 647 7979

Sinoatrial (SA)node

Bachman's
bundle

Atrioventricular
(AV) node

Left Bundle
Branch

Atrioventricular
bundle
(Bundle of His)

Left Posterior
Fascicle

Right Bundle Branch

Left Anterior
Fascicle

Purkinje Fibers

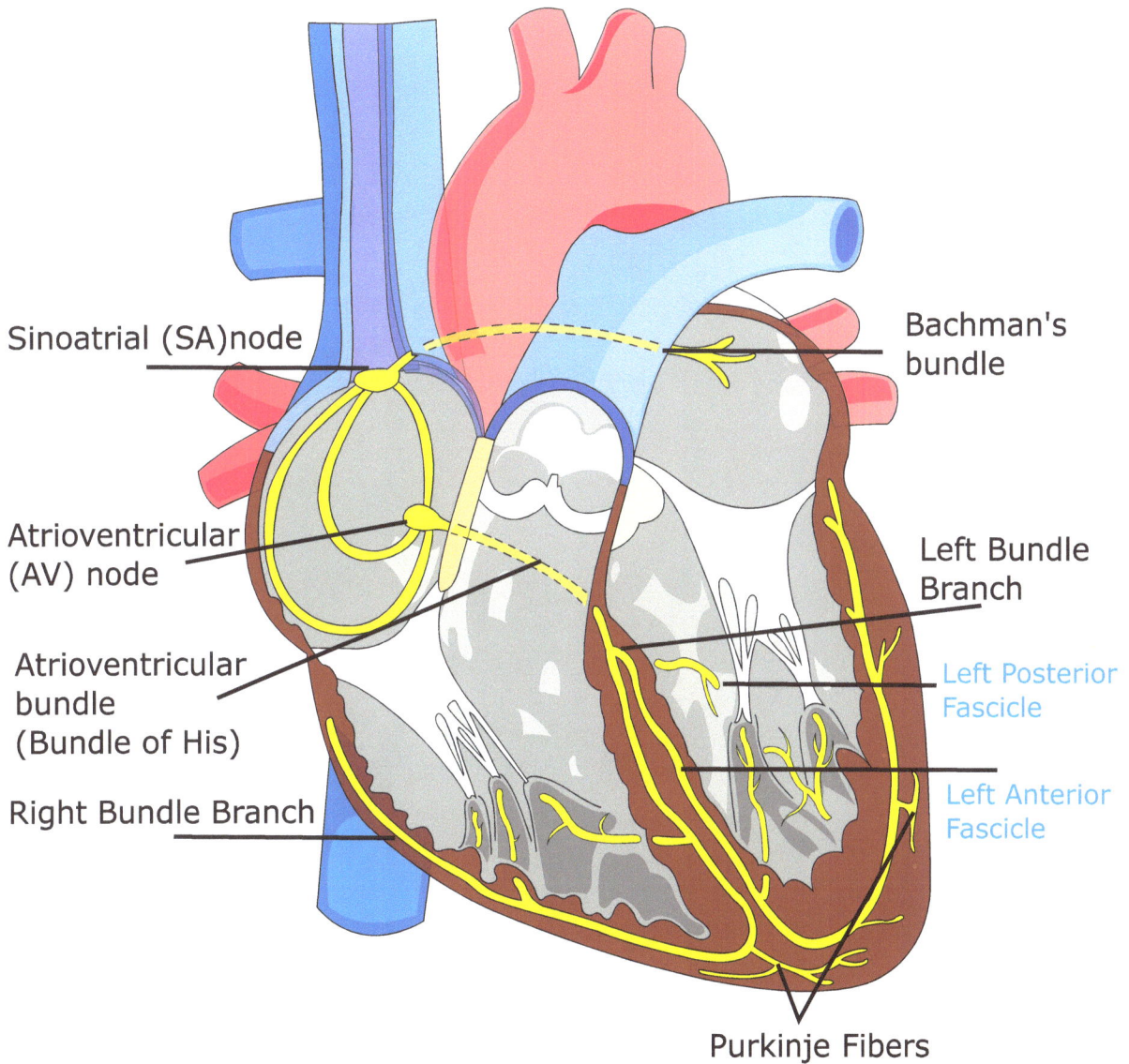

Figure A. Conduction System of the Heart

IMAGE ATLAS – HEART CYCLE

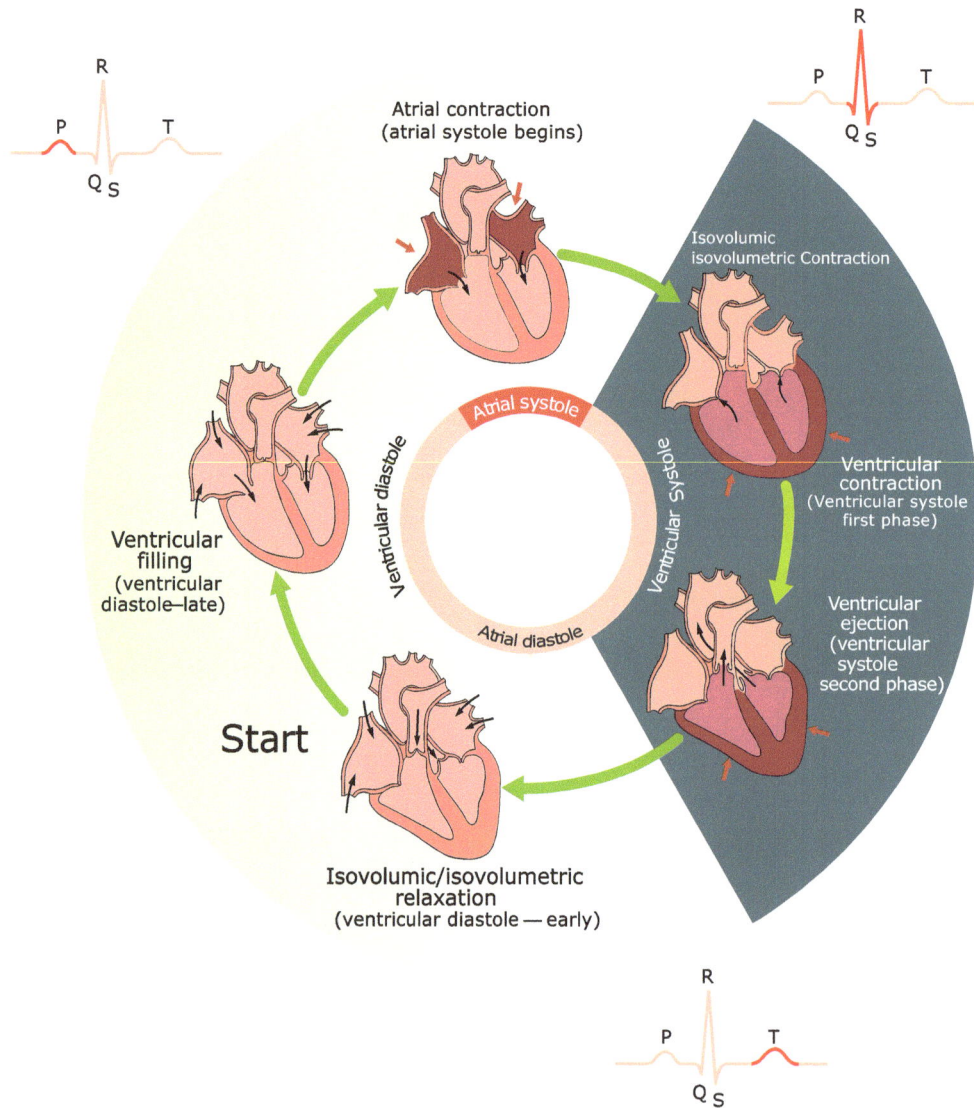

Figure B. The cardiac cycle begins with atrial systole and progresses to ventricular systole, atrial diastole, and ventricular diastole, when the cycle begins again. Correlations to the EKG are highlighted.

IMAGE ATLAS - AXIS

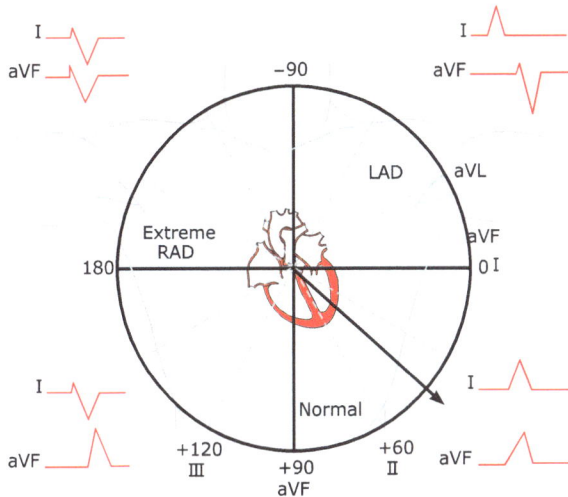

Figure C. Circle of Axes

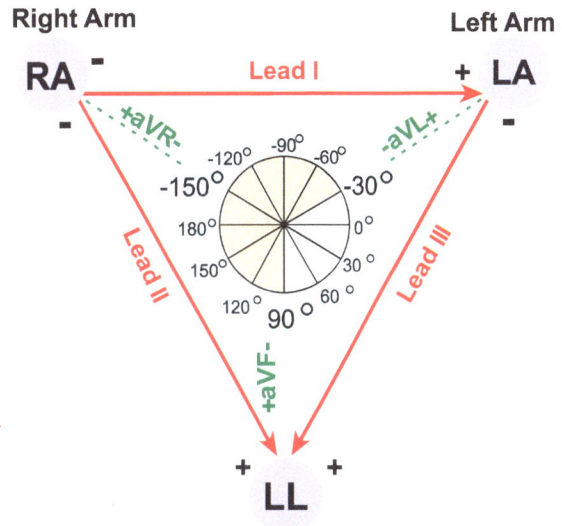

Figure D. Einthoven's Triangle

- The cardiac axis refers to the mean direction of the wave of ventricular depolarization in the vertical plane, as measured from a zero reference point. The zero axis is parallel to lead I. A normal heart axis is between -30 and +90 degrees.

- Left Axis Deviation (LAD) is present when the QRS in lead I is positive and negative in II (between -30 and -90 degrees).

- Right Axis Deviation (RAD) is present when lead I is negative and AVF positive (between +90 and +180).

- Extreme Right Axis Deviation, also known as " North West axis" is present when both I and AVF are negative. (Axis between -90 and +180 degrees).

ACRONYM AND ABBREVIATIONS

AET - Atrial Ectopic Tachycardia

AF - Atrial Fibrillation

AHCM - Apical Hypertrophic Cardiomyopathy

AICD - Automatic Implantable Cardioverter Defibrillator

AIVR - Accelerated Idioventricular Rhythm

AJR - Accelerated Junctional Rhythm

AMI - Anterior Myocardial Infarction

APB - Atrial Premature Beat

APC - Atrial Premature Contraction

Apps - application

ARVC - Arrhythmogenic Right Ventricular Cardiomyopathy

ASD - Atrial Septal Defect

AT - Atrial Tachycardia

AV - Atrioventricular (node)

AVNRT - AV Nodal Reentrant Tachycardia

AVRT - Atrioventricular Reentrant Tachycardia

BP - blood pressure

bpm - beats per minute

CACP - Cocaine Associated Chest Pain

CAD - Coronary Artery Disease

CHF - Congestive Heart Failure

COPD - Chronic Obstructive Pulmonary Disease

CPVT - Catecholaminergic Polymorphic Ventricular Tachycardia

CT - Computed Tomography

DM - Diabetes Mellitus

EKG and ECG - Electrocardiogram

ER - Early Repolarization

ER - Emergency Room

HCM - Hypertrophic Cardiomyopathy

HTN - Hypertension

ICD - Implantable Cardioverter-Defibrillator

ICU - Intensive Care Unit

IV - Intravenous

IVCD - Interventricular Conduction Delay

LAD - Left Anterior Descending Artery

LAD - Left Axis Deviation

LAFB - Left Anterior Fascicular Block

LBBB - Left Bundle Branch Block

LCA - Left Coronary Artery

LMA - Left Marginal Artery

LMCA - Left Main Coronary Artery

LPFB - Left Posterior Fascicular Block

LQTS - Long QT Syndrome

LV - Left Ventricle

LVH - Left ventricular hypertrophy

MAT - Multifocal Atrial Tachycardia

MI - Myocardial Infarction

MRI - Magnetic Resonance Imaging

ms (msec) - millisecond

NSVT- Non-Sustained Ventricular Tachycardia

PAC - Premature Atrial Contraction

PDA - Posterior Descending Artery

PE - Pulmonary Embolism

PIV - Posterior Interventricular Artery

PJRT - Permanent Junctional Reciprocating Tachycardia

PMI - Posterior Myocardial Infarction

PSVT - Paroxysmal Supraventricular Tachycardia

RAD - Right Axis Deviation

RBBB - Right Bundle Branch Block

RCA - Right Coronary Artery

RMA - Right Marginal Artery

RV - Right Ventricle

RVH – Right ventricular hypertrophy

RVOT - Right Ventricular Outflow Tract (Tachycardia)

SA - Sinoatrial (node)

SCD - Sudden Cardiac Death

sec - second

STE - ST Elevation

STEMI - ST Elevation Myocardial Infarction

SVT - Supraventricular Tachycardia

TCM - Takotsubo Cardiomyopathy

TdP - Torsades de Pointes

TEE - Transesophageal Echocardiography

TTE - Transthoracic Echocardiogram

VSD - Ventricular Septal Defect

WAP - Wandering Atrial Pacemaker

WPW - Wolff–Parkinson–White (syndrome)

TABLE OF CONTENTS

EKG Case 1

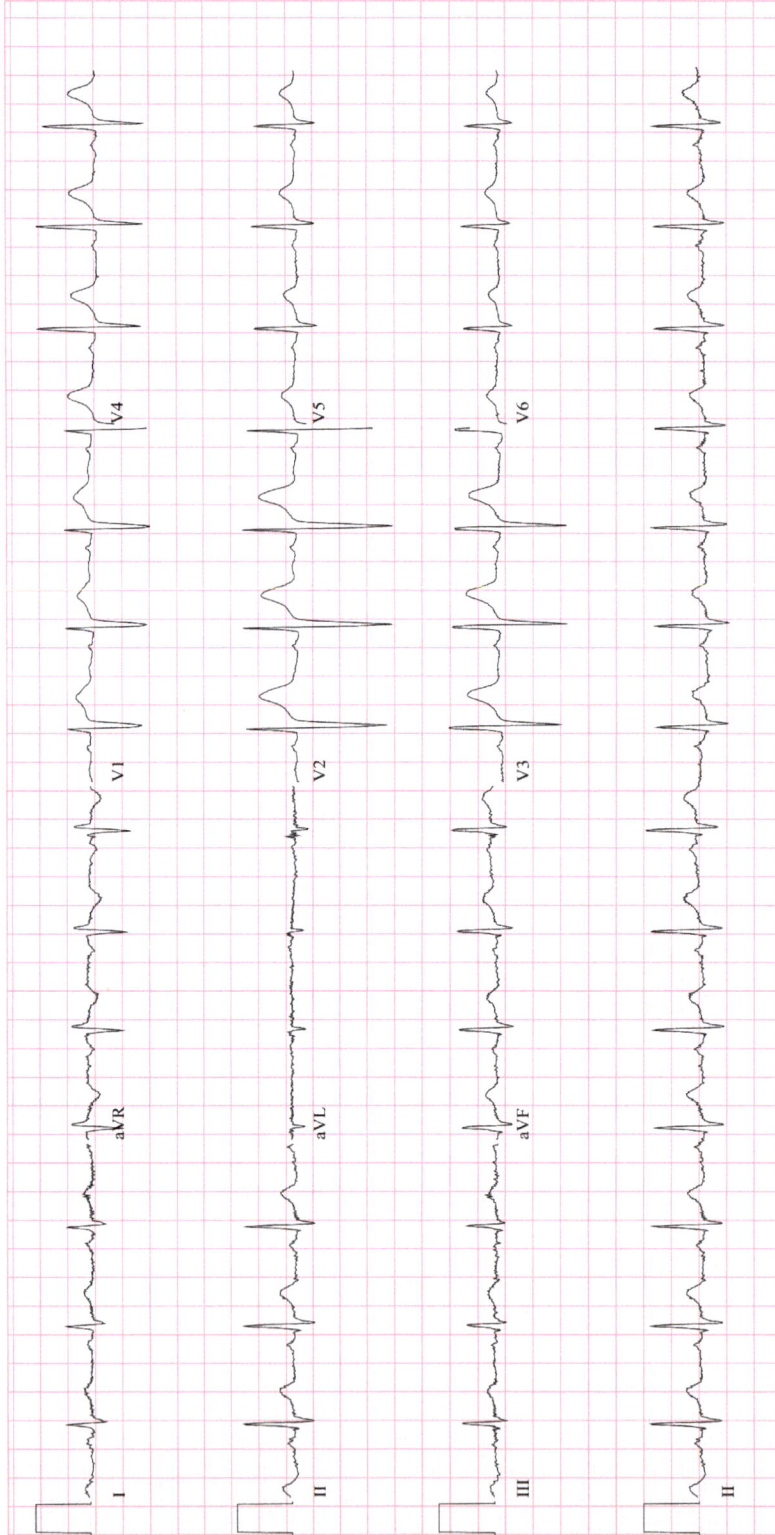

A 25 year-old male is brought to the hospital after motor vehicle accident. Patient denies chest pain or shortness of breath. Labs and CT scan of chest are within normal limits. An EKG is obtained. What does it show?

DIAGNOSIS: Normal Sinus Rhythm

This EKG is within normal limits. The rhythm is sinus at a rate of about 80 beats per minute. PR interval 132 ms (normal 120 – 200 ms), QRS duration 88 ms (normal 70 -100 ms), and QT interval 372 ms. The mean QRS axis is about +30 degrees. The P wave morphology and duration are normal. There is no evidence of left or right ventricular hypertrophy. R wave progression is normal in the precordial leads, and T wave axis in the frontal and horizontal planes is normal. ST segments are also normal.

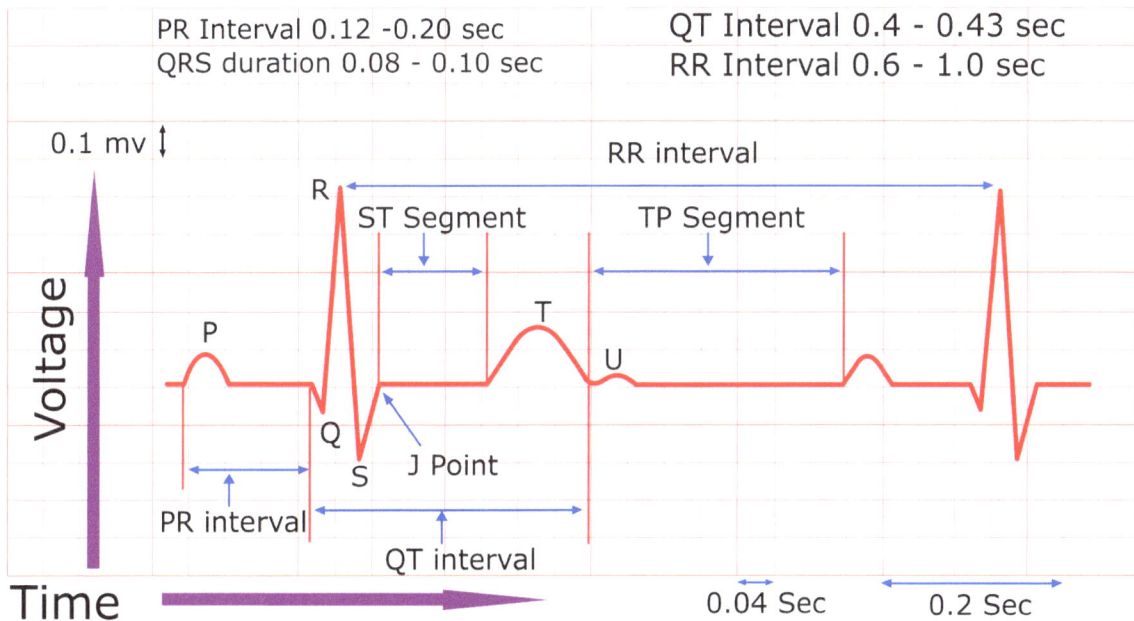

Figure: A normal EKG tracing showing various waves and intervals.

Characteristics of normal sinus rhythm: Regular rhythm at a rate of 60 -100 bpm at rest (or age-appropriate rate in children). Each QRS complex is preceded by a normal P wave. Normal P wave axis: P waves should be upright in leads I and II, inverted in aVR.

EKG Case 2

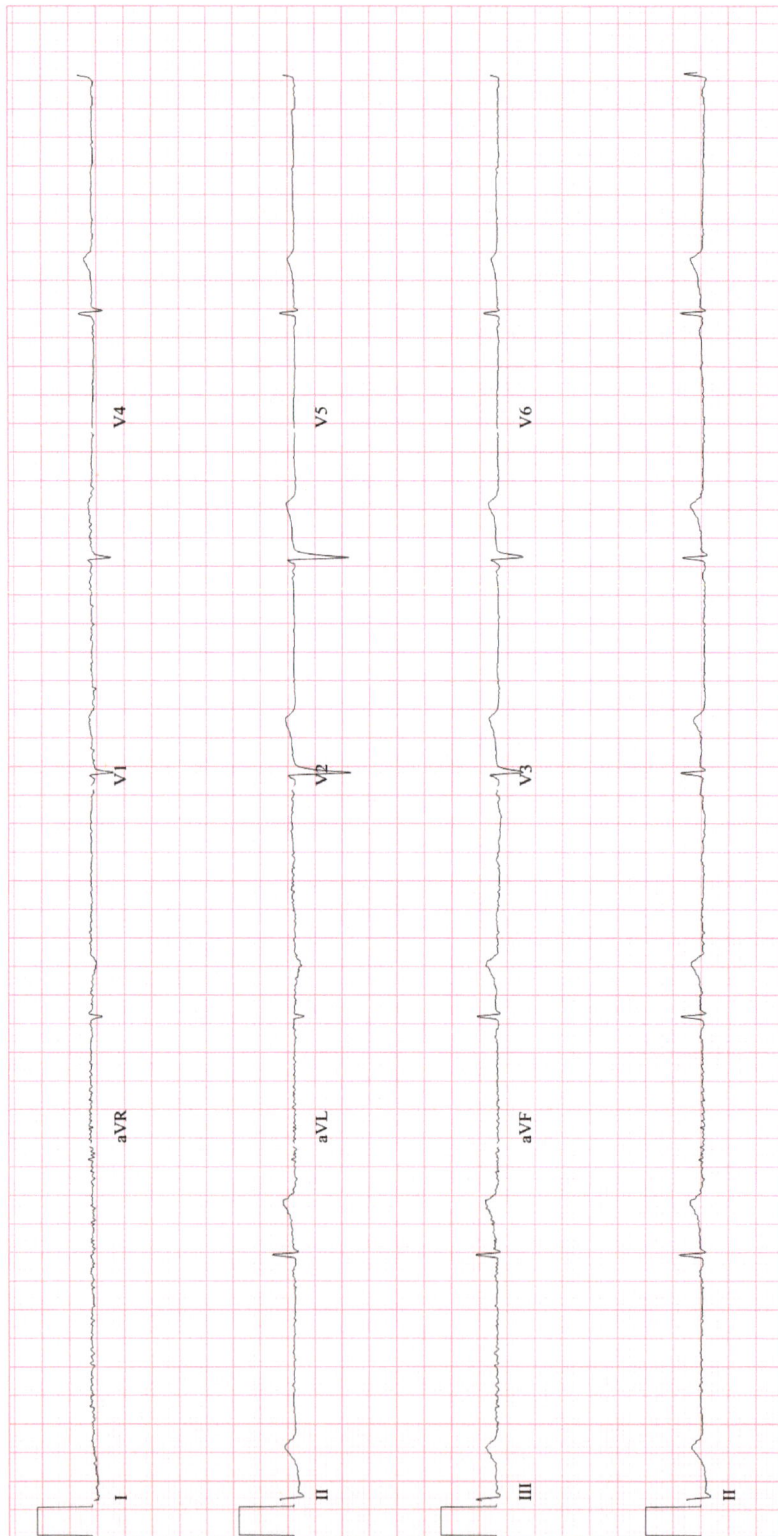

A 30-year old overweight female with a history of anorexia nervosa is brought to the ER with complaints of nausea and vomiting. What does the EKG show?

DIAGNOSIS: Sinus Bradycardia in Anorexia Nervosa patient

Sinus bradycardia is defined as sinus rhythm with a resting heart rate of < 60 bpm in adults, or below the normal range for age in children.

There are several ways of measuring heart rate. For sinus bradycardia, we recommend using the "300" method. Check that the EKG has been recorded at the standard US paper speed of 25 mm/s. One minute of EKG tracing covers 300 large squares. If the rhythm is regular, count the number of large squares between 2 consecutive QRS complexes and divide 300 by the number of large squares. In our case, we have 8 large squares between consecutive QRS complexes, which translates into a heart rate of 300/8 or ~38 bpm.

Number of Large Boxes	Rate / Min
1	300
2	150
3	100
4	75
5	60
6	50
7	43
8	38
9	33
10	30

The differential diagnosis of sinus bradycardia includes: resting or sleeping, increased vagal tone (e.g, athletes), vagal stimulation (e.g, pain), inferior myocardial infarction, sinus node disease, hypothyroidism, hypothermia, anorexia nervosa, electrolyte abnormalities – hyperkalemia, hypermagnesaemia, brainstem herniation (the Cushing reflex), and medications such as beta-blockers, nondihydropyridine calcium channel blockers, clonidine and lithium, etc.

Sinus bradycardia occurs in about 95% of patients with anorexia nervosa and is the most common EKG feature associated with this condition. It is important to appreciate the significance of sinus bradycardia in this clinical setting because it may be associated with sudden death, especially in the presence of other arrhythmias or EKG abnormalities, such as QT/QTc interval prolongation due to electrolyte disturbances.

EKG Case 3

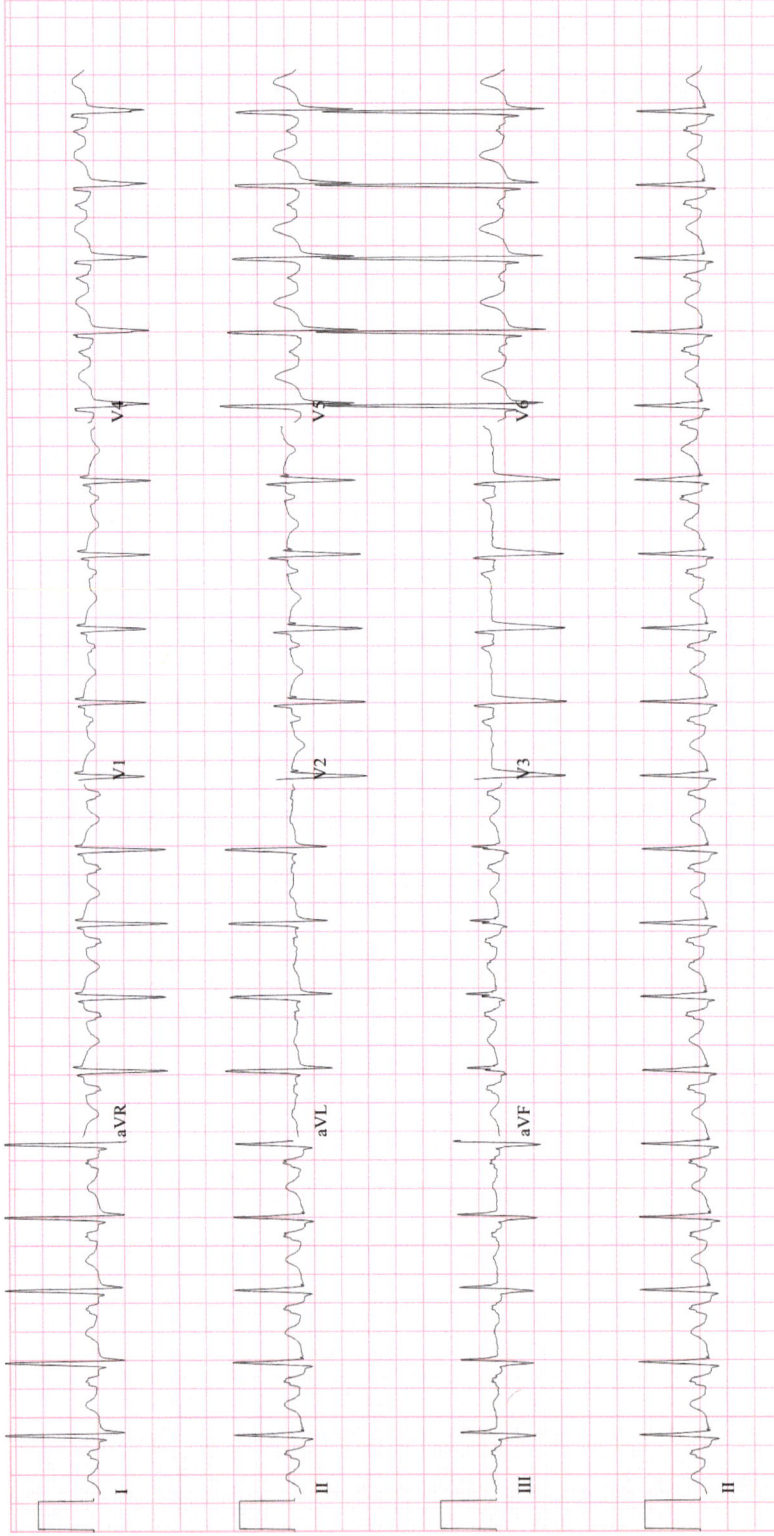

A 65-year old woman with a history of coronary artery disease is admitted to the ICU with septic shock. Her BP is 60/40 and she is on an IV norepinephrine drip. An EKG is obtained. What does it show?

DIAGNOSIS: Sinus Tachycardia

This EKG shows sinus tachycardia at 130 bpm. Left ventricular hypertrophy by voltage criteria (the Cornell-criterion for LVH). M shaped P waves in lead II with p prominent terminal negative component to P wave in lead V1 signifying left atrial abnormality.

- Sinus Tachycardia (Heart rate calculation is described in previous case).
- Sinus tachycardia is sinus rhythm with a rate of > 100 bpm.
- Sinus tachycardia is an example of a supraventricular rhythm. In sinus tachycardia, the sinus node fires at a rate above 100 bpm, which is faster than normal at rest. The maximal sinus rate that can be achieved decreases with age and can be estimated by subtracting the age in years from 220.
- Sinus tachycardia normally has a gradual onset and offset.
- Most often sinus tachycardia is caused by an increase in the body's demand for oxygen, such as during exercise, stress, infection, blood loss, and hyperthyroidism. It can also represent a compensatory mechanism for reduced stroke volume, as in the case of cardiomyopathy.

Some of the causes of sinus tachycardia include:

Exercise, anxiety, alcohol, caffeine use and drugs (e.g, beta-agonists like dobutamine), fever, hypotension, hypoxia, systolic congestive heart failure, anemia, hyperthyroidism and myocarditis etc. When no clear explanation for persistent sinus tachycardia can be found, the condition is termed "Inappropriate sinus tachycardia".

- LVH, Inferior wall MI, and atrial abnormalities are described further in the book.

EKG Case 4

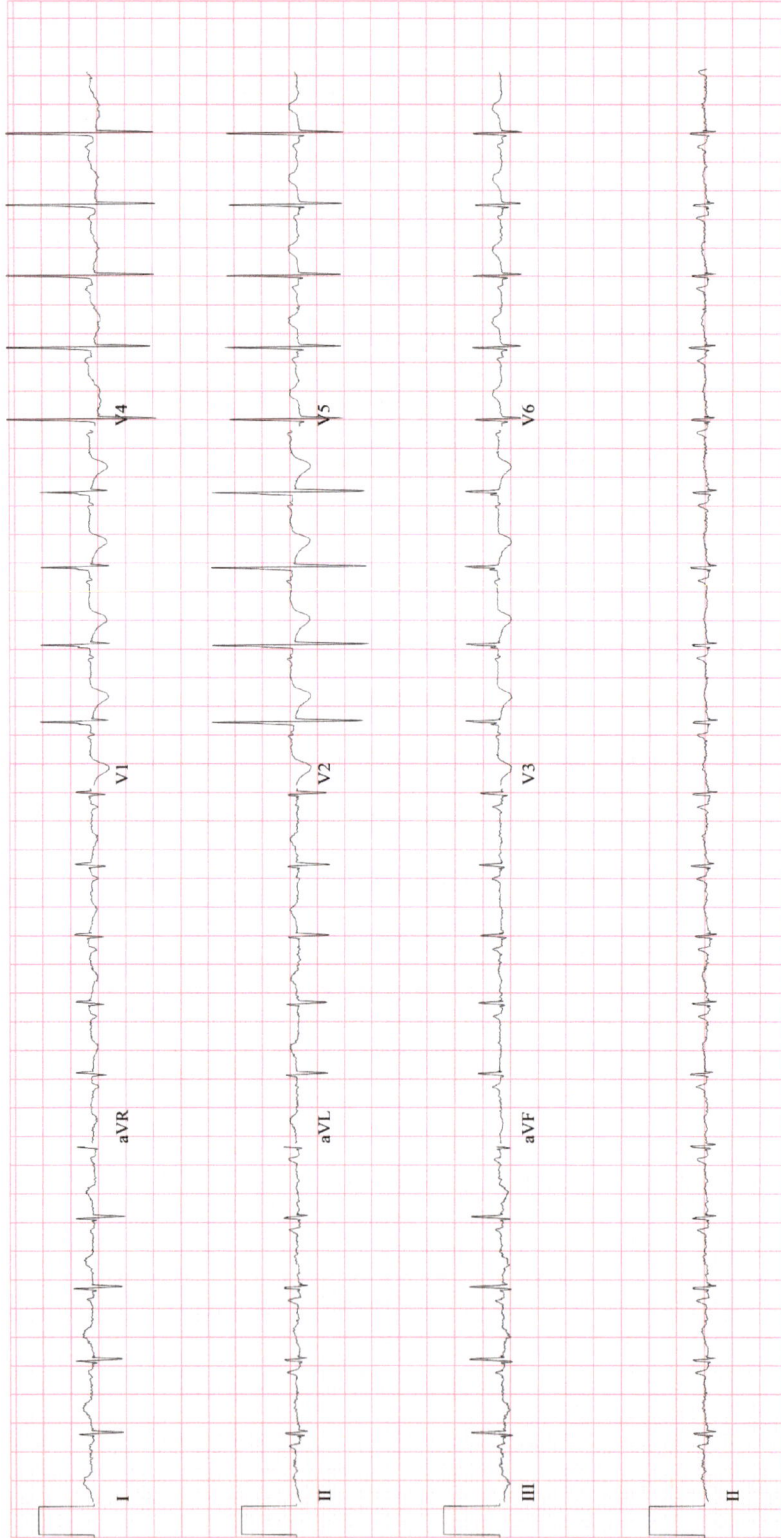

An EKG is recorded on a 2- day-old female neonate who is admitted in ICU with respiratory distress syndrome. What does the EKG show?

DIAGNOSIS: Normal Pediatrics EKG

This is a normal pediatrics EKG with normal sinus rhythm at 120 bpm.

- At birth, the right ventricle is larger and thicker than the left ventricle, reflecting the greater physiological stresses placed upon it in utero (i.e, pumping blood through the relatively high-resistance pulmonary circulation).

- This produces an EKG pattern suggestive of right ventricular hypertrophy in the adult, i.e, marked rightward axis, dominant R wave in V1, and T-wave inversions in V1-V3.

- Conduction intervals (PR interval, QRS duration) are shorter than those of adults due to the smaller cardiac size.

- Heart rates are much faster in neonates and infants, decreasing as the child grows older.

Common normal electrocardiographic features on the Pediatrics EKG

- Heart rate > 100 bpm
- Rightward QRS axis > +90°
- T wave inversions in V1-3 ("juvenile T-wave pattern")
- Dominant R wave in V1
- RSR' pattern in V1
- Marked sinus arrhythmia
- Short PR interval (< 120ms) and QRS duration (< 80ms)
- Slightly peaked P waves (< 3mm in height is normal if ≤ 6 months)
- Q waves in the inferior and left precordial leads

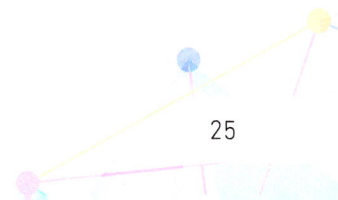

EKG Case 5

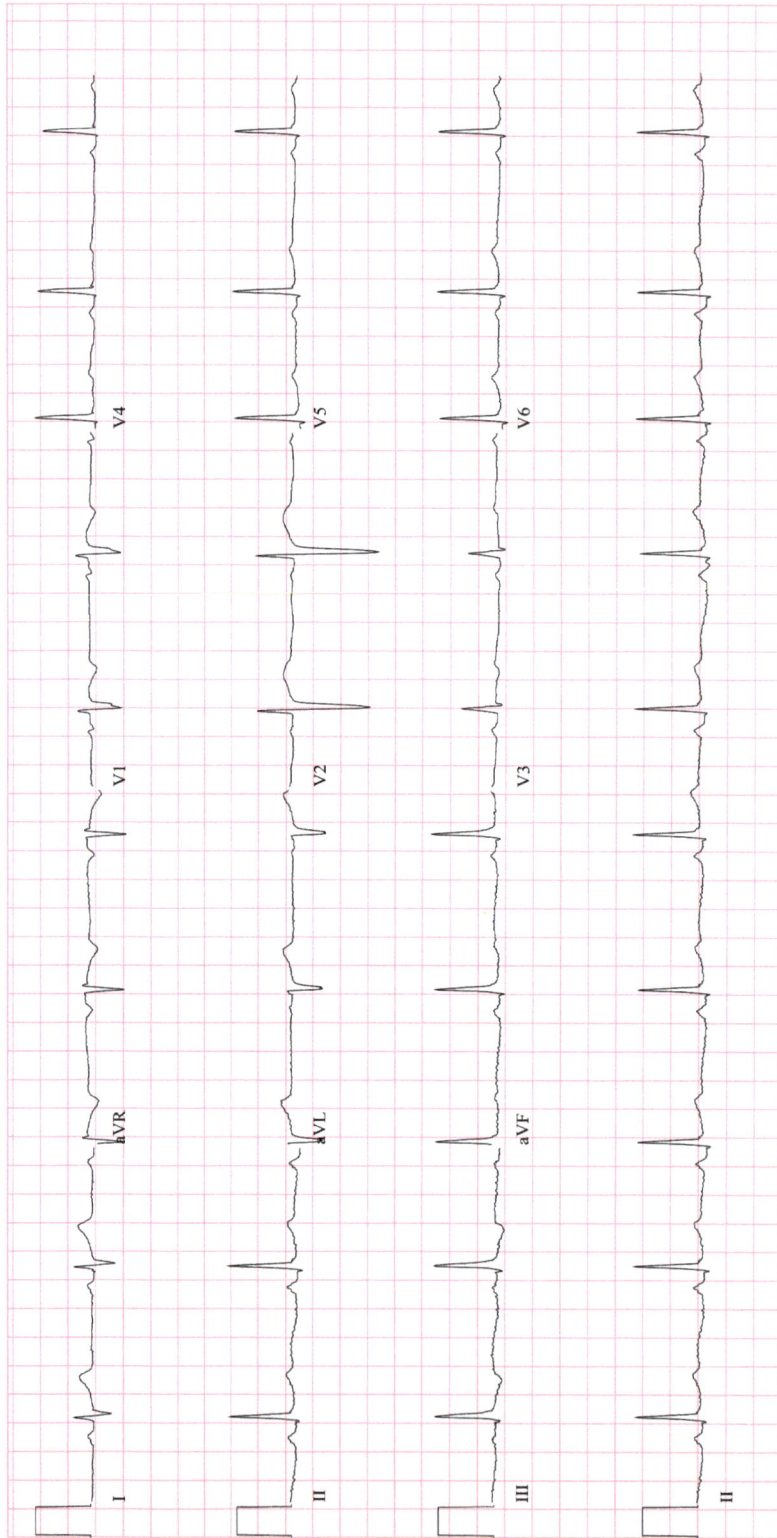

A 20-year-old female is seen in the office for an annual regular visit. She is found to have an irregular pulse. Should she be concerned about this arrhythmia?

DIAGNOSIS: Sinus Arrhythmia

This EKG shows normal sinus rhythm at 60 bpm with variable RR Interval.

- Sinus arrhythmia is a variant of sinus rhythm with a beat-to-beat variation in the R-R interval (> 0.16 sec) variation, producing an irregular ventricular rate with a pattern of cyclic acceleration and deceleration.

- The R-R interval gradually lengthens and shortens in a cyclical fashion, usually corresponding to the phases of the respiratory cycle.

- Normal sinus P waves with a constant morphology (i.e, no evidence of premature atrial contractions). Constant P-R interval (i.e, no evidence of Mobitz I AV block).

- Sinus arrhythmia is a normal physiological phenomenon, most commonly seen in young, healthy people. The heart rate varies due to reflex changes in vagal tone during the different stages of the respiratory cycle. Inspiration increases the heart rate by decreasing vagal tone. With the onset of expiration, vagal tone is restored, leading to a subsequent decrease in heart rate.

- The incidence of sinus arrhythmia decreases with age, presumably due to age-related decreases in carotid baroreceptor reflex sensitivity.

- Sinus arrhythmia can be very pronounced in patients with a high vagal tone or vasovagal syncope.

EKG Case 6

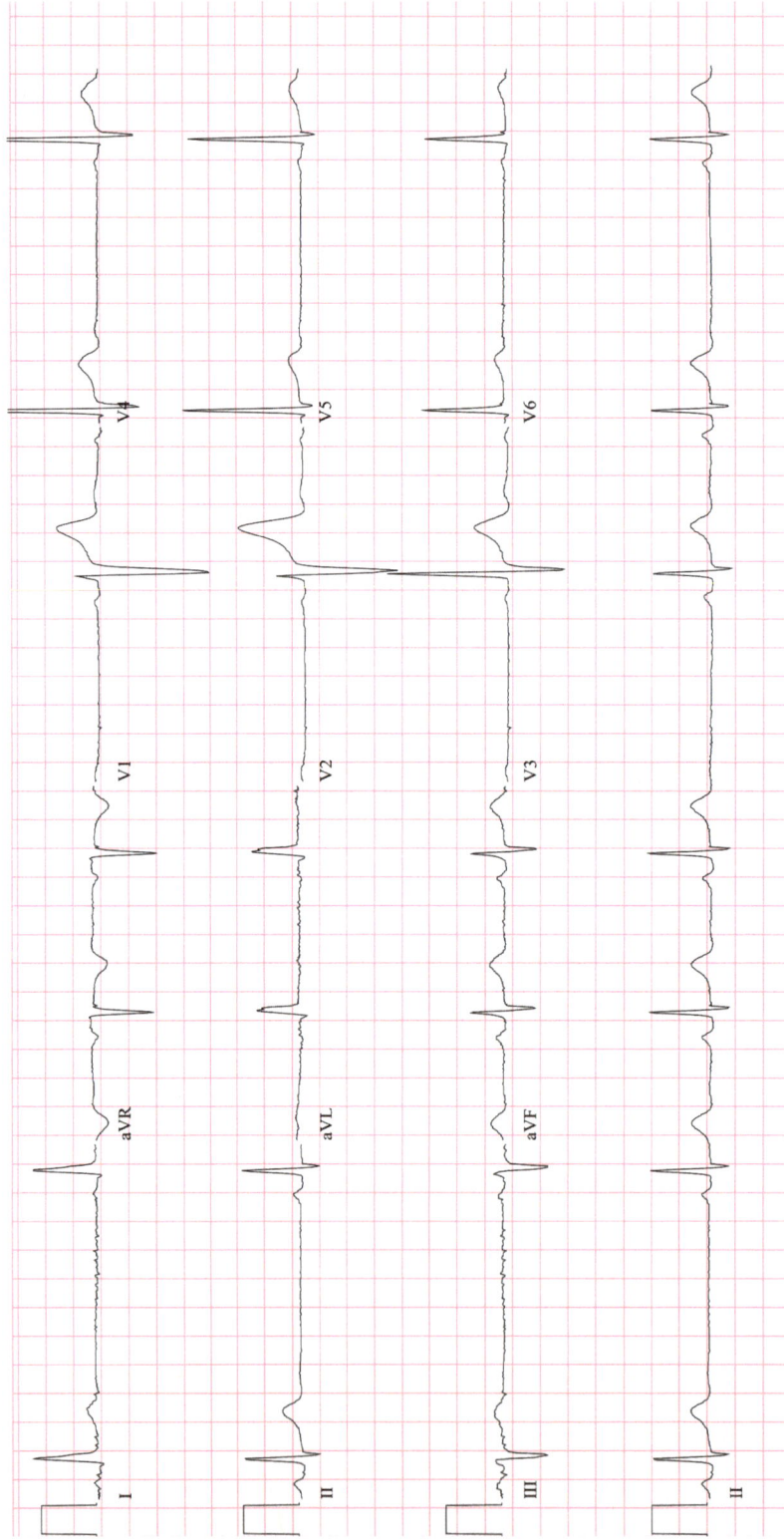

A 70-year-old man presented to the outpatient clinic with a sensation of "fluttering" in his chest. He also has lightheadedness and dizziness during these episodes. An EKG was obtained. What does it show?

DIAGNOSIS: Sinus Pause

This EKG shows sinus bradycardia with three sinus pauses. Heart rate is 55. The first and third sinus pauses are 2 seconds in duration whereas the second sinus pause is ~ 1.96 seconds in duration. The pauses are followed by resumption of sinus node activity. There is absence of P wave activity for a variable and unpredictable period of time that is not a multiple of the ambient sinus rate.

- EKG features include an absence of P wave due to transient failure of sinus node impulse generation; the next P wave does not appear where expected. The P-P interval of the pause is not a multiple of the baseline (normal) P-P interval in case of sinus pause/arrest. This feature is used to differentiate sinus pause/arrest from sinoatrial block where the P-P interval of the pause is a multiple of the normal P-P interval.

- The sinus node fails to produce an impulse on time and there is an absence of electrical activity for an unpredictable period of time. If there is no impulse for a prolonged period of time (> 3s) then it is termed sinus arrest. The pause is followed by resumption of sinus node activity and a P wave; however in case of a prolonged pause, a subsidiary pacemaker (usually the AV node) takes over.

- Causes of sinus pause/arrest are excessive vagal inhibition, infarction, fibrosis, myocarditis, drugs (beta-blockers, digoxin, procainamide, quinidine) and amyloidosis.

- Differential diagnosis of sinus pause/arrest are marked sinus arrhythmia, blocked premature atrial impulses and single reciprocating ("echo") P waves.

- If asymptomatic, then no treatment is indicated, although offending drugs should be withdrawn. Symptomatic patients may need to be admitted for continuous cardiac monitoring and should be evaluated for possible permanent pacemaker implantation.

EKG Case 7

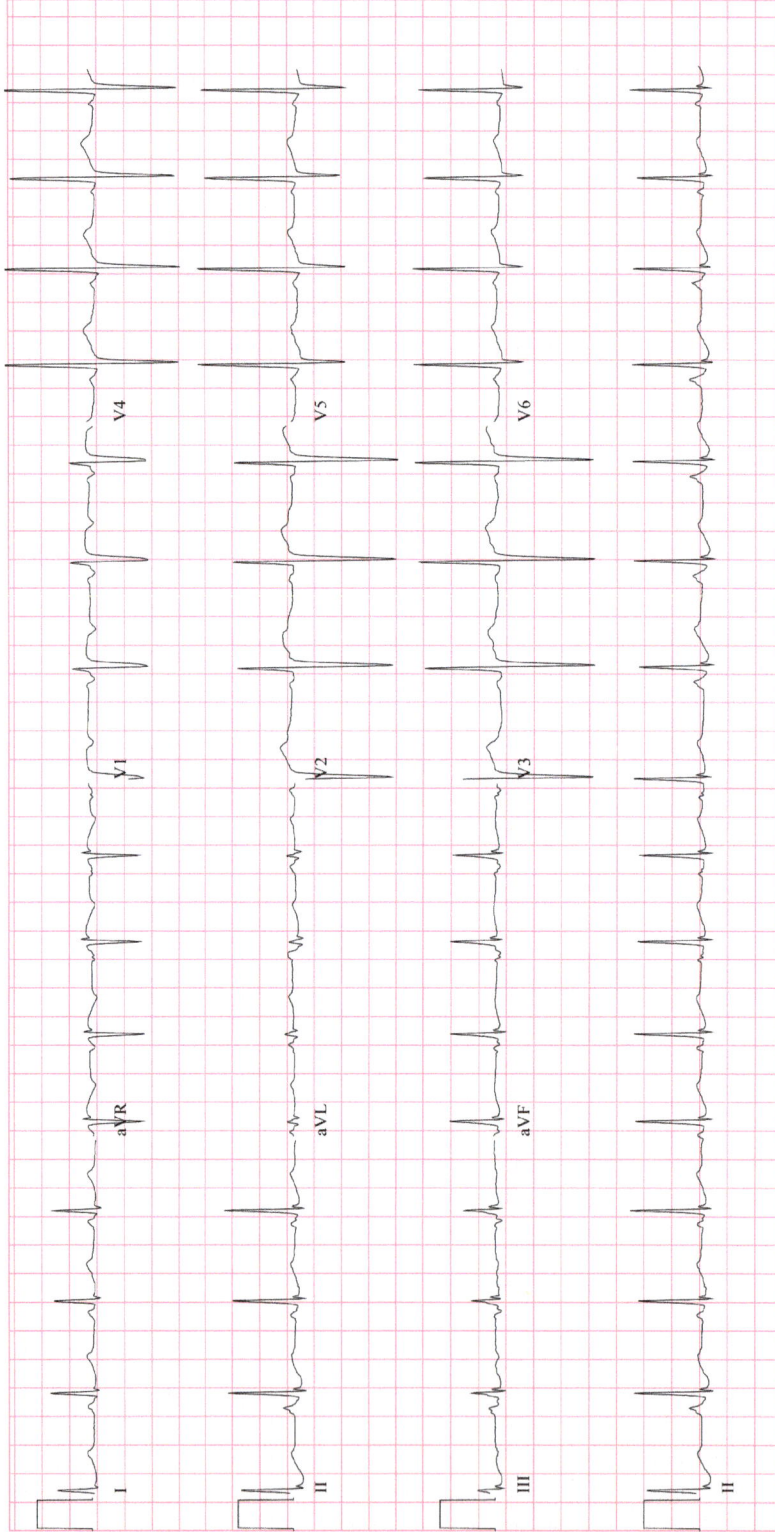

65-year-old female with a history of hypertension presents to the office for pre-op clearance for an elective knee replacement surgery. The patient has no complaints. An EKG is obtained. What does it show?

DIAGNOSIS: Wandering Atrial Pacemaker (WAP)

This EKG shows atrial rhytm with variable P wave morphologies at a rate of 90 bpm.

- P-wave morphology in otherwise regular sinus rhythm was initially described by Schamroth and Goldberg[1] in 1972.

- Wandering atrial pacemaker (WAP) is an atrial arrhythmia that occurs when the natural cardiac pacemaker site shifts between the sinoatrial node, the atria, and/or the atrioventricular node.

- The shifting of the pacemaker from the SA node to adjacent tissue is identifiable on the EKG lead II by morphological changes in the P-waves; sinus beats have smooth upright P-waves, while the atrial beats have flattened, notched, or biphasic P-waves. WAP is usually caused by varying vagal tone. With increased vagal tone, the SA node slows down, allowing for ectopic pacemaker sites in the atria or AV node to generate impulses. Once vagal tone decreases, the SA node resumes its faster pace and takes over again. Similarly, sympathomimetic drugs are known to induce WAP.

- In WAP, the RR intervals have variable cycle lengths since the ectopic foci exhibit differences in automaticity (rate of impulse generation). Therefore, the rhythm is irregular and may be confused with atrial fibrillation (AF). However, in contrast to AF, distinct P-waves are present before each QRS complex in WAP. Sinus arrhythmia may also exhibit an irregular rhythm however, one P-wave morphology and PR interval is seen in this situation[2]. WAP may also be confused with sinus rhythm with multifocal premature atrial contractions, although in this situation a dominant sinus P-wave morphology can be identified and there are periods of RR interval regularity.

- Patients with WAP are usually asymptomatic and treatment is usually not warranted.

- In WAP, the heart rate is less than 100 bpm. If it exceeds 100 bpm, the rhythm is known as multifocal atrial tachycardia (MAT).

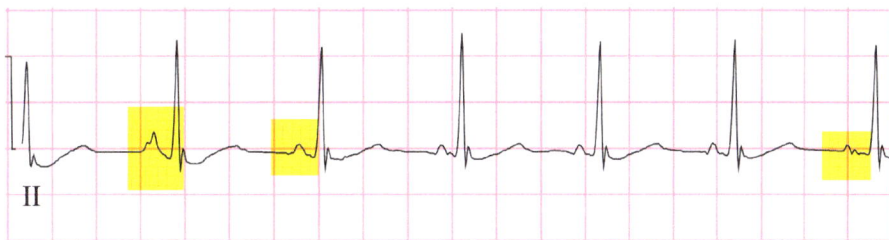

Figure: Three different P wave morphologies are highlighted above. Tented, normal, biphasic

---

1   The concept of a wandering pacemaker. Heart Lung. 1972;1(4):519–522

2   Hannibal, Gerard B. "Wandering atrial pacemaker and multifocal ectopic atrial tachycardia." *AACN advanced critical care* 26, no. 1 (2015): 73-76

EKG Case 8

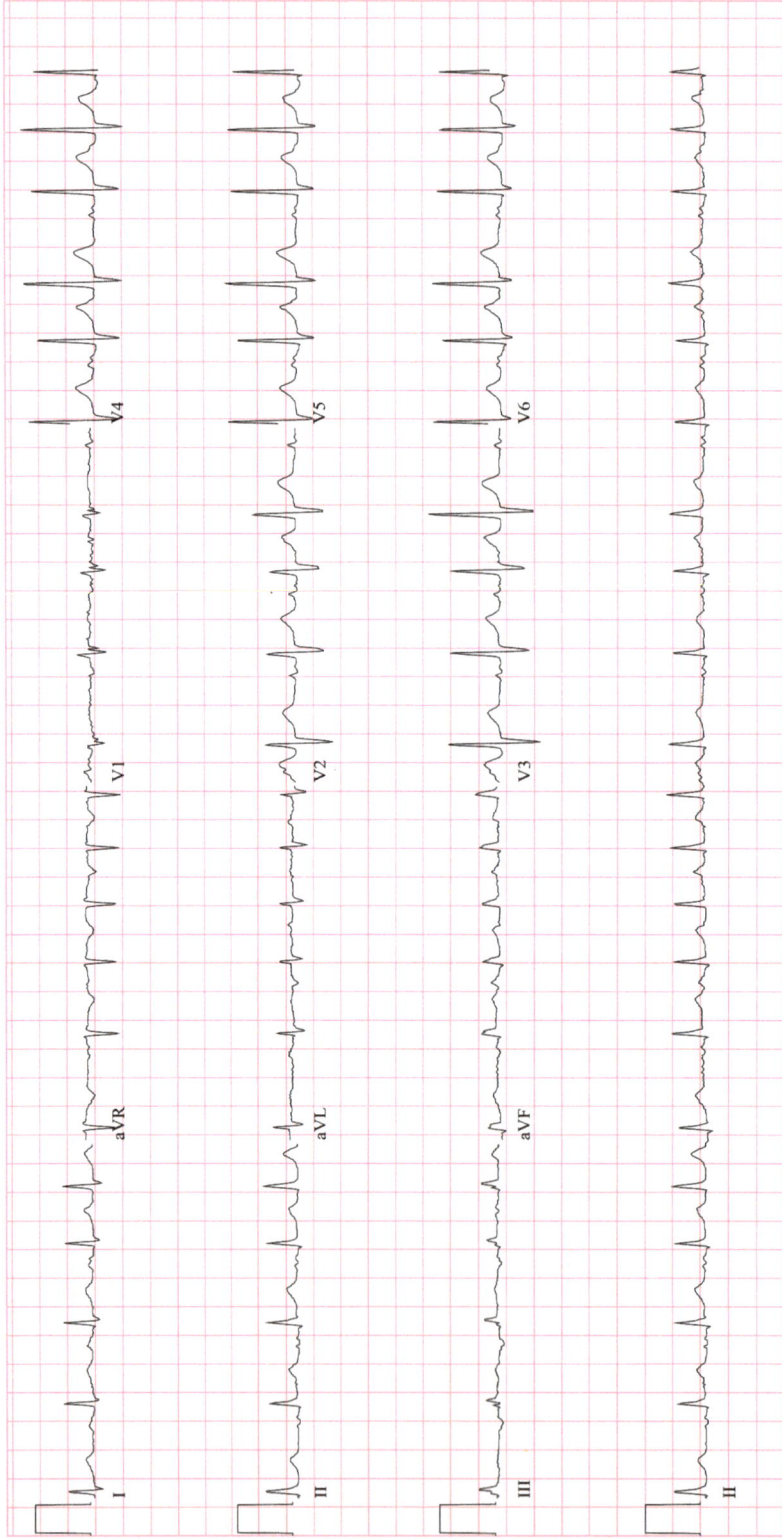

A 90-year-old male with a history of COPD and CHF is admitted to the hospital with shortness of breath. Nurse reports an irregular heart rate and an EKG is obtained. What does it show?

DIAGNOSIS: Multifocal Atrial Tachycardia (MAT), also known as Chaotic Atrial Tachycardia

- A rapid, irregular atrial rhythm arising from multiple ectopic foci within the atria.

- MAT is associated with significant lung disease, most commonly with COPD or congestive heart failure, in about 60% of cases.

- It is typically a transitional rhythm between frequent premature atrial complexes (PACs) and atrial fibrillation.

- Diagnostic criteria include:
    - Heart rate > 100 bpm (usually 100 -150 bpm; may be as high as 250 bpm).
    - Irregularly irregular rhythm with varying PP, PR and RR intervals.
    - At least three distinct P-wave morphologies in the same lead.
    - Isoelectric baseline between P-waves (i.e, no atrial flutter waves).
    - Absence of a single dominant atrial pacemaker (i.e, not just sinus rhythm with frequent PACs).

- Some P waves may be non-conducted; others may be aberrantly conducted to the ventricles.

- Patients with multiple P wave morphologies but a normal heart rate (60 to 100 bmp) are considered to have a "wandering atrial pacemaker", since the heart rate does not meet criteria for a tachycardia.

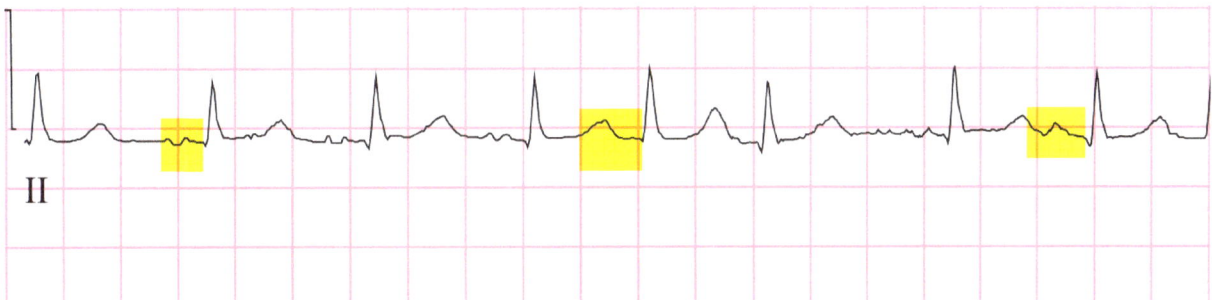

Figure: Multifocal atrial tachycardia in above patient. Rapid, irregular rhythm with multiple P-wave morphologies. The diagnostic criteria include an average atrial rate above 100 bpm.

EKG Case 9

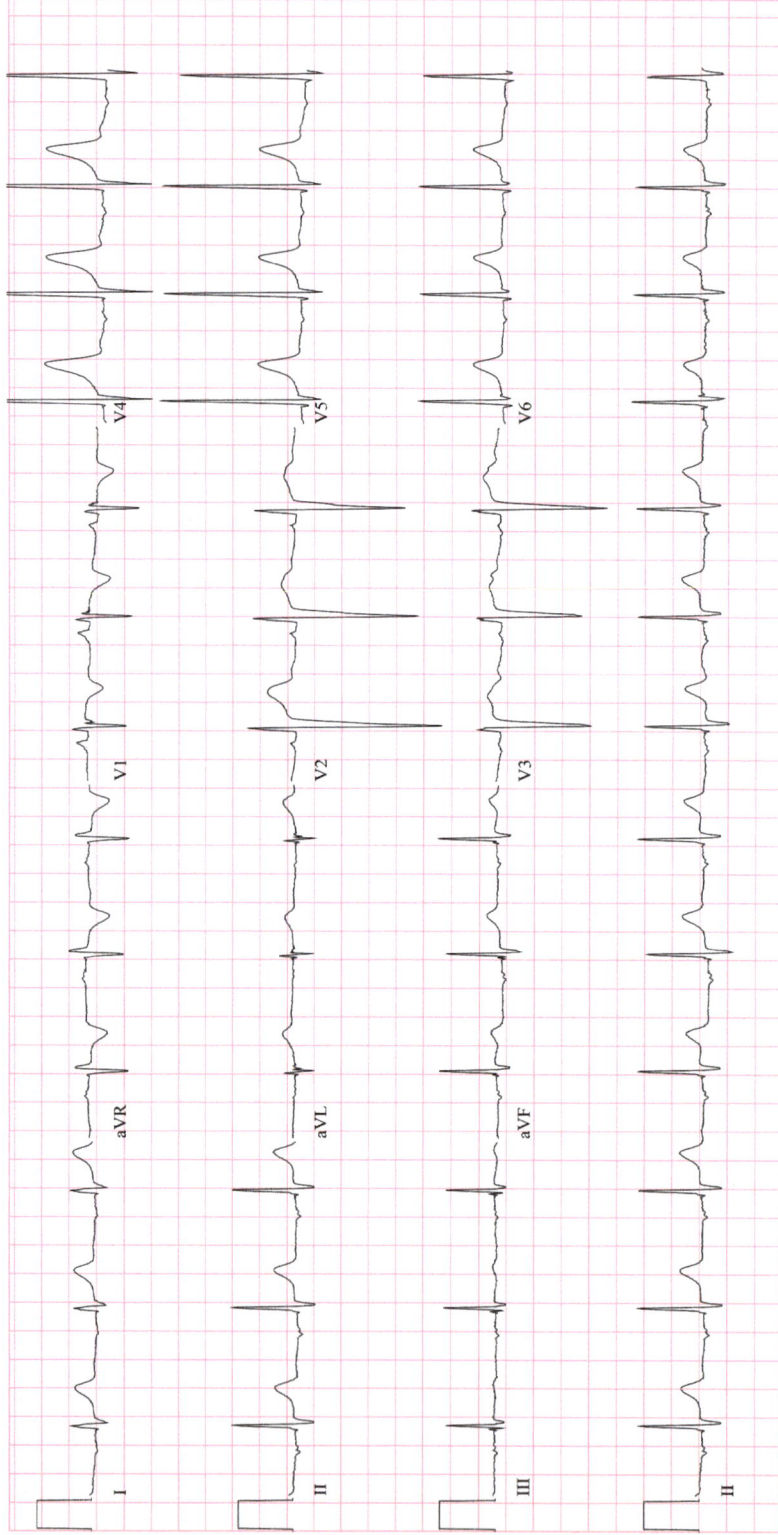

A 15-year-old female needs to undergo urgent knee surgery after a motor vehicle accident. An EKG is obtained for pre-op clearance. What does it show?

DIAGNOSIS: Ectopic Atrial Rhythm likely arising in left atrium

This EKG shows ectopic regular rhythm with ventricular rate of 75 bpm. On close inspection, the P waves are upright in lead V1 and inverted in leads II, III, aVF, V5, and V6.

- Left atrial rhythm is characterized by a left-to-right spread of atrial depolarization[1]. The most frequent electrocardiographic pattern of this rhythm consists of upright or isoelectric P waves in lead I and inverted P waves in lead V6.

- A negative P wave in lead V6 is the most sensitive and the most specific sign of left atrial rhythm.

- There is no contraindication to urgent surgery in above patient. Ectopic atrial rhythm is usually transient and should be followed up by serial EKGs.

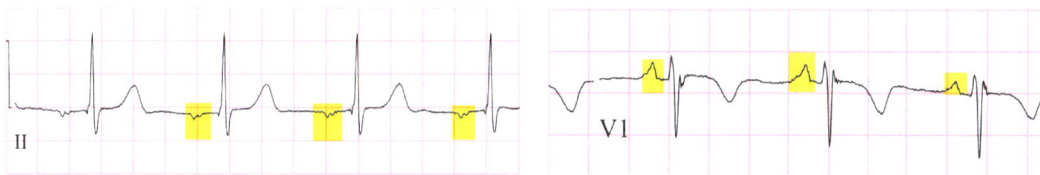

1   Mirowski, M. "Left atrial rhythm: diagnostic criteria and differentiation from nodal arrhythmias."
     The American Journal of Cardiology 17, no. 2 (1966): 203-210

EKG Case 10

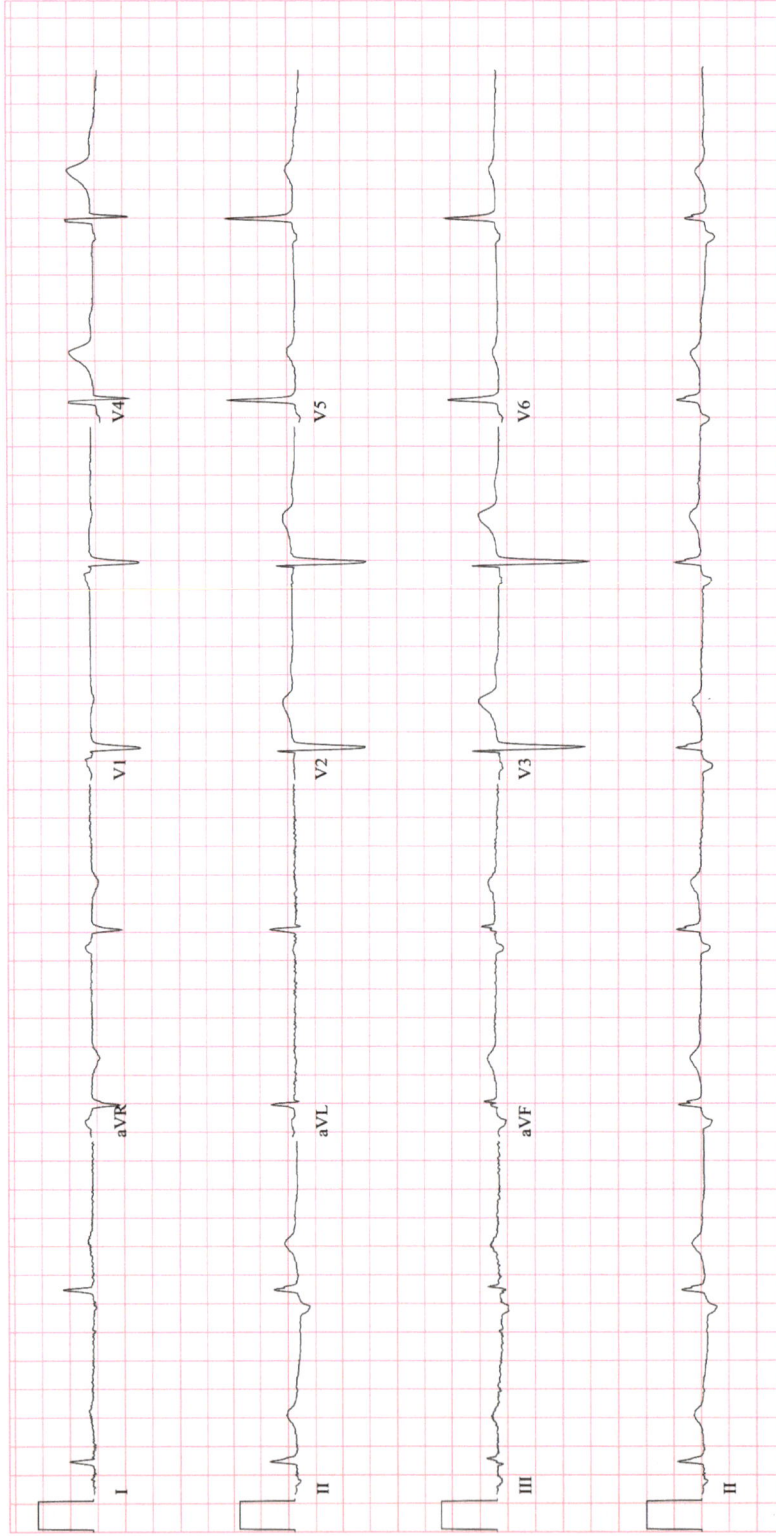

A 65-year-old male with a history of hypertension on metoprolol presents for a routine office visit. An EKG is obtained. What does it show?

DIAGNOSIS: Ectopic Atrial Rhythm – Bradycardia

The EKG shows regular ectopic atrial rhythm at 50 bpm. Note markedly inverted P waves in lead II, III, and aVF.

- In ectopic atrial rhythm, also known as ectopic atrial pacemaker, the atrial rate is less than 100 bpm and PR interval is within normal limits.

- Since the origin of electrical activity is not from the sinus node, the P wave would often not have its normal sinus appearance (upright in lead II and biphasic in V1). When the ectopic pacemaker is located in the lower atrium (as in this case), the P waves are inverted in the inferior leads and the rhythm may be mistaken for AV junctional rhythm.

- Ectopic atrial rhythm is often transient and is seen in people with or without structural heart disease.

- The more common version of uniform and regular ectopic atrial rhythm is Atrial ectopic tachycardia (AET). See case 11.

EKG Case 11

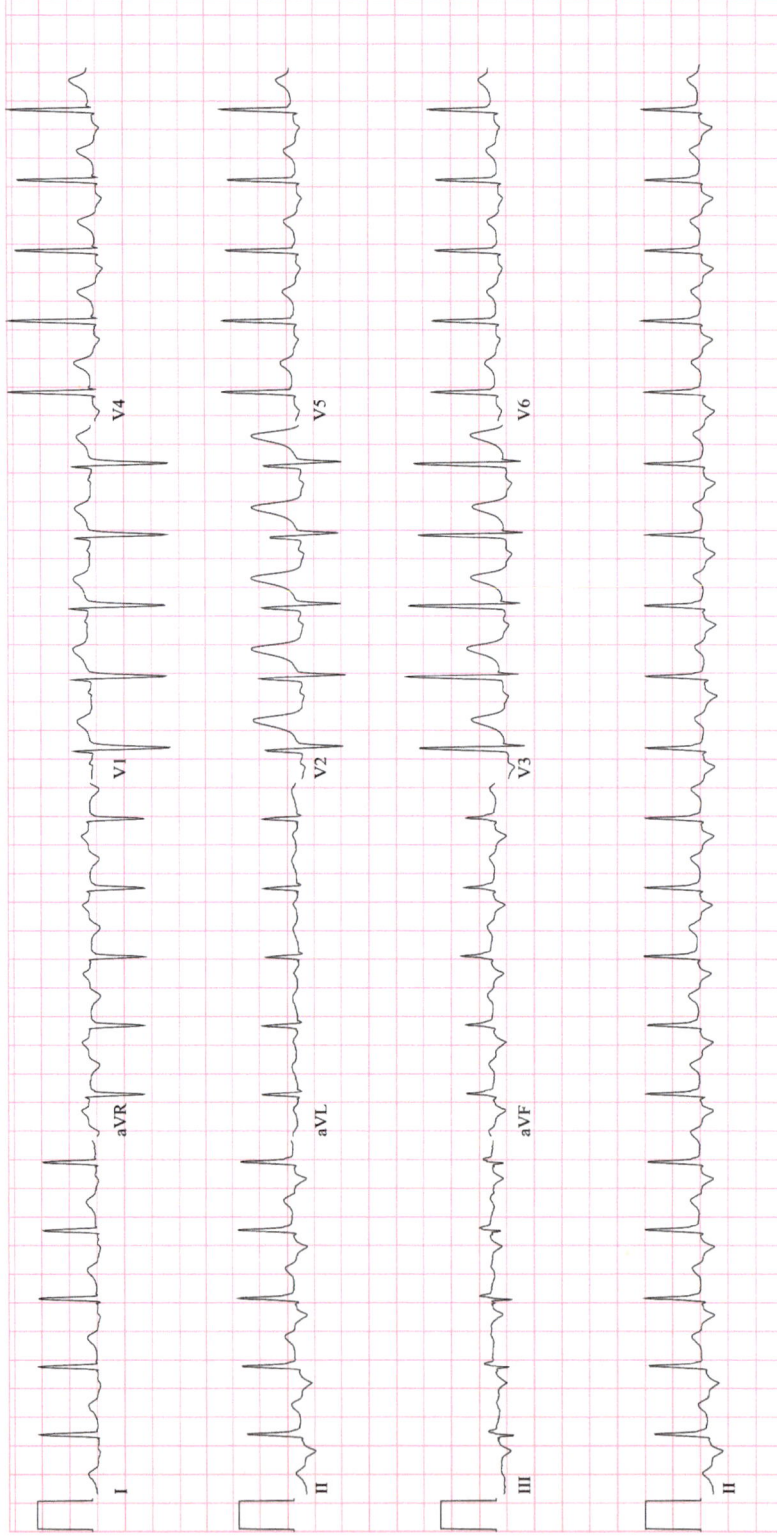

A 30-year-old male presents to the office with complaints of occasional palpitations and fatigue. An EKG is obtained. What does it show?

DIAGNOSIS: Atrial Ectopic Tachycardia (AET)

This EKG shows atrial ectopic tachycardia at 130 bpm. Note markedly inverted P waves in lead II, III, and AVF (Long RP Narrow complex tachycardia).

- Atrial ectopic tachycardia (AET) is a rare arrhythmia; however, it is the most common form of incessant supraventricular tachycardia (SVT) in young adults.

- AET originates within the atria but outside of the sinus node. It is usually of a single ectopic focus.

- It may be transient, paroxysmal, sustained, or incessant. The tachycardia is considered sustained when it lasts longer than 30 seconds.

- The underlying mechanism can involve reentry, triggered activity, or increased automaticity.

- Multiple causes including digoxin toxicity, atrial scarring, catecholamine excess, congenital abnormalities; the condition may also be idiopathic.

- Chronic persistent atrial tachycardias are less common but are frequently disabling and can lead to tachycardia-induced cardiomyopathy.

- Differential diagnosis may include Paroxysmal Reciprocating Junctional Tachycardia (PJRT) and atypical AVNRT.

EKG features include:

- Regular atrial rate above 100 bpm.

- Onset: sudden and is initiated by atrial premature depolarization.

- Termination: usually abrupt.

- P waves morphology is different from sinus P wave due to ectopic origin.

- Inverted P waves best seen in leads II, unless originating high in atria. Normal P waves are positive in II and biphasic in V1.

- At least three consecutive identical ectopic P waves.

- Isoelectric baseline (unlike atrial flutter).

- As with sinus tachycardia, ST segment depression and T wave inversion may be seen during AET.

EKG Case 12

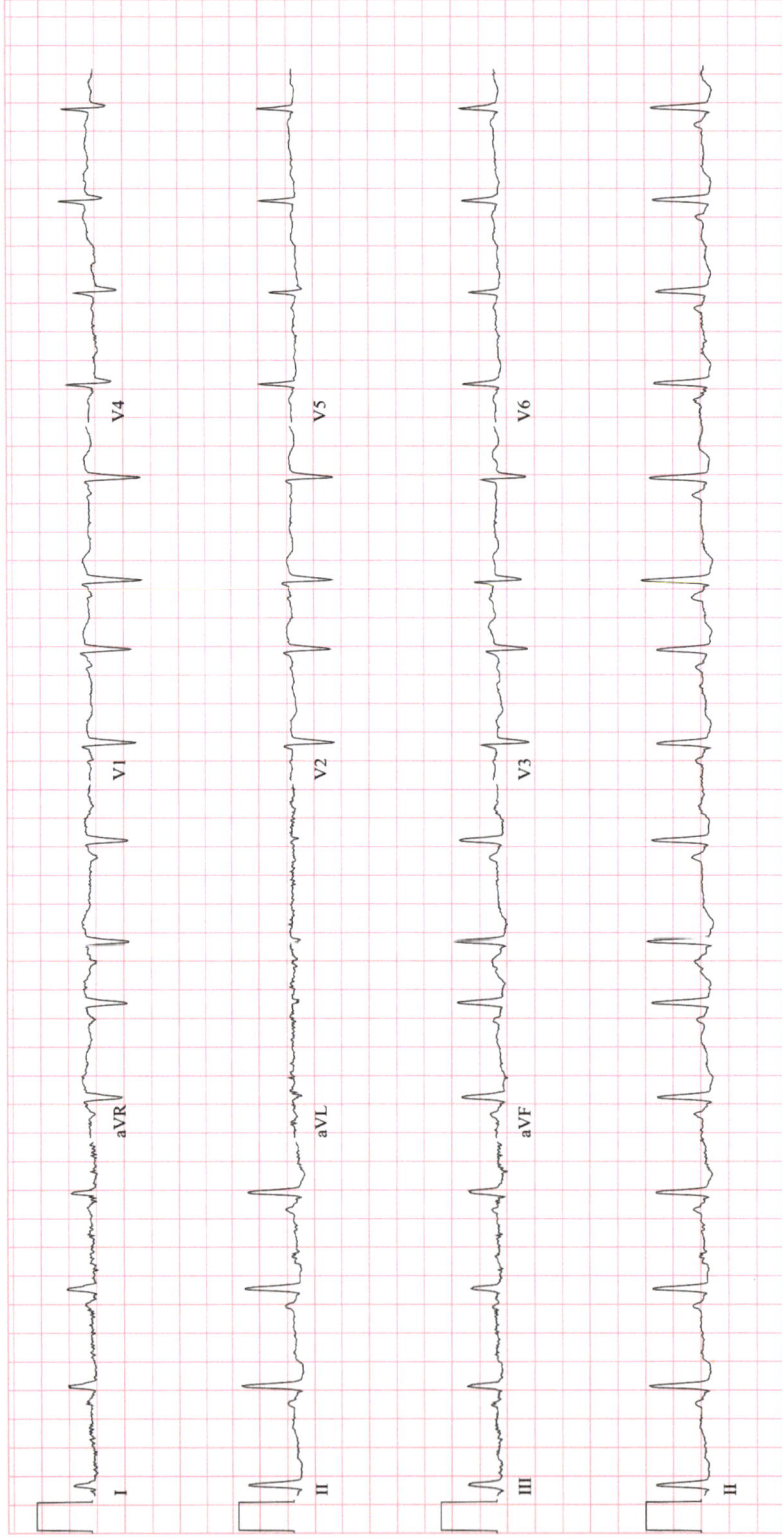

An EKG obtained from a 75-year-old male with a history of COPD. What does it show?

DIAGNOSIS: Premature Atrial Complexes (PAC), also known as Atrial \ Premature Complexes (APC)

Atrial premature beats (APB), atrial extra systoles, or atrial premature depolarization

- PACs commonly occur in healthy young and elderly people with or without heart disease, and by themselves are not considered an abnormal finding.

- Common dysrhythmia characterized by a premature beat originating from an ectopic focus within the atria. Normally, a group of pacemaker cells in the sinus node are capable of spontaneous depolarization, leading to normal sinus rhythm. Ectopic impulses from subsidiary pacemakers are normally suppressed by more rapid impulses from sinus node. However, if an ectopic focus depolarizes early enough before the arrival of the next sinus impulse - it may "capture" the atria and possibly the ventricles, producing a premature contraction.

- The P wave may or may not have a different morphology than the sinus P wave depending on site of origin of PAC in the atria.

- The abnormal P wave may be hidden in the preceding T wave, producing a "peaked" or "camel hump" appearance - if this is not noticed, the PAC may be mistaken for a PJC (premature junctional contraction).

- Low atrial ectopic beats, i.e, PACs arising close to the AV node activate the atria retrogradely, producing an inverted P wave in the inferior leads with a relatively short PR interval (often <120 msec). PACs that reach the SA node may depolarize it, causing the SA node to "reset". This results in a longer-than-normal interval before the next sinus beat is generated ("post-extra systolic pause"). Unlike with PVCs, this pause is usually not equal to twice the preceding RR interval, i.e, not a "full compensatory pause".

- PACs arriving early in the cycle may be conducted aberrantly, usually with a RBBB morphology (as the right bundle branch has a longer refractory period than the left bundle branch). They can be differentiated from PVCs by the presence of a preceding P wave. If very premature, a PAC may not conduct to the ventricles (blocked PAC).

- In most cases, no treatment other than reassurance is needed for PACs, although medications such as beta blockers can reduce the frequency of symptomatic PACs.

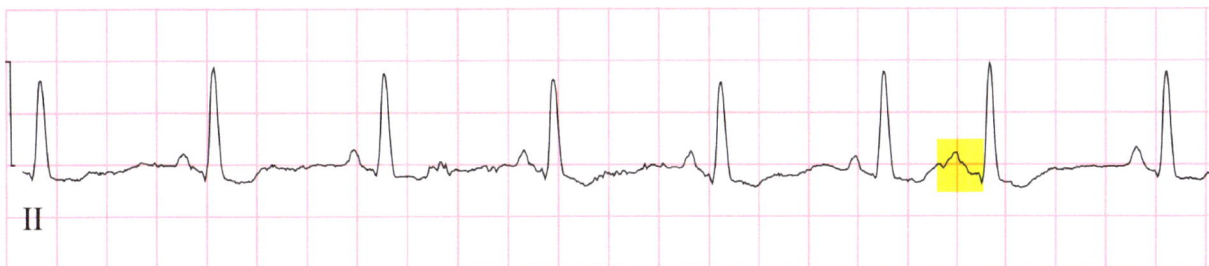

Figure: The seventh beat is an atrial premature beat. The P wave is shaped differently from the other, somewhat unusual-looking P waves, and the beat is clearly premature.

EKG Case 13

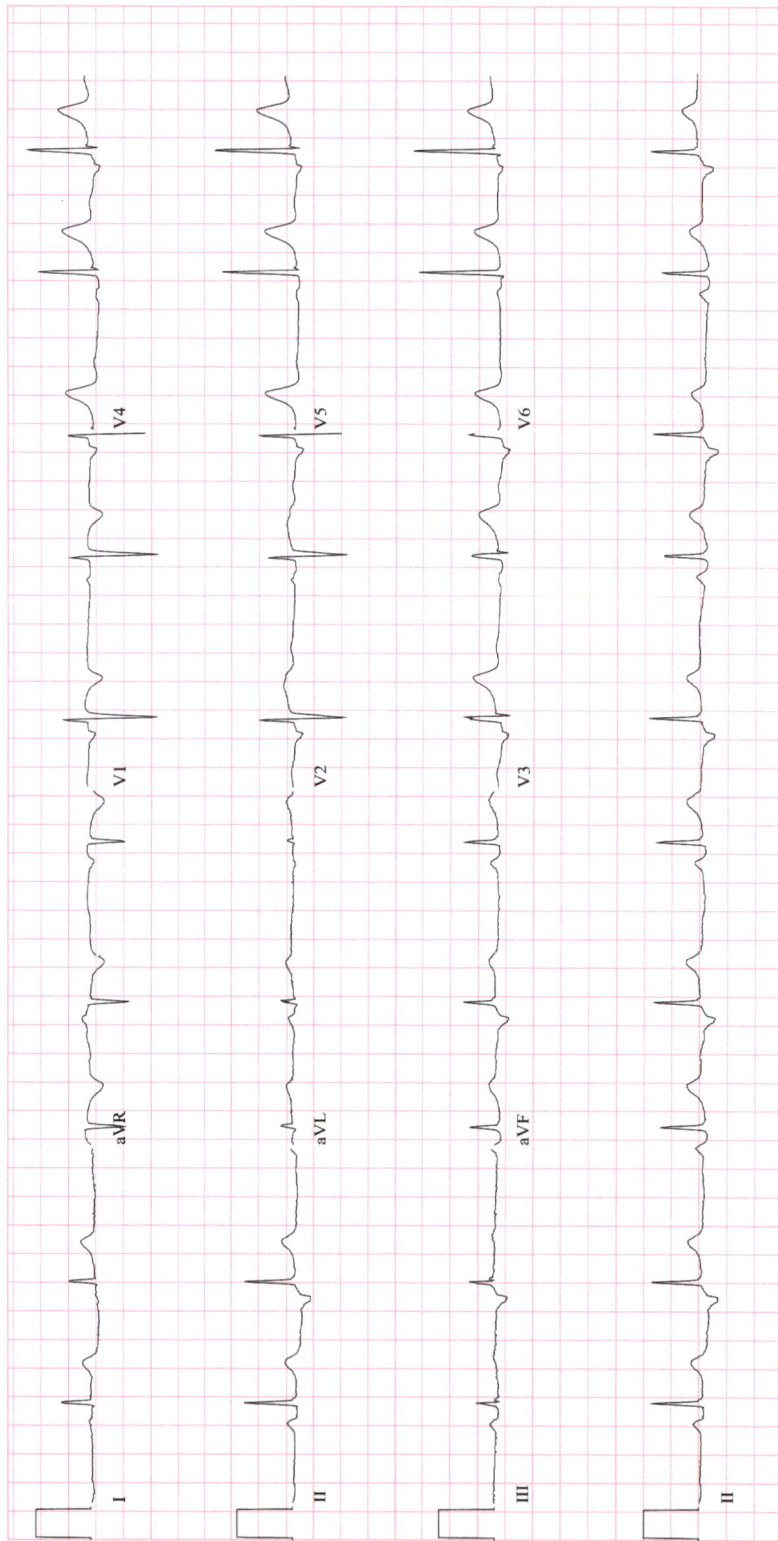

An EKG is obtained from a 55-year-old male with a history of hypertension at a regular office visit. What does the EKG show?

DIAGNOSIS: Atrial Bigeminy

In atrial bigeminy, a premature atrial beat follows each sinus beat. The coupling of the PAC to the previous sinus P wave is usually fixed, leading to a regularly irregular rhythm. Close inspection of the P-QRS relationship in lead II (below) reveals two findings: all P waves have associated QRS complexes (therefore there is no AV block) and the P waves are not all of the same morphology, i.e, there are both normal sinus wave marked as P and inverted ectopic beat marked as P'. Every other beat (wave 2,4,6,8 etc.) features a P' wave. When a PAC follows every sinus beat, the rhythm is termed atrial bigeminy; if every third beat is a PAC, the term used is atrial trigeminy; and if every fourth beat is a PAC, the rhythm is atrial quadrigeminy. These are all regularly irregular rhythms.

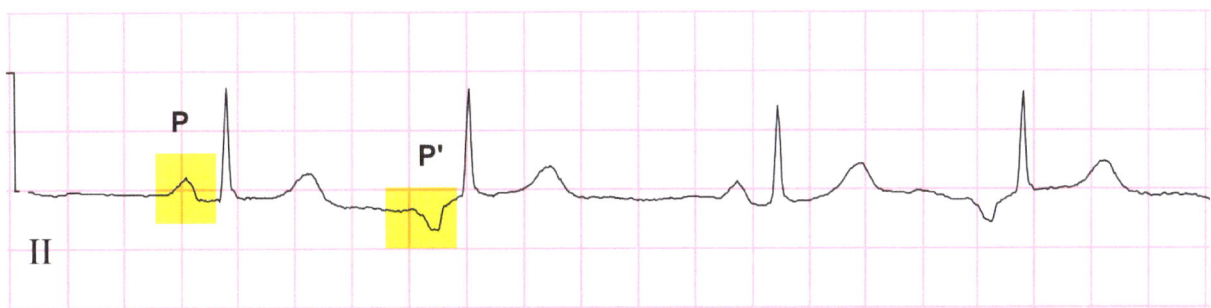

Figure: Atrial Bigeminy

EKG Case 14

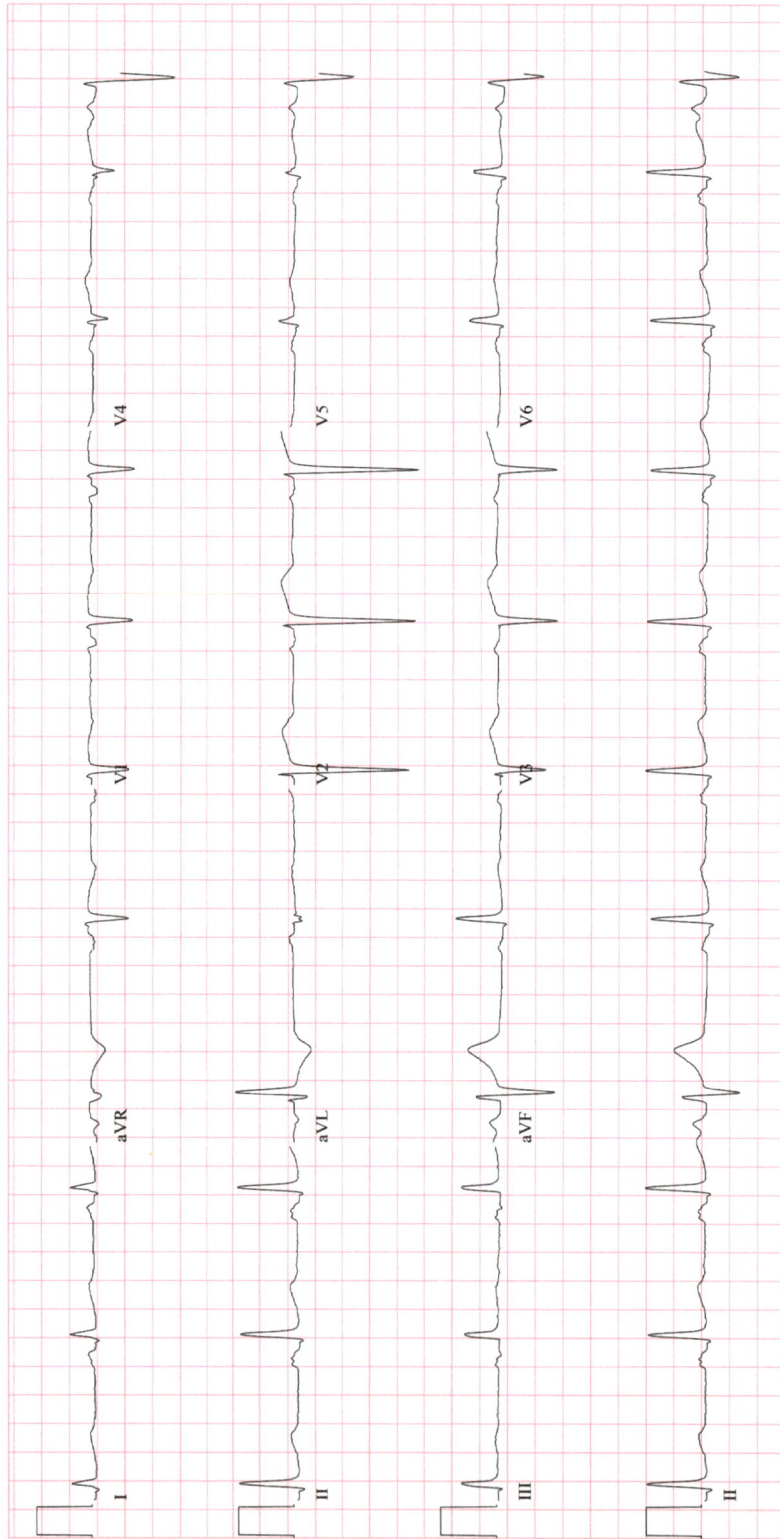

A 49-year-old male who is otherwise asymptomatic, complains of missing or skipped heart beats. What does the EKG show?

DIAGNOSIS: Aberrantly conducted Premature Atrial Contraction (PAC)

- PACs have three different outcomes.

1. Normal conduction: similar to normal QRS complexes in the EKG.

2. Non-conducted: no QRS complex because the PAC meets the AV node when still refractory.

3. Conducted with aberration: the PAC makes it into the His Purkinje system but finds one or more of its fascicles or bundle branches refractory, hence the resulting QRS is usually different.

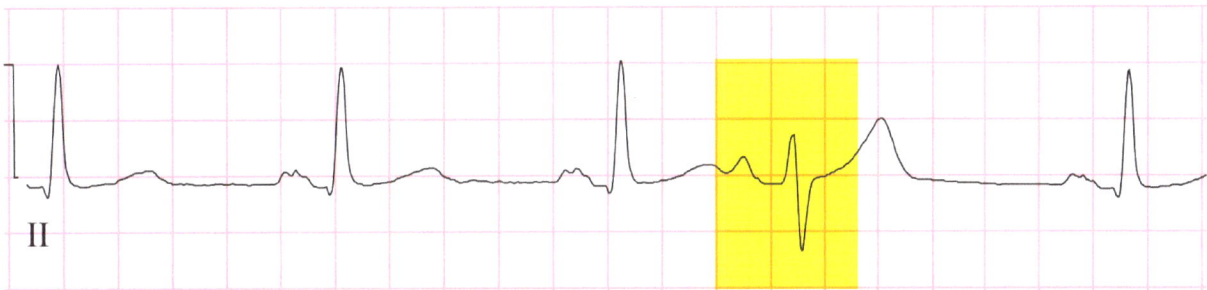

In the above example, the fourth (and eleventh beat) is premature atrial contraction with a preceding abnormal P' wave (notched positive compared to the biphasic P waves of each sinus beat). It conducts with a longer PR interval compared to sinus rhythm and with a wider QRS complex. The wide QRS complex following the PAC is not a PVC. The morphology of the wider QRS complex is different from the rest of the beats because of aberrant condution (slower or blocked conduction down a fascicle or bundle branch). Aberrant PACs mostly have a RBBB morphology as the right bundle branch has a longer refractory period than the left bundle branch at slower rates.

EKG Case 15

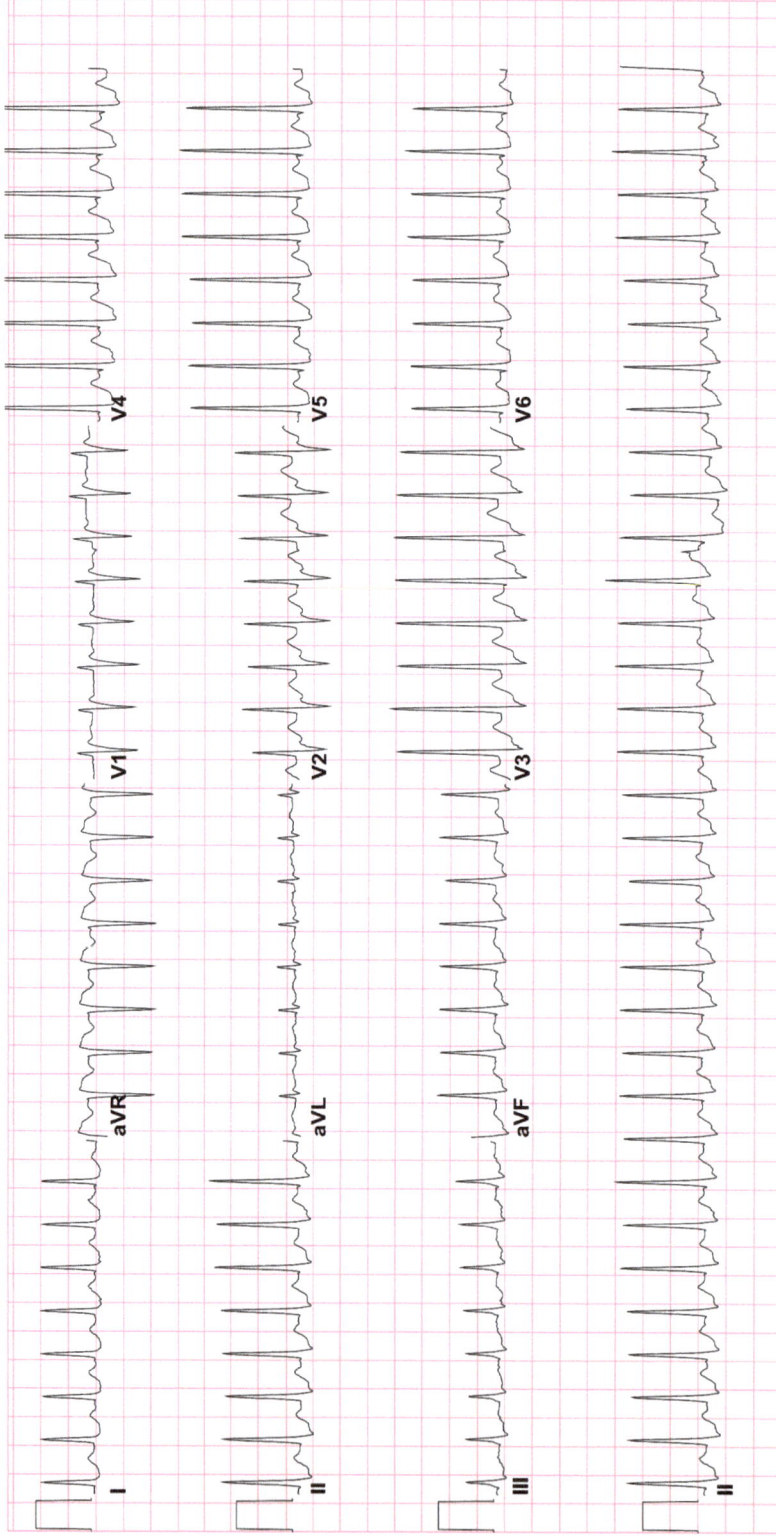

A 45-year-old male presents to the hospital with sudden onset of shortness of breath and palpitations over the last one hour. He reports previous episodes of palpitations. An EKG is obtained. What does it show?

46

DIAGNOSIS: Supraventricular Tachycardia, likely AV Nodal Re-entry Tachycardia (AVNRT)

This EKG shows narrow complex supraventricular tachycardia (AVNRT) at rate of 250 bpm. Differential diagnosis includes sinus tachycardia, but the rate is too fast for sinus tachycardia.

- The term supraventricular tachycardia (SVT), while often used synonymously with AV nodal re-entry tachycardia (AVNRT), can be used to refer to any tachyarrhythmia arising from above the level of the Bundle of His.

- Different types of SVT arise from or are propagated by the atria or AV node, typically producing a *narrow-complex tachycardia* (unless aberrant conduction is present).

- *Paroxysmal SVT* (pSVT) describes an SVT with abrupt onset and offset - characteristically seen with re-entrant tachycardia involving the AV node, such as AVNRT or atrioventricular re-entry tachycardia (AVRT).

- Regular narrow QRS complex tachyarrhythmias includes the following:

	Regular	Irregular
Atrial	Sinus tachycardia Atrial tachycardia (AT) Atrial flutter (fixed AV block) Inappropriate sinus tachycardia Sinus atrial node re-entrant tachycardia (SANRT)	Atrial fibrillation Atrial flutter with variable block Multifocal atrial tachycardia
Atrioventricular	Atrioventricular re-entry tachycardia (AVRT) AV nodal re-entry tachycardia (AVNRT) Automatic junctional tachycardia and Paroxysmal Junctional Reciprocating Tachycardia (PJRT)	

AVNRT is the most common mechanism of SVT in adults with structurally normal hearts. It is typically paroxysmal and may occur spontaneously or upon provocation with exertion, caffeine, alcohol, beta-agonists (Albuterol), or sympathomimetics (amphetamines). In comparison to AVRT, which involves an *anatomical* re-entrant circuit using an accessory pathway (Bundle of Kent), AVNRT utilizes the slow and fast AV nodal pathways

In AVNRT, there are two pathways within the AV node:

- The slow pathway (*alpha*): a slowly-conducting pathway with a shorter refractory period.
- The fast pathway (*beta*): a rapidly-conducting pathway with a longer refractory period.

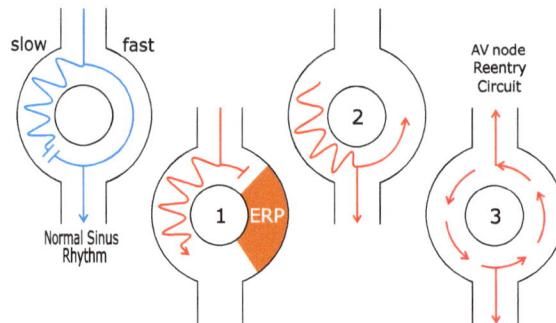

Initiation of re-entry

- During sinus rhythm, electrical impulses travel down both pathways simultaneously. The impulse transmitted down the fast pathway enters the distal end of the slow pathway and the two impulses collide in the slow pathway.

- When a premature atrial contraction (PAC) occurs, the electrical impulse is blocked in the fast pathway and conducts slowly down the slow pathway, given the difference in refractory periods between the two pathways (1).

- By the time the premature impulse reaches the end of the slow pathway, the fast pathway is no longer refractory (2). Hence the impulse can conduct retrogradely up the fast pathway.

- This creates a circus movement whereby the impulse continually cycles around the two pathways, activating the Bundle of His anterogradely and the atria retrogradely (3). The short cycle length is responsible for the rapid heart rate.

- This is the most common type of SVT in adults and is termed Slow-Fast (or typical) AVNRT.

- Because the retrograde conduction is via the fast pathway, stimulation of the atria (which produces the inverted P wave) will occur at the same time as stimulation of the ventricles (which causes the QRS complex). As a result, the inverted P wave is usually not seen on the surface EKG since it is buried within the QRS complexes. Often the retrograde P-wave is visible at the tail-end of the QRS complex, appearing as a "pseudo R prime" wave in lead V1 or a "pseudo S" wave in the inferior leads.

- The fast and slow pathways should not be confused with the accessory pathways that give rise to Wolff-Parkinson-White syndrome (WPW syndrome)

- Atypical AVRNT is an SVT where conduction is in the opposite direction compared to typical AVRNT, i.e, down the fast pathway and up the slow pathway

---

1   Image Courtesy – Lifeinthefastlane.com - modified and reproduced with permission

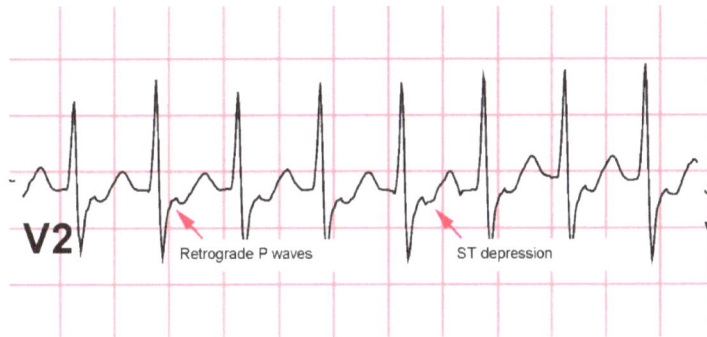

V2

Retrograde P waves   ST depression

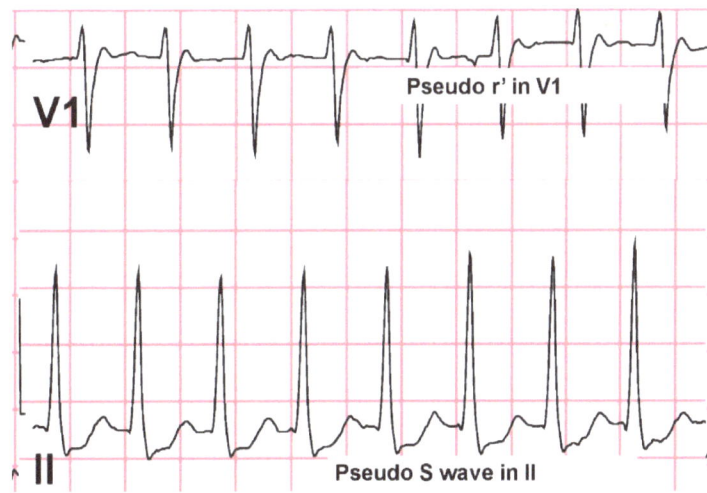

Pseudo r' in V1

V1

II   **Pseudo S wave in II**

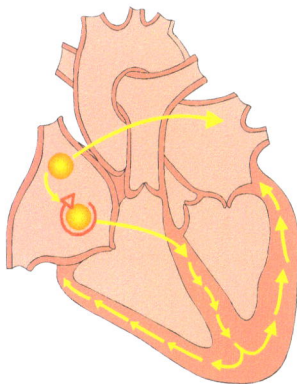

AVNRT

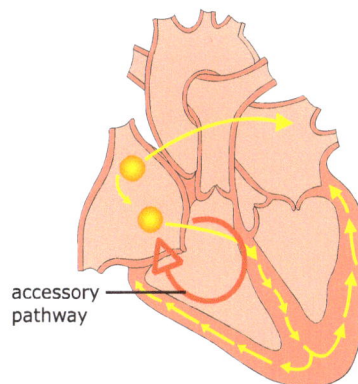

accessory pathway

AVRT

EKG Case 16

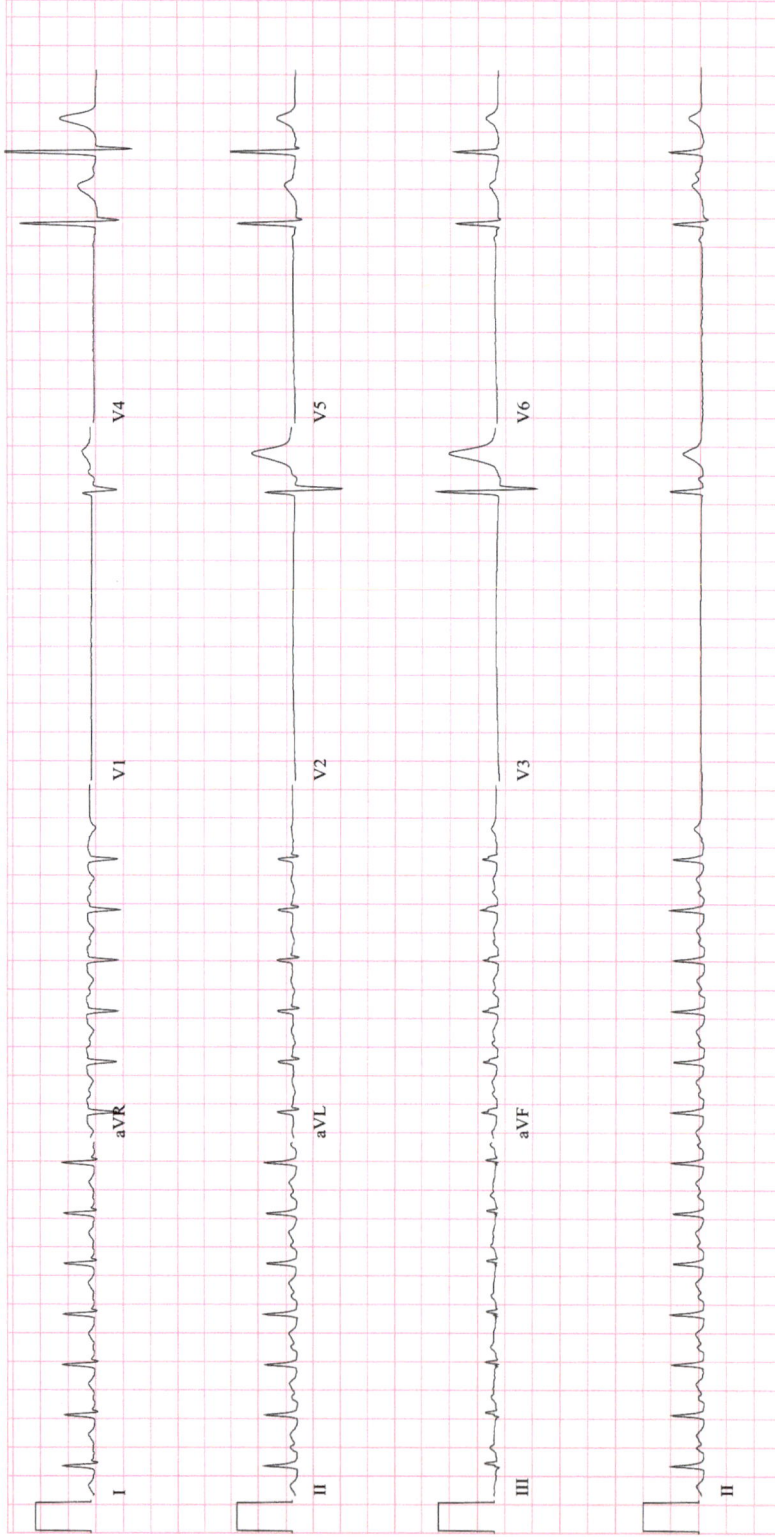

A 45 year male with a history of palpitations is receiving a carotid sinus massage in the ER while an EKG is being obtained. What does the EKG show?

DIAGNOSIS: SVT, Sinus Pause, Junctional Escape Beat

This EKG shows the followings: supraventricular tachycardia (SVT) followed by a sinus pause, a junctional escape beat, and finally a sinus beat. Last beat on rhythm strip likely represents a premature atrial contraction (PAC).

The above patient presented with supraventricular tachycardia and received carotid sinus massage (CSM), which increases the vagal tone and often slows down, or even terminates as in this case, the SVT mechanism. The effect of the CSM on the sinus node is clear in the long pause that follows.

Treatment of SVT:

The first-line acute treatment in hemodynamically stable patients is vagal maneuvers, e.g, breath holding and Valsalva maneuver. Carotid massage is another vagal maneuver that can terminate arrhythmias, particularly if the SVT mechanism is AV nodal dependent. Massage the carotid sinus for a few seconds on the side of non-dominant cerebral hemisphere after ensuring that there is no bruit by auscultation. When SVT is not terminated by vagal maneuvers, short-term management involves intravenous adenosine or calcium channel blockers. Adenosine is a short-acting drug that blocks the AV nodal conduction; it terminates 90% of tachycardia due to AVNRT or AVRT. DC cardioversion is rarely required for patients who do not respond to above measures or are hemodynamically unstable in SVT. Long term anti-arrhythmic drug management or catheter ablation may be considered for recurrent episodes that are not amenable to medical treatment.

EKG Case 17

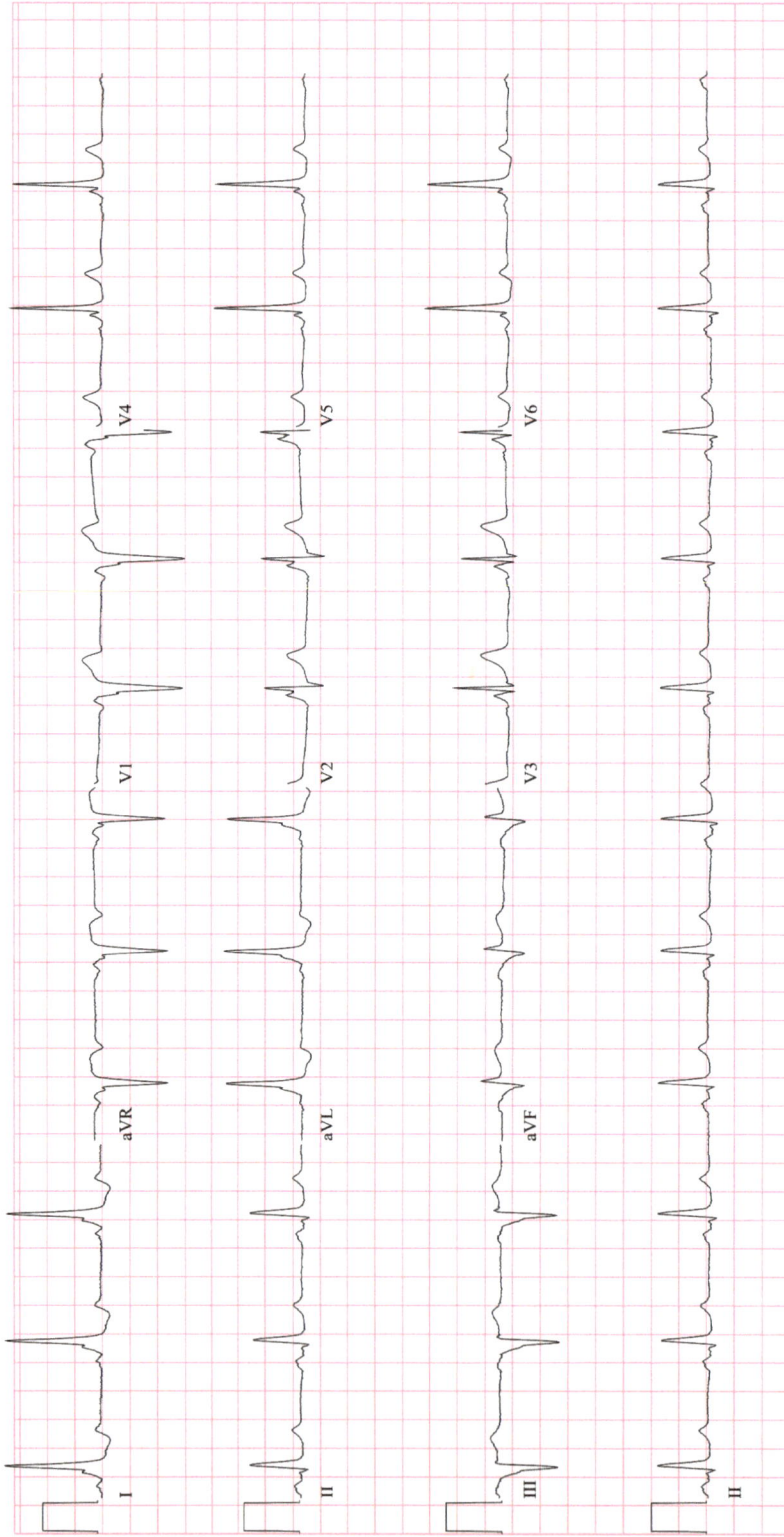

A 45-year-old male with a history of palpitations, is referred to you by his primary care doctor with concerns about silent heart attack and conduction abnormalities. What does the EKG show?

DIAGNOSIS: Type - B WPW (Wolff-Parkinson-White) syndrome

- Sinus rhythm with very short PR interval (< 120 ms).

- Broad QRS complexes with a slurred initial component of the QRS complexes - the delta wave.

- Dominant S wave in V1 - this pattern is known as "Type B" WPW and indicates a right-sided accessory pathway.

- Tall R waves and inverted T waves in V4-6 mimic the appearance of left ventricular hypertrophy (not seen in this case) - this is due to WPW and does not indicate underlying LVH.

- Negative delta waves in leads III and aVF simulate the Q waves of prior inferior MI. This is referred to as the "pseudo-infarction" pattern. It localized the accessory pathway to the posterior-septal area.

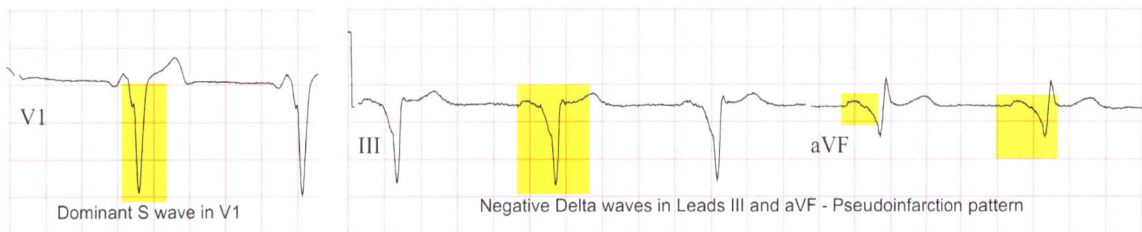

V1

Dominant S wave in V1

III   aVF

Negative Delta waves in Leads III and aVF - Pseudoinfarction pattern

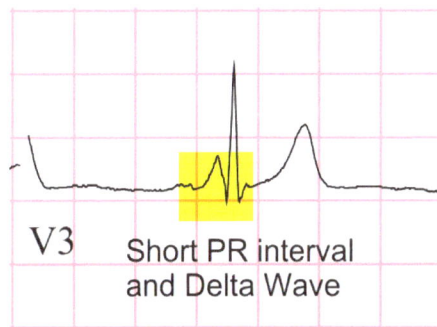

V3   Short PR interval
and Delta Wave

EKG Case 18

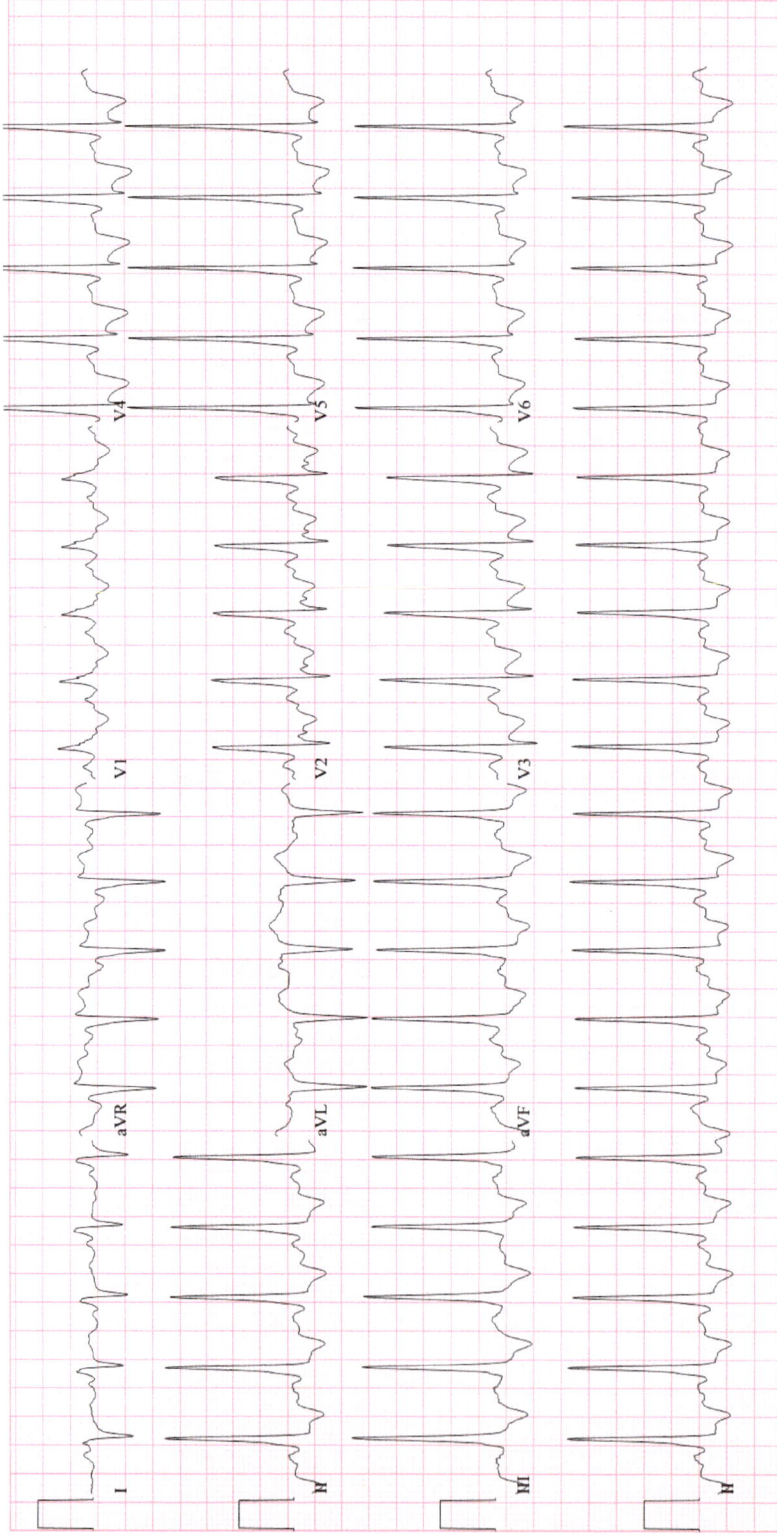

A 46-year-old male is brought to the ER after a syncope. Patient has since then, regained consciousness and is complaining of palpitations and shortness of breath. He had a similar event six months ago. What does the EKG show?

54

DIAGNOSIS: Type - A WPW (Wolff-Parkinson-White) syndrome

- Sinus tachycardia with a very short PR interval (< 120 ms).

- Broad QRS complexes with a slurred upstroke to the QRS complex - the delta wave.

- Dominant R wave in V1 - this pattern is known as "Type A" WPW and is associated with a left-sided accessory pathway.

- Tall R waves and inverted T waves in V1-3 mimicking right ventricular hypertrophy - these changes are due to WPW and do not indicate underlying RVH.

- Negative delta wave in aVL simulating the Q waves of lateral infarction - this is referred to as the "pseudo-infarction" pattern, consistent with a left lateral accessory pathway.

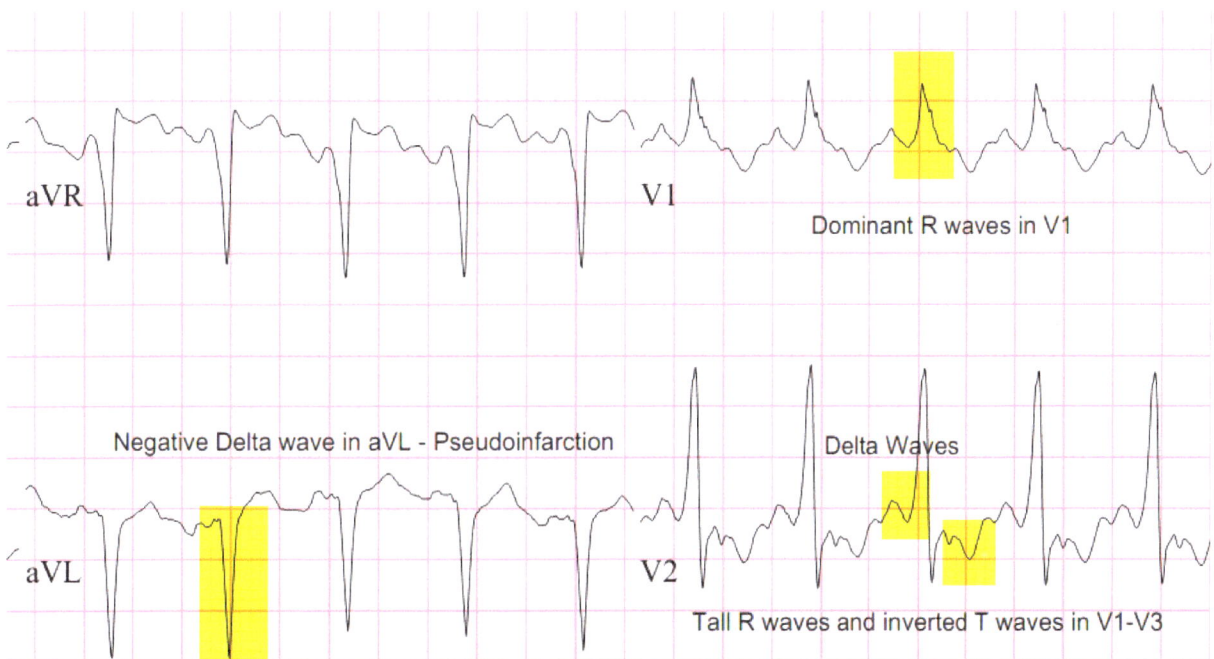

aVR

V1

Dominant R waves in V1

Negative Delta wave in aVL - Pseudoinfarction

aVL

Delta Waves

V2

Tall R waves and inverted T waves in V1-V3

EKG Case 19

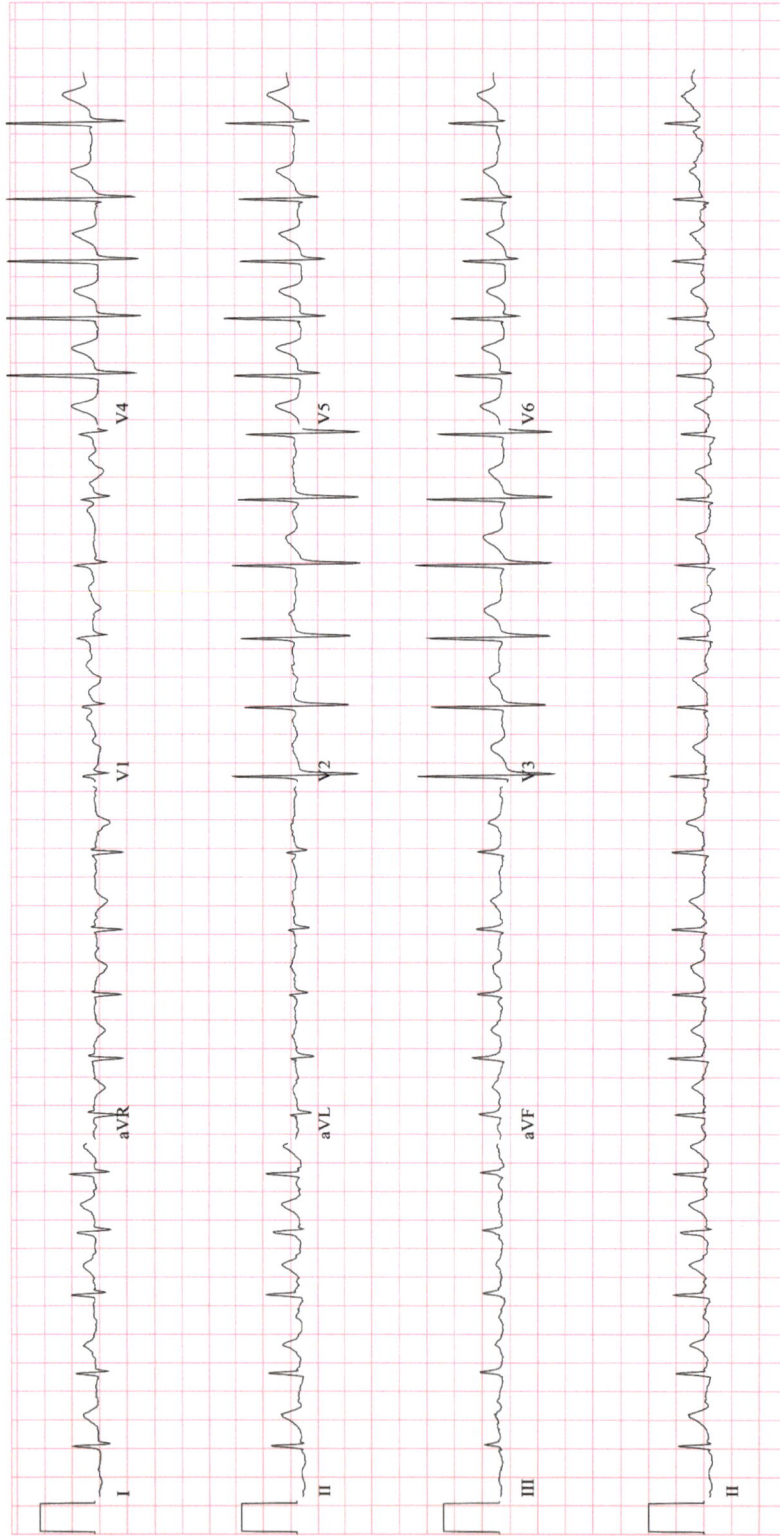

A 67-year-old female with a history of obstructive sleep apnea presents to the hospital with complaint a of new onset palpitations. An EKG is obtained. What does it show?

DIAGNOSIS: Atrial Fibrillation (AFib) with Rapid Ventricular Response (RVR)

The EKG shows an irregularly irregular rhythm with no P waves. At times, the rhythm appears "regular" but upon close inspection it shows subtle irregular RR intervals. The ventricular response is at 130 bpm. The atrial (f) waves are best seen in lead II with varying morphology and a very short cycle length. Some of the fibrillatory (f) waves also mimic true P waves.

- Atrial Fibrillation (AF) is the most common sustained arrhythmia. The incidence and prevalence of AF is increasing because of the aging population. Complications of fast AF include hemodynamic instability, cardiomyopathy, heart failure, and embolic events such as stroke.

EKG Features of Atrial Fibrillation Include:

- Irregularly irregular QRS complexes.

- Absent P waves.

- Absence of an isoelectric baseline.

- Variable ventricular rate.

- QRS complexes usually < 120 ms unless pre-existing bundle branch block, accessory pathway, or rate-related aberrant conduction.

- Fibrillatory waves may be present and can be either fine (amplitude < 0.5mm) or coarse (amplitude >0.5mm).

- Fibrillatory waves may mimic P waves leading to misdiagnosis.

- Commonly AF is associated with a ventricular rate ~ 110 - 160.

- AF is often described as having "rapid ventricular response" once the ventricular rate is > 100 bpm.

- "Slow" AF is a term often used to describe AF with a ventricular rate of < 60 bpm.

EKG Case 20

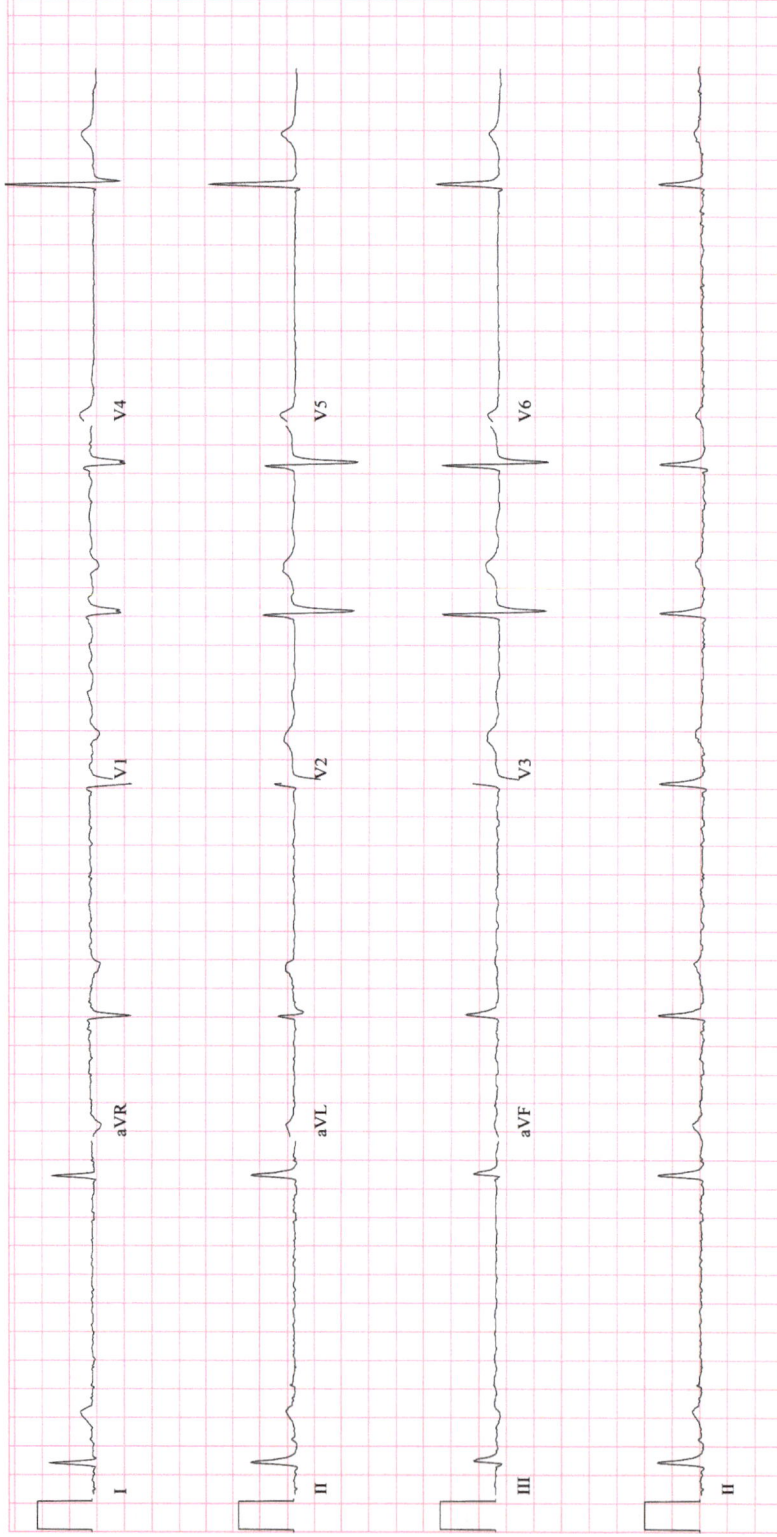

A 85-year-old male is admitted to the hospital from a nursing home with fatigue, generalized weakness, and failure to thrive. An EKG is obtained on admission. What is the atrial mechanism? What is the likely AV relationship?

DIAGNOSIS: Atrial Fibrillation with Slow Ventricular Response

This EKG shows atrial fibrillation slow ventricular response at about 40 bpm. Fine fibrillatory waves can be seen in lead II.

- There is no agreement on the definition of atrial fibrillation (AF) with a slow ventricular response. The condition may be characterized as an AF with slow resting heart rate, or as an AF with normal resting heart rate but with prolonged ventricular pauses.

- Irregular heart rate with no evidence of organized atrial activity.

- Fine fibrillatory waves in V1.

- Slow ventricular response is seen in patients on AV nodal blocking agents such as beta-blockers, calcium channel blockers, digoxin etc. Other causes include AV node conduction abnormalities, hypothermia, and ischemia.

- Although non-specific, symptoms of asthenia, easy fatigue, and dyspnea may be attributable to low cardiac output due to a slow heart rate. Cardiac pauses may be responsible for neurologic symptoms such as presyncope or syncope.

- In above patient, if no reversible cause(s) of symptomatic bradycardia can be found, the patient may require an implanted ventricular pacemaker.

EKG Case 21

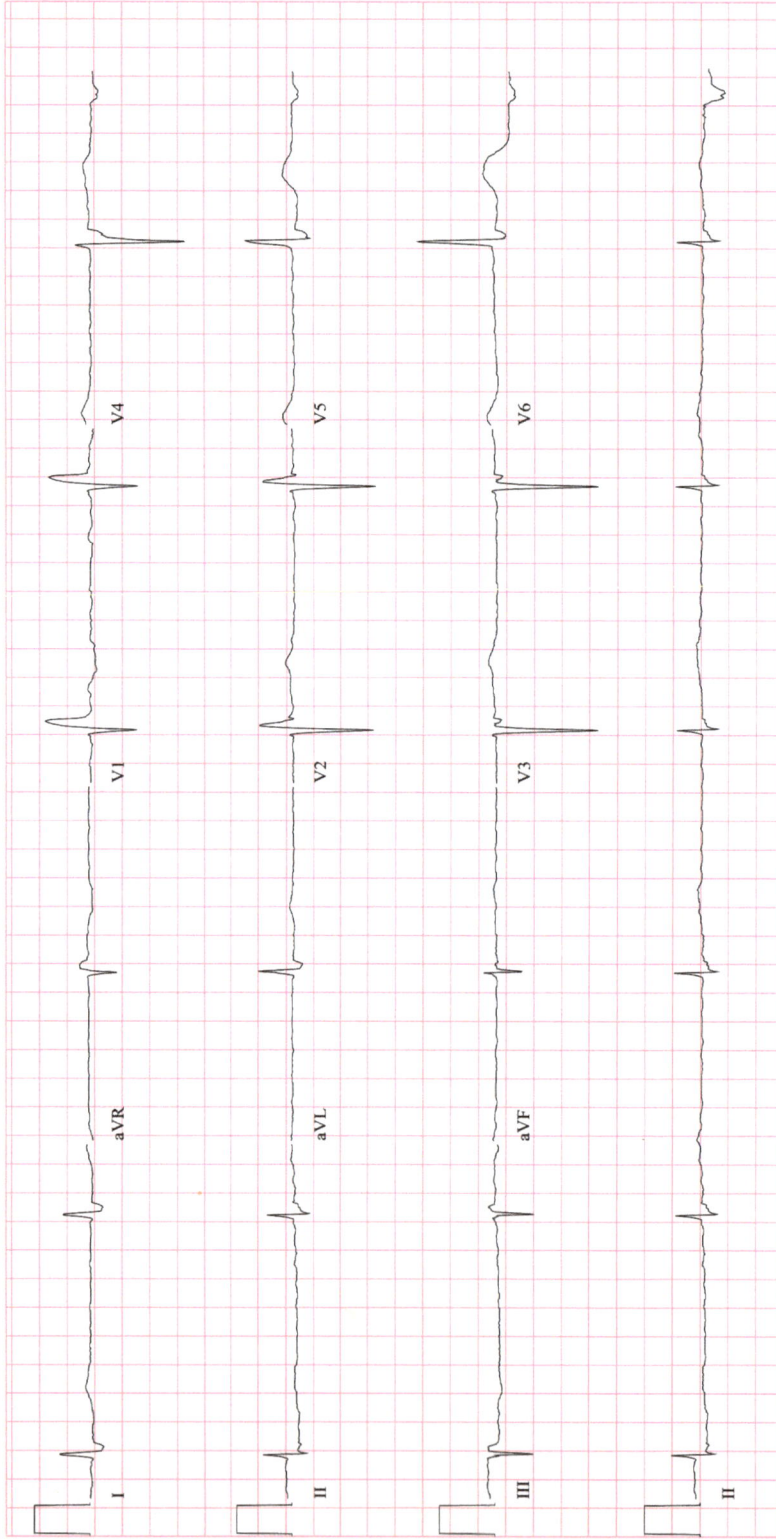

A 85-year-old male with a long-standing history of atrial fibrillation is being evaluated in the ER for dizziness. An EKG is obtained. What does it show?

DIAGNOSIS: Atrial Fibrillation with Complete Heart Block and Junctional Escape Rhythm

- The combination of atrial fibrillation with a regular rhythm ("regularized AF") indicates that none of the atrial impulses are conducted to the ventricles, i.e, complete heart block is present.

- The regular narrow complex rhythm (< 120 ms) at 35 bpm is therefore a junctional escape rhythm.

- Regularized AF is characteristically seen as a consequence of digoxin toxicity.

- The presence of Q waves in anterior leads (V1-V3) indicate an old anterior myocardial infarction. RSR' in lead V1 indicates RBBB.

EKG Case 22

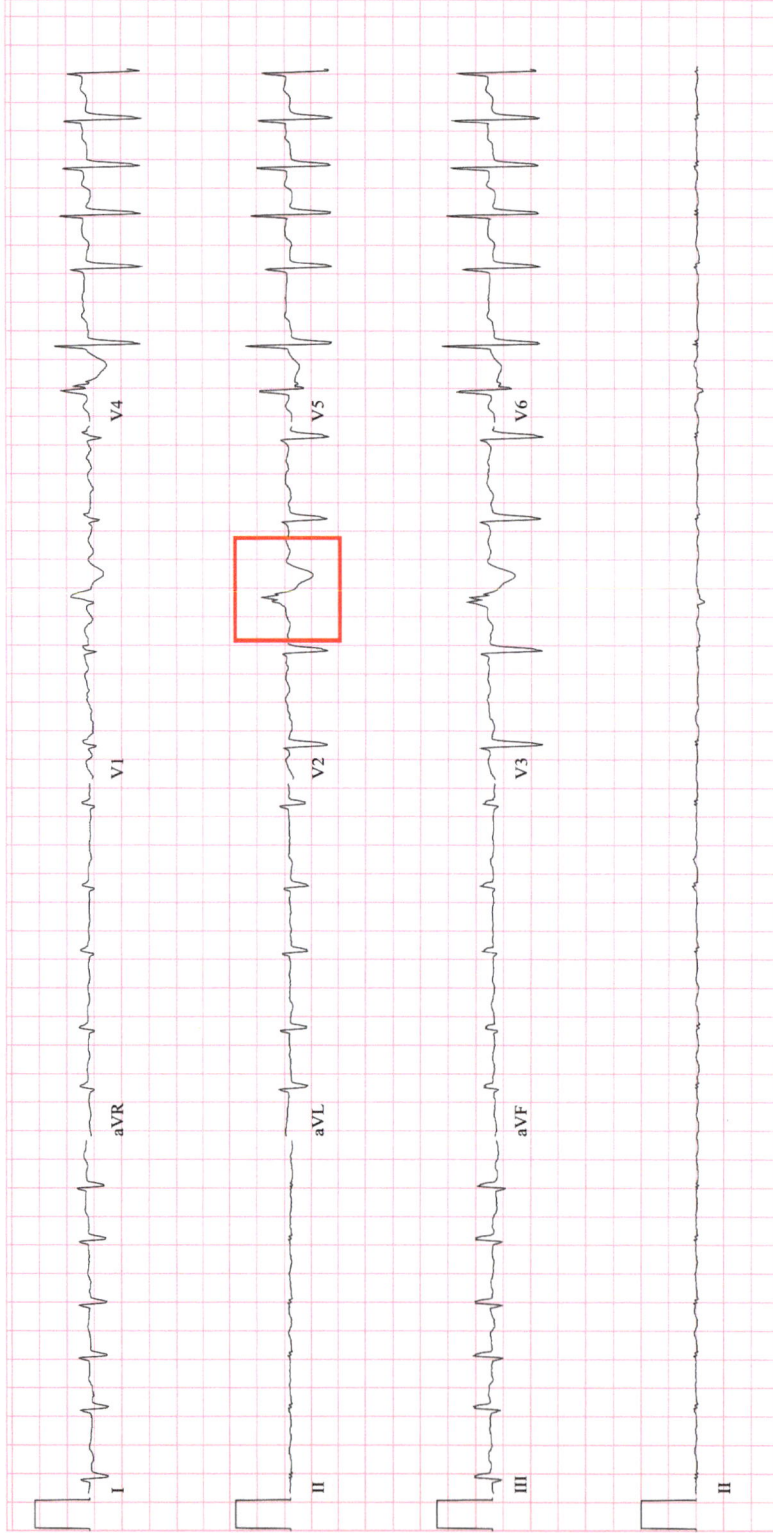

An EKG is obtained from an 85-year-old male with a known history of atrial fibrillation. What conduction pattern is highlighted?

DIAGNOSIS: Ashman's Phenomenon in Atrial Fibrillation

In the presence of atrial fibrillation, impulses of supraventricular origin that are transmitted to the ventricles during periods of relative refractoriness to impulse conduction exhibit anomalous configurations called aberrancy. These "aberrant beats" can be difficult to distinguish from ventricular ectopic beats, and groups of aberrant beats may be mistaken for ventricular tachycardia. Richard Ashman, PhD, a physiologist at Louisiana State University School of Medicine in New Orleans, noted that ventricular refractoriness varied with the lengths of the preceding cardiac cycle (i.e, the longer the preceding RR interval, the longer the refractory period); that aberrant beats typically featured short cycles following long cycles; and that aberrant beats often have a right bundle branch block configuration (because the right bundle usually has a longer refractory period than the left bundle at slower rates). The observation shown in the present EKG is known as the "Ashman phenomenon". Its recognition may allow clinicians to distinguish aberrant beats from ventricular ectopy.[1]

1   Kennedy, L. B., W. Leefe, and B. R. Leslie. "The Ashman phenomenon." *The Journal of the Louisiana State Medical Society: official organ of the Louisiana State Medical Society* 156, no. 3 (2003): 159-162.

EKG Case 23

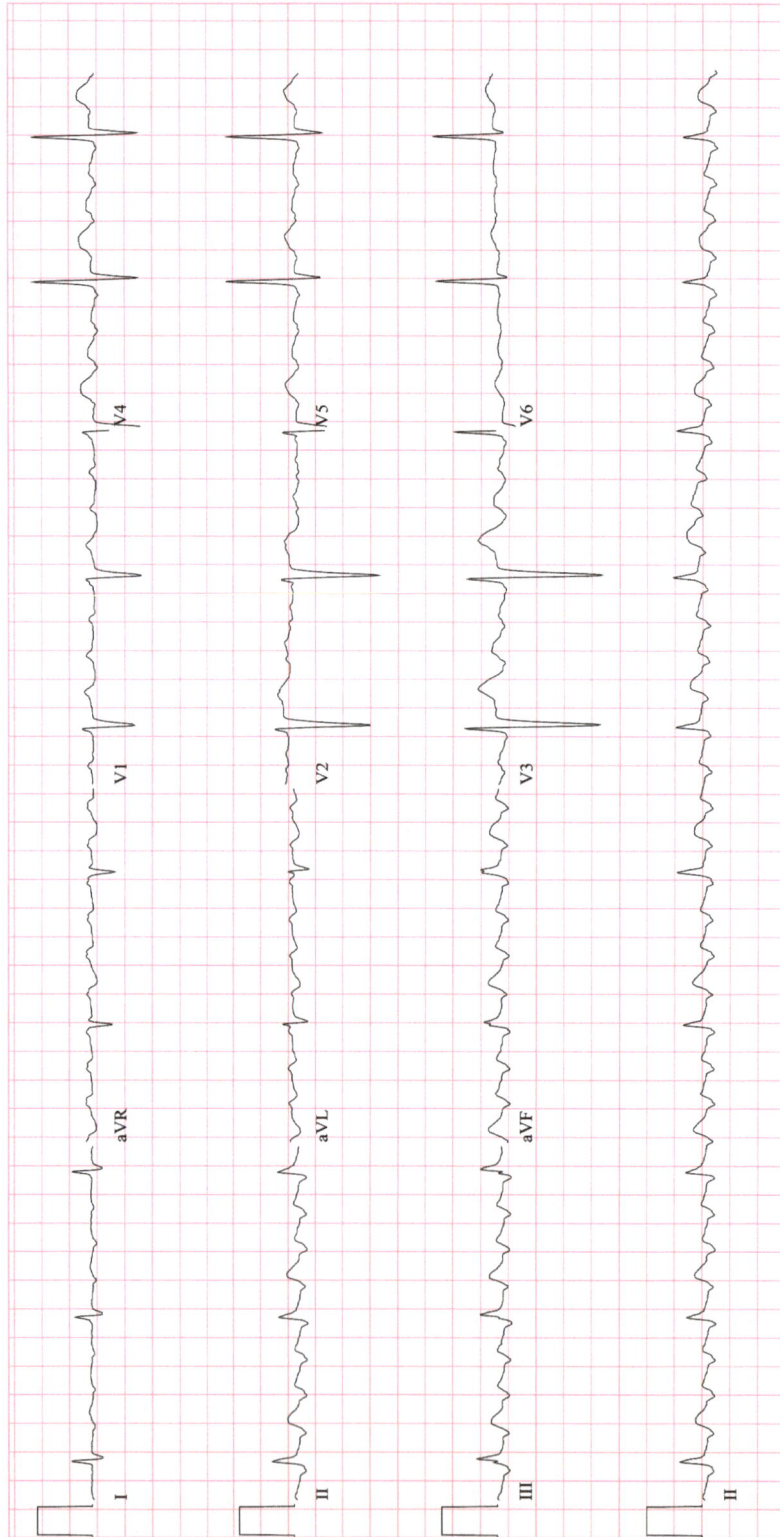

A 65-year-old female with a history of atrial fibrillation and hypertension presents to the hospital with palpitations. What does the EKG show?

DIAGNOSIS: Typical Right Atrial Flutter Counterclockwise with 4:1 AV Block

The EKG shows counterclockwise typical atrial flutter with atrial rate of ~ 300 bpm. Typical P waves are absent and atrial activity is seen as saw tooth-like oscillations (also called F waves), best seen in the inferior leads. Typically, flutter waves are negative in II, III, and aVF, and positive in V1, indicating counterclockwise pattern. Opposite flutter wave orientations are seen in clockwise typical flutter.

- Typical atrial flutter is a type of supraventricular tachycardia caused by a re-entry circuit within the right atrium. The length of the re-entry circuit corresponds to the size of the right atrium, resulting in a fairly predictable atrial rate of around 300 bpm.

- Ventricular rate is determined by the AV conduction ratio ("degree of AV block").

- The most common AV ratio is 2:1, resulting in a ventricular rate of ~150 bpm.

- Ventricular rate is determined by ratio of AV conduction, e.g, 2:1 block = 150 bpm, 3:1 block = 100 bpm, 4:1 block = 75 bpm. Variable block may be seen in some patients.

- Atrial flutter with 1:1 conduction can occur due to sympathetic stimulation, parasympathetic withdrawal, and the use of antiarrhythmic drug therapy such as Class IA or IC agents without concomitantly using AV nodal blocking agents. The presence of an accessory bypass tract leads to pre-excited atrial flutter. Atrial flutter with 1:1 conduction is often associated with hemodynamic instability.

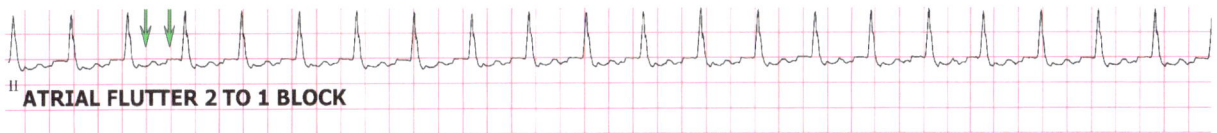

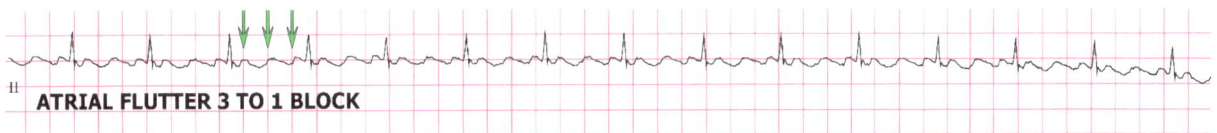

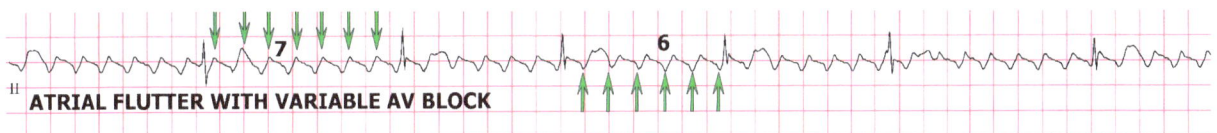

ATRIAL FLUTTER 2 TO 1 BLOCK

ATRIAL FLUTTER 3 TO 1 BLOCK

ATRIAL FLUTTER WITH VARIABLE AV BLOCK

EKG Case 24

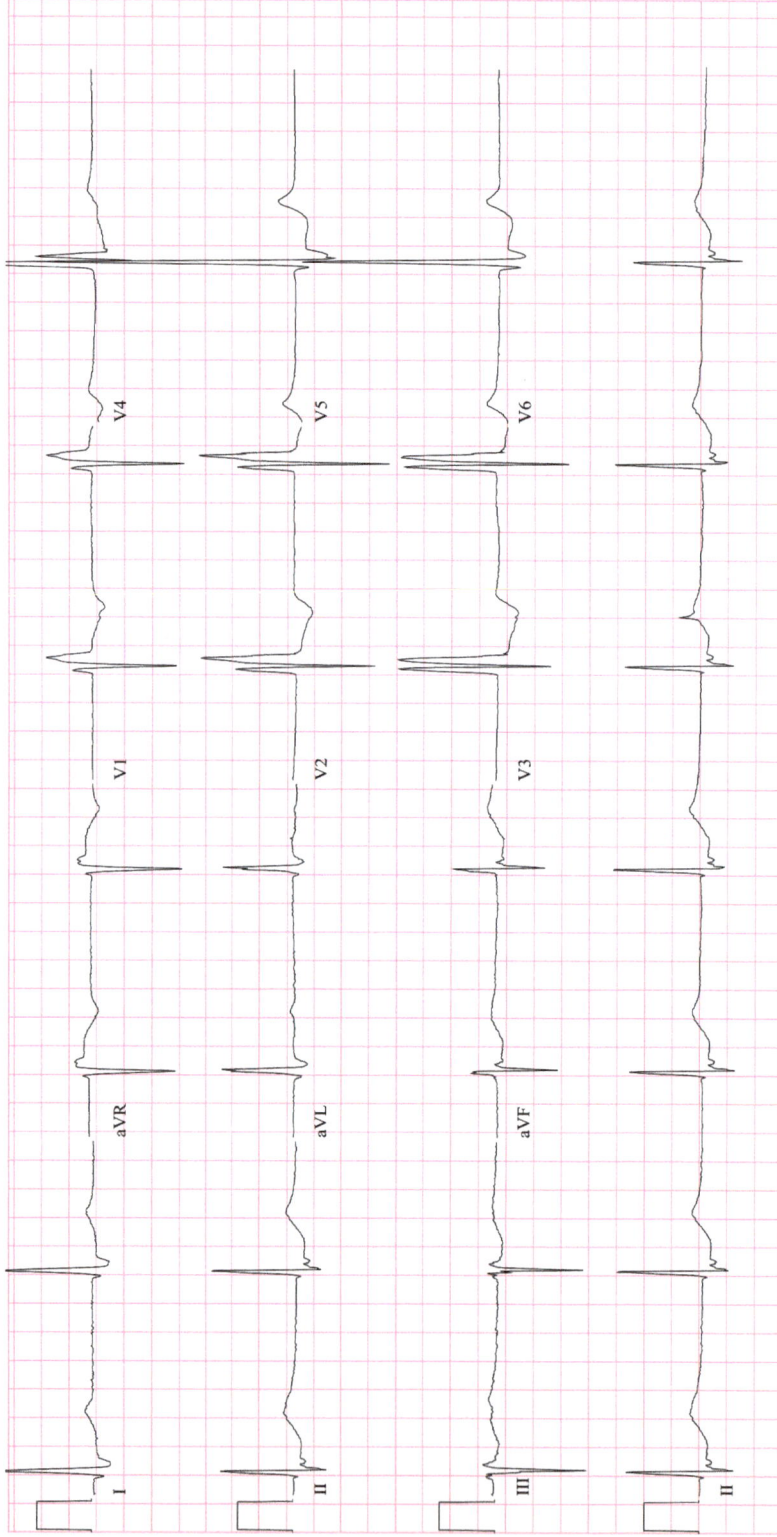

A 65-year-old male with a history of hypertension on beta-blocker and calcium-channel blocker presents for a routine checkup. An EKG is obtained. What does it show?

DIAGNOSIS: Junctional Escape Rhythm

This EKG shows junctional escape rhythm with ventricular response of 40 bpm. There is an absence of P waves preceeding the QRS complex, but retrograde atrial activation could be seen with inverted P waves in leads II, III, and aVF. The EKG also shows an rsR' pattern in lead V1 indicating RBBB.

- The rate of spontaneous depolarization of pacemaker cells decreases down the conducting system. SA node (60 -100 bpm). Atria (< 60 bpm)- AV node (40-60 bpm)- Ventricles (20-40 bpm).

- Junctional and ventricular escape rhythms arise when the rate of supraventricular impulses arriving at the AV node or ventricle is less than the intrinsic rate of the ectopic pacemaker.

- A junctional rhythm is a narrow complex (< 120ms) rhythm with a rate of 40 - 60 bpm. There is no relationship between the QRS complexes and any preceding atrial activity (e.g, P-waves, flutter waves).

- Retrograde P waves may be present and can appear before, during, or after the QRS complex. Retrograde P waves are usually inverted in the inferior leads (II, III, aVF), and upright in leads aVR and V1.

- Conditions leading to the emergence of a junctional or ventricular escape rhythm include: severe sinus bradycardia, sinus arrest, sino-atrial exit block, high-grade second degree AV block, third degree AV block, hyperkalemia, and drugs like beta-blockers, calcium-channel blockers, or digoxin.

Terminology of junctional rhythms include:

- Junctional bradycardia = junctional rhythm at a rate of < 40 bpm.

- Junctional escape rhythm = junctional rhythm at a rate of 40 -60 bpm.

- Accelerated junctional rhythm = junctional rhythm at 60 -100 bpm.

- Junctional tachycardia = junctional rhythm at > 100 bpm.

EKG Case 25

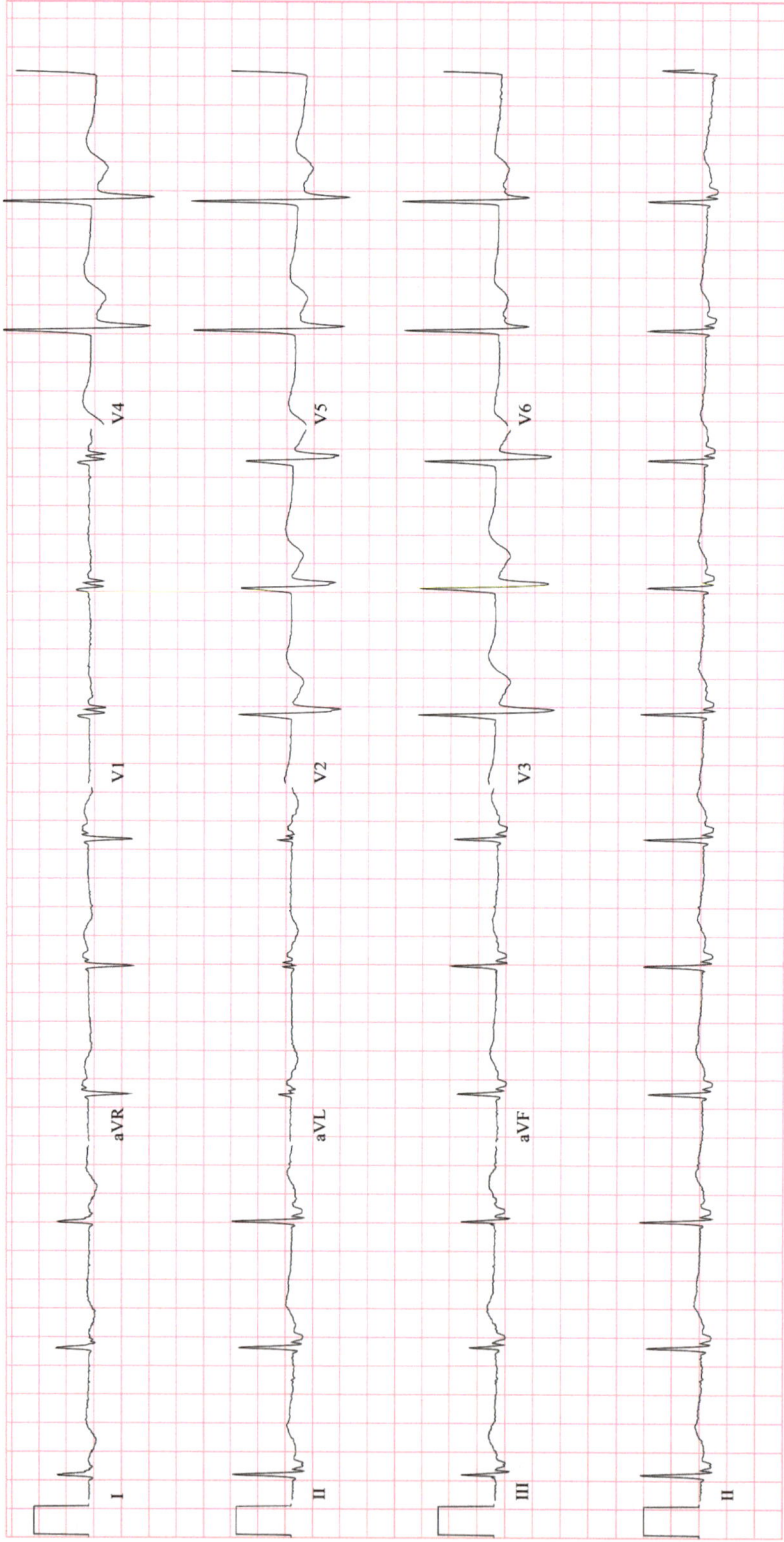

A 72-year-old male with history of coronary artery disease, hypertension, and heart failure presents with dizziness. An EKG is obtained. What does it show?

DIAGNOSIS: Accelerated Junctional Rhythm (AJR)

This EKG shows narrow QRS complexes at a rate of 70 bpm. Retrograde inverted P waves could be identified in lead II, III and aVF, and upright retrograde P waves are seen in aVR and V1. Lateral leads demonstrate "scooping" of ST segment as seen with digoxin effect.

- Accelerated junctional rhythm (AJR) occurs when the rate of an AV junctional pacemaker exceeds that of the sinus node. This situation arises when there is *increased automaticity* in the AV node coupled with *decreased automaticity* in the sinus node.

- Junctional rhythms are arbitrarily classified by their rate, Junctional Escape Rhythm 40-60 bpm , Accelerated Junctional Rhythm 60-100 bpm and Junctional Tachycardia > 100 bpm.

- The most common causes of AJR include digoxin toxicity, use of beta-agonists (e.g, epinephrine), myocardial ischemia, myocarditis, and cardiac surgery.

EKG Features of AJR Include:

- Narrow complex rhythm with QRS duration < 120ms (unless pre-existing bundle branch block or rate-related aberrant conduction).

- Ventricular rate between 60 -100 bpm.

- Retrograde P waves may be present and can appear before, during, or after the QRS complex.

- Retrograde P waves are usually inverted in the inferior leads (II, III, aVF); upright in aVR and V1.

- AV dissociation may be present with the ventricular rate usually greater than the atrial rate.

- There may be associated EKG features of digoxin effect or toxicity.

- The ectopic rhythm lacks the sudden onset and termination that are characteristic of the paroxysmal SVTs.

EKG Case 26

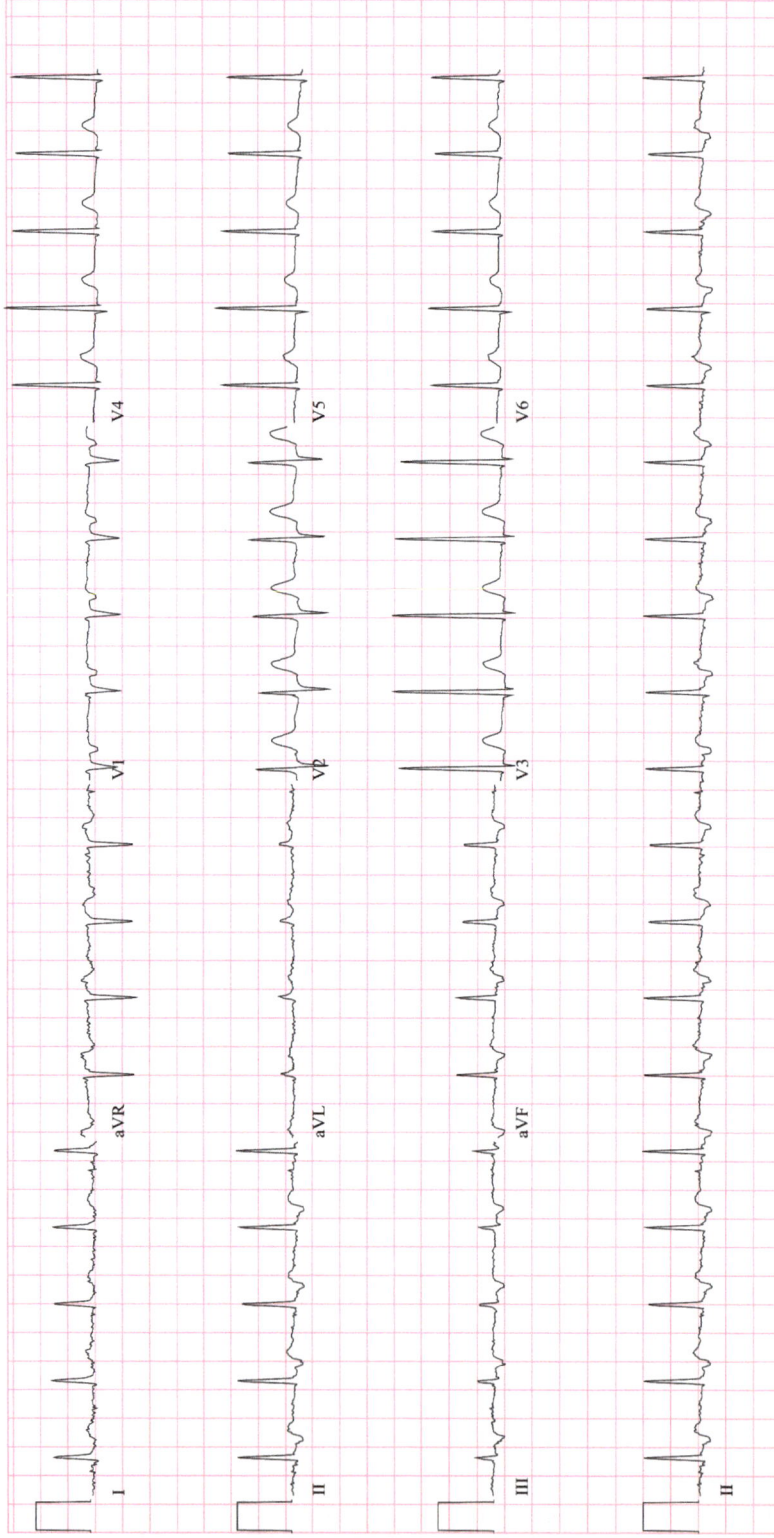

A 56-year-old male with a history of atrial fibrillation on digoxin presents with shortness of breath and palpitations. An EKG is obtained. What does the EKG show?

DIAGNOSIS: Junctional Tachycardia

This EKG shows narrow complex tachycardia at 115 bpm. Retrograde inverted P waves in II, III, and aVF; upright P waves in aVR - suggestive of junctional tachycardia.

EKG Features of Junctional Tachycardia include:

- Narrow complex rhythm; QRS duration < 120 ms (unless pre-existing bundle branch block or rate-related aberrant conduction).

- Ventricular rate > 100 bpm.

- Retrograde P waves may be present and can appear before, during, or after the QRS complex. Retrograde P waves are usually inverted in the inferior leads (II, III, aVF), upright in aVR.

- AV dissociation may be present with the ventricular rate usually greater than the atrial rate.

- There may be associated EKG features of digoxin effect or toxicity.

- Similar rhythm with heart rate between 60 -100 is termed as accelerated junctional rhythm, as discussed in previous case (Case # 25).

EKG Case 27

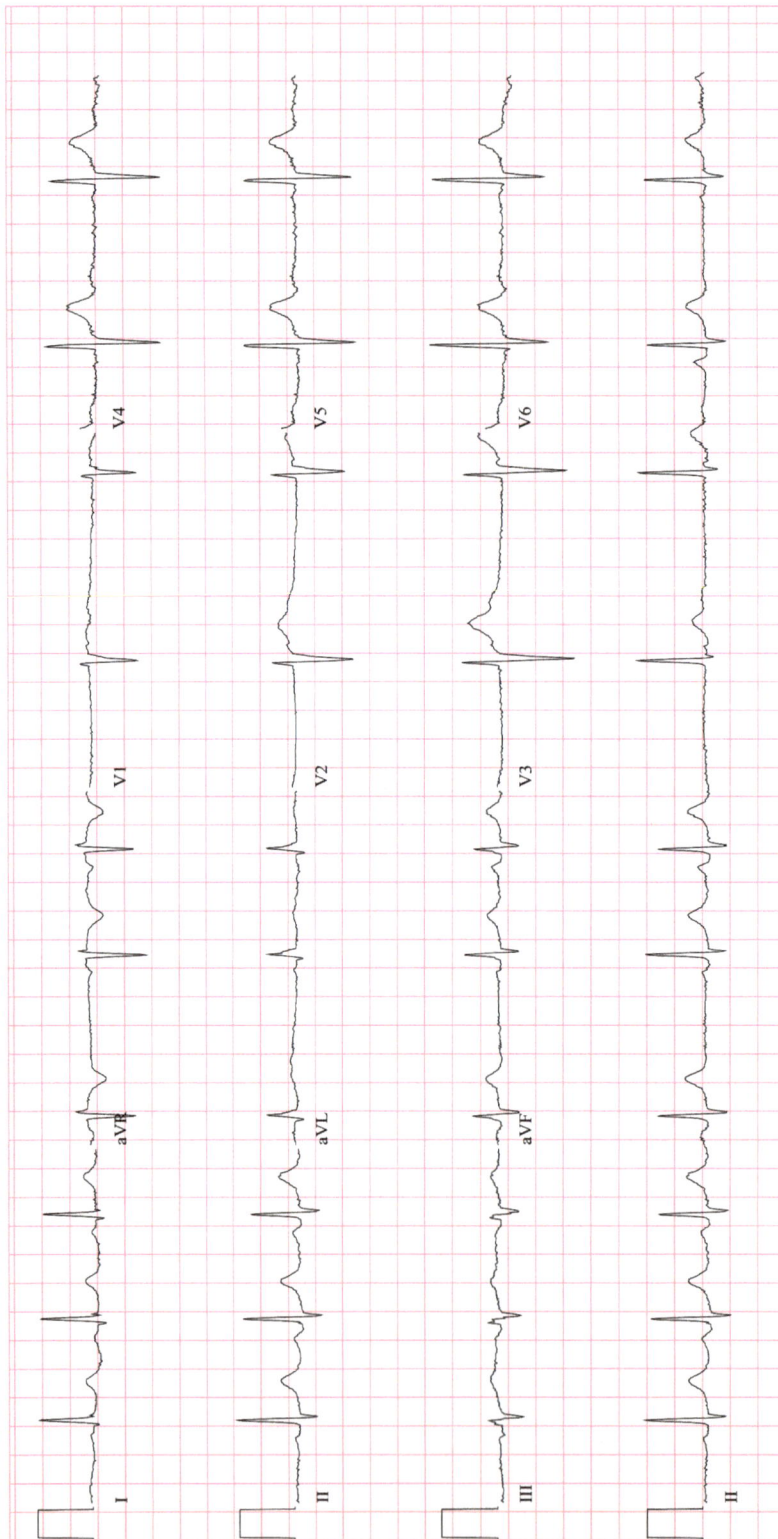

A 65-year-old female with history of hypertension and congestive heart failure has a pre-op EKG performed. What does it reveal?

DIAGNOSIS: Sinus Arrhythmias and Junctional Escape

The above EKG reveals normal sinus rhythm with fluctuating RR intervals in the first cardiac cycles, suggestive of sinusarrhythmias. This is followed by a delayed sinus discharge and normal QRS complex (5th beat). The 7th and the 8th beats do not have a preceding P waves and are of normal (< 120 ms) QRS morphology suggestive of junctional escape beats. The prolonged pause after 6th beat prompted the AV node to discharge electrical impulse, resulting in junctional escape. The rate of spontaneous depolarization of pacemaker cells decreases down the conducting system. SA node (60- 100 bpm). Atria (< 60 bpm), AV node (40-60 bpm), Ventricles (20-40 bpm).

Junctional escape rhythms arise when the rate of supraventricular impulses arriving at the sinus node is less than the intrinsic rate of the ectopic pacemaker, or - in case of complete heart block when the AV node discharges at its intrinsic rate to depolarize the ventricles. Junctional escape can be transient (one or few beats) or sustained (with complete heart block).

For junctional escape rhythm, see Case # 24.

EKG Case 28

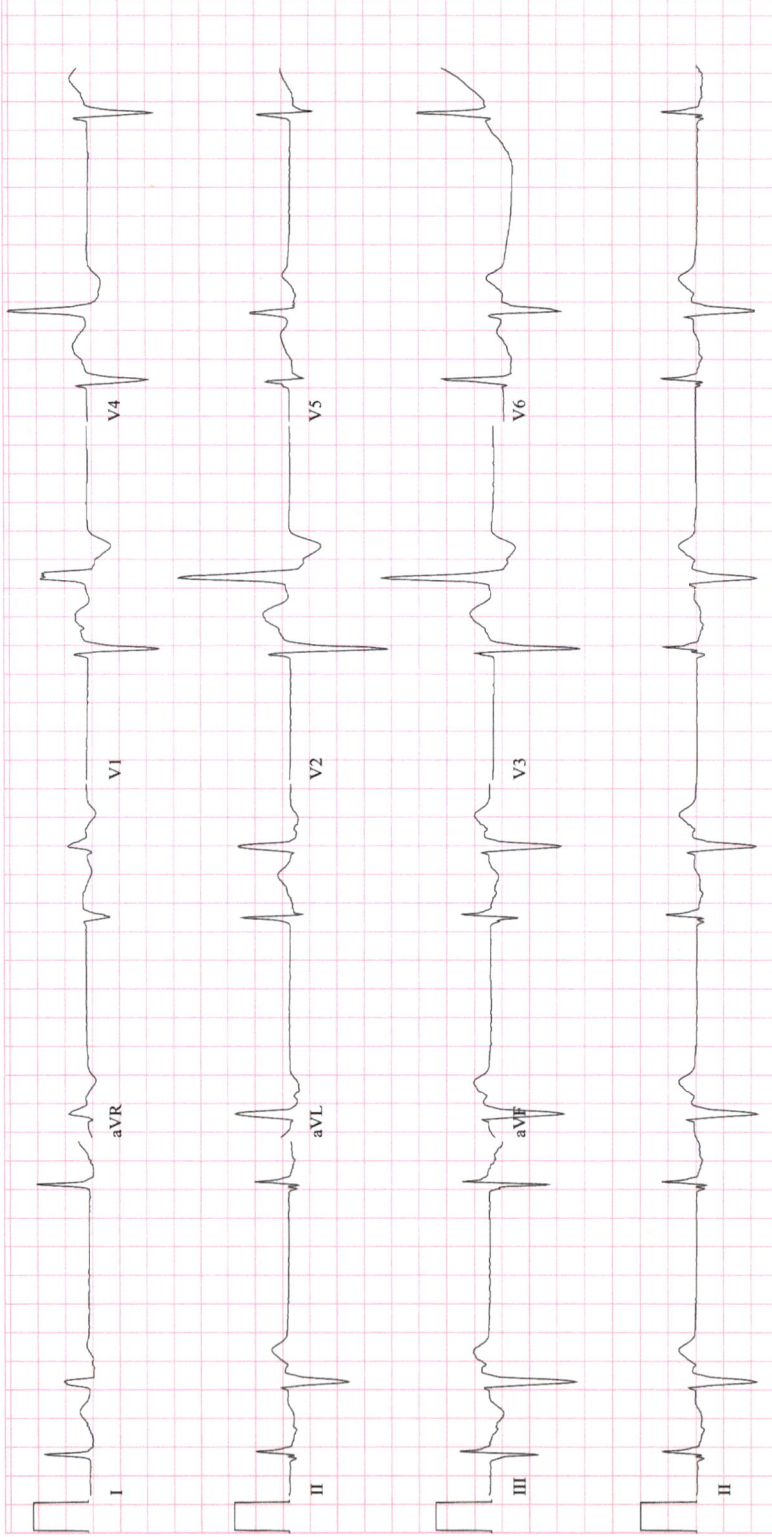

A 85-year-old male with a history of coronary artery disease presents with occasional palpitations. EKG is shown. What does it reveal?

DIAGNOSIS: Junctional Escape Rhythm with Retrograde Conduction to the Atria and Premature Ventricular Contractions in a Bigeminal Pattern

Premature contractions ("ectopic") are classified by their origin - atrial (PACs), junctional (PJCs), or ventricular (PVCs).

- Premature Ventricular Contractions (PVC) are abnormal beats that originate from an ectopic focus within the ventricles. Characteristics include wide QRS width (≥ 120 ms), and ST segments and T waves directed opposite to the main vector of the QRS complex. In the above example, the origin of PVC is in the left ventricle leading to RBBB morphology.

- The long compensatory pause after each PVC leads to junctional escape beat, presumably because of depressed sinus node automaticity.

EKG Case 29

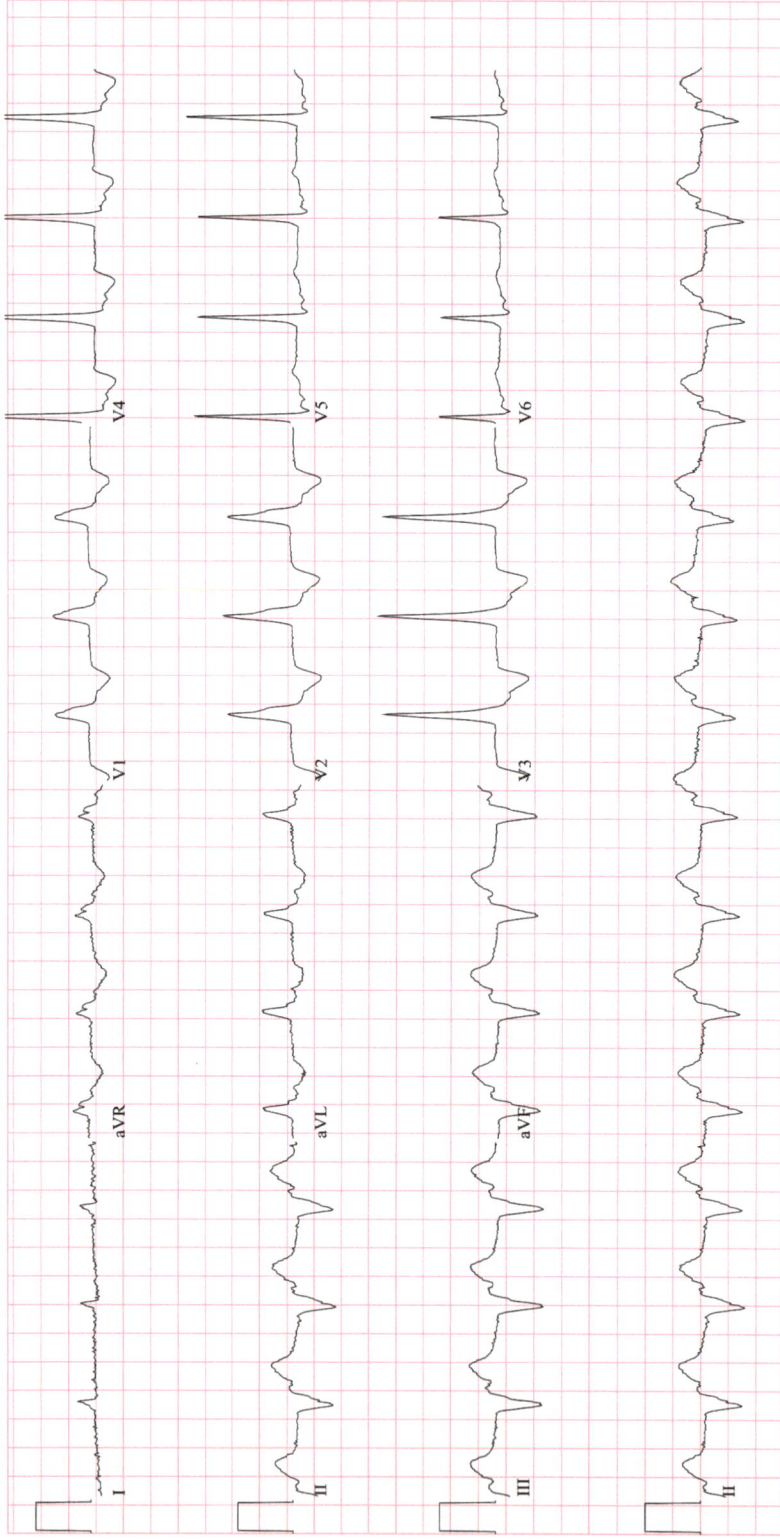

A 80-year-old male with a history of hypertension and recent myocardial infarction presents with chest tightness. An EKG is obtained. What does it show?

DIAGNOSIS: Accelerated Idioventricular Rhythm (AIVR), also known as Accelerated Ventricular Rhythm

This EKG shows wide complex (QRS 140 ms) rhythm at 70bpm with retrograde atrial activation, left axis deviation, RBBB (indicating origin of ectopic focus from left ventricle), and deep Q waves in inferior leads.

- In accelerated idioventricular rhythm, the QRS complexes are wide (> 120ms) and appear in a regular rhythm occurring at a rate of 60 - 100 bpm.

- It results when the rate of impulse generated by the ectopic ventricular focus exceeds that of the sinus node.

- Rate of AIVR distinguishes it from other rhythms of similar morphology. Rates < 50 bpm are consistent with a ventricular escape rhythm and rates > 100 bpm are consistent with ventricular tachycardia.

- AIVR is often associated with increased vagal tone, decreased sympathetic tone, acute myocardial ischemia, hypoxia, return of spontaneous circulation (ROSC) following cardiac arrest, or digoxin toxicity.

- AIVR is classically seen in the first two days of acute myocardial infarction, or in the reperfusion phase after acute STEMI, e.g, post thrombolysis.

- Rhythm is usually well-tolerated, benign, and self-limiting. Treatment is warranted when AIVR transforms to VT or VF or when the patient is hemodynamically unstable.

EKG Case 30

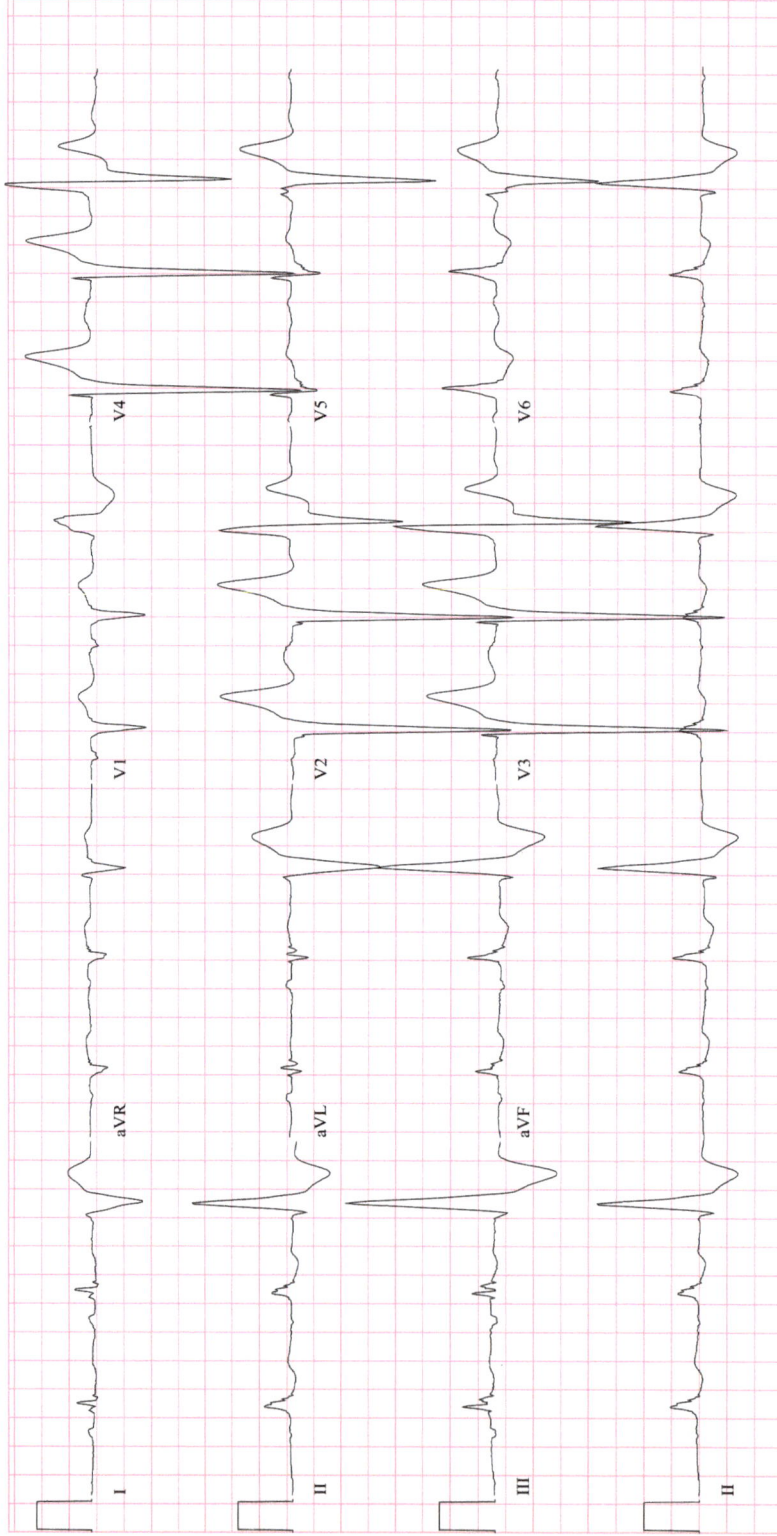

A 28-year-old college student presents to the office with a complaint of occasional palpitations and "skipping heart beat". Patient is stressed out due to upcoming semester exams and is consuming more coffee than usual. What does the EKG show?

DIAGNOSIS: Ventricular Trigeminy

This EKG shows normal sinus rhythm with broad QRS complexes with LBBB morphology and PVC's in a pattern of trigeminy.

- Premature Ventricular Contraction (PVC) is an abnormal beat that originates from an ectopic focus within the ventricles.

- Characteristics include: wide abnormal width (≥ 120 ms) QRS, premature and discordant ST segment, and T wave, that are directed opposite to the main vector of the QRS complex. Usually PVCs are followed by a compensatory pause.

- Frequency: PVC's can occur in different patterns: ventricular bigeminy is noted when every other beat is a PVC (example below), while ventricular trigeminy is when every third beat is a PVC, and ventricular quadrigeminy is when every fourth beat is a PVC. PVCs can also present in pairs (two consecutive PVCs) known as couplet, or with three consecutive PVCs known as triplet.

- Origin: morphology of QRS complex determines its site origin. PVCs originating from the same site are unifocal. PVCs arising from two or more foci leading to multiple QRS morphologies are termed multifocal.

- Location: vector of PVC determines location of origin as electricity travelling in direction of lead gives a positive deflection in that lead and the converse is also true. e.g, PVCs arising from the right ventricle or LV septum can have a left bundle branch block morphology (dominant S wave in V1). PVCs arising from the left ventricle usually have a right bundle branch block morphology (dominant R wave in V1).

- It is important to differentiate between PVC's and PAC's with aberrancy. Aberrant PACs distort the QRS less and the QRS axis tends to be similar to that of normal beats. Aberrant PACs are usually preceded by P wave and have typical patterns of RBBB, LBBB, LAFB, or LPFB.

- In patients with underlying predispositions (e.g, ischemic heart disease, WPW), a PVC may trigger the onset of a re-entrant tachydysrhythmia - e.g, VT, AVNRT/AVRT.

- Anxiety, stress, and the use of coffee can act as triggers to frequent PVCs. In the presence of frequent PVCs, it is important to rule out structural heart abnormalities with a cardiac echocardiogram or cardiac MRI.

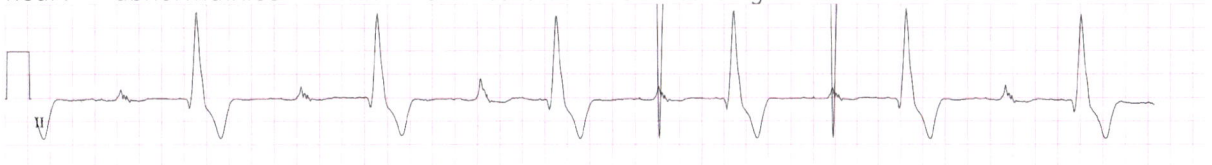

Figure: An example of bigeminy (PVC appears every second beat)

EKG Case 31

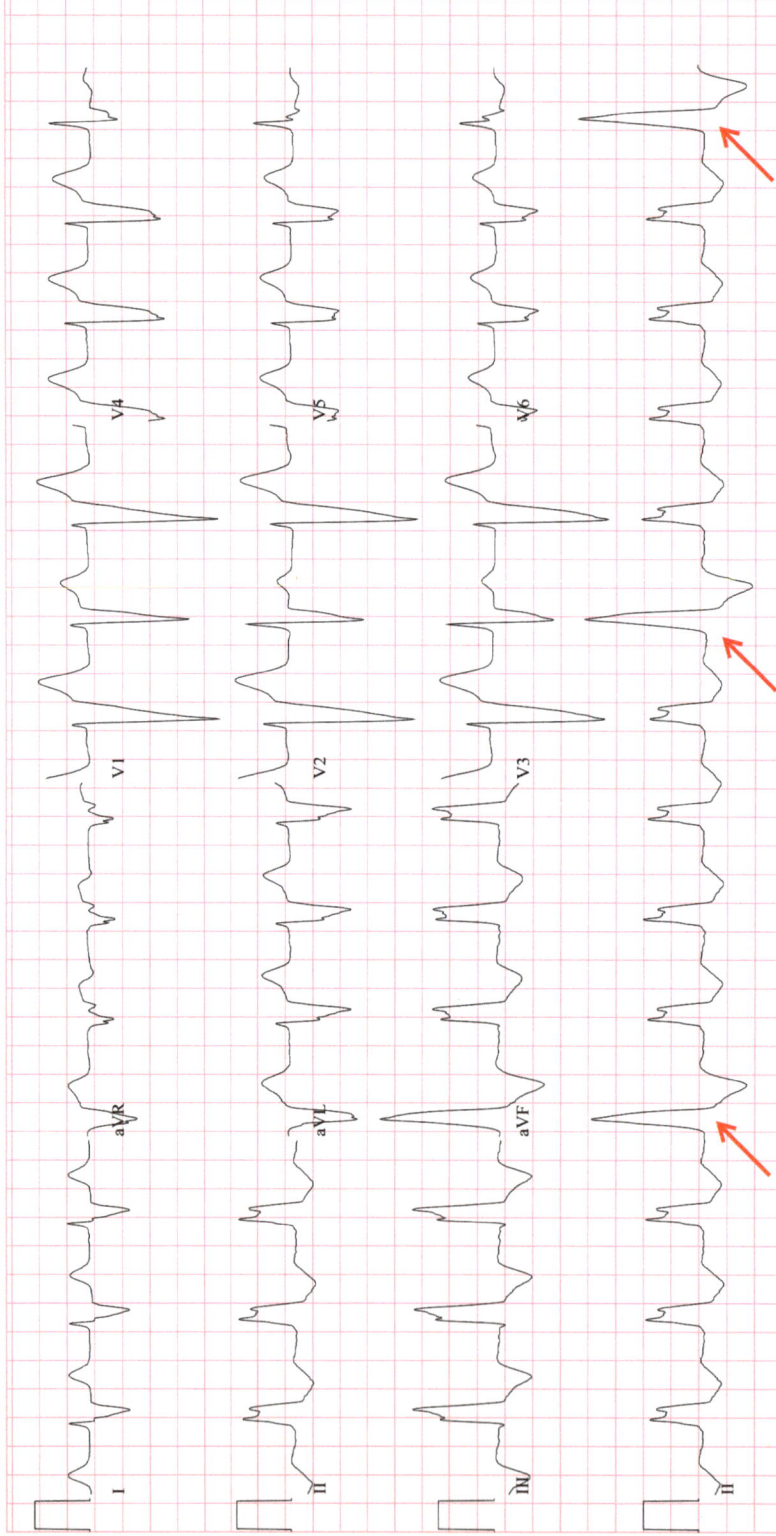

A 75-year-old male with a history of coronary artery disease and heart failure is brought to the ER with shortness of breath. Physical exam reveals bilateral pulmonary crackles and +2 pedal edema. Chest x-ray is consistent with congestive heart failure. An EKG is obtained that shows wide complex rhythm. What is the rhythm and what do the 4th, 9th, and 14th QRS complex represent?

DIAGNOSIS: Accelerated Idioventricular Rhythm (AIVR) with Frequent Parasystole

This EKG shows wide complex (QRS 192 ms) rhythm at 85 bpm - consistent with accelerated idioventricular rhythm. The EKG also shows right axis deviation, LBBB (indicating origin of ectopic focus from right ventricle or septum), and 4th, 9th and 14th beats representing frequent parasystole.

EKG Case 32

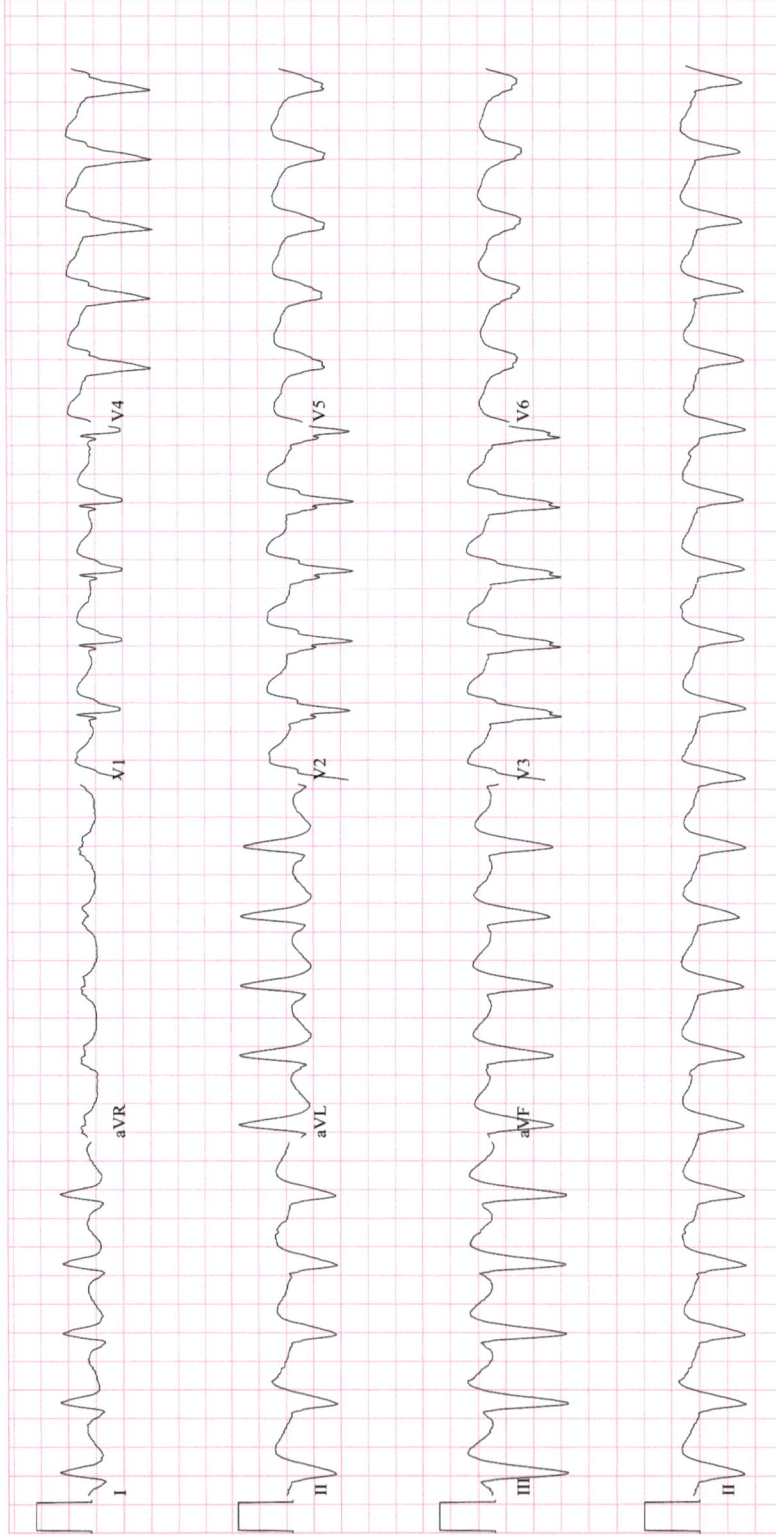

A 75-year-old male with a history of coronary artery disease is admitted to ICU for unstable angina. Patient suddenly becomes cold and clammy, and nurse reports a change in mental status. BP is 60/30 mm hg – An EKG is recorded. What does it show?

DIAGNOSIS: Monomorphic Ventricular Tachycardia

- Given the history of CAD, the presence of wide complex tachycardia is indicative of VT until proven otherwise.

- This EKG shows classic monomorphic VT with uniform broad QRS complexes (~ 200 ms).

- The main features of this wide QRS tachycardia that indicates its ventricular origin is the negative concordance of QRS complexes' in the precordial leads (all are pointing in the negative direction).

- Other features, not seen in our case includes extreme axis deviation ("northwest axis") - QRS is positive in aVR and negative in aVF. rS complex in V6 (tiny R wave, deep S wave). RSR' complexes with a taller left rabbit ear. This is in contrast to typical RBBB, where the right rabbit ear is taller.

- **Brugada's sign:** The distance from the onset of the QRS complex to the nadir of the S wave is > 100 ms, here best seen in aVF.

- **Josephson's sign:** Notching near the nadir of the S wave , best seen in V2.

- An immediate DC cardioversion is needed in circulatory failure due to ventricular tachycardia, as in this patient.

- For difficult cases, the Brugada algorithm can be used to distinguish between VT and SVT with aberrancy.

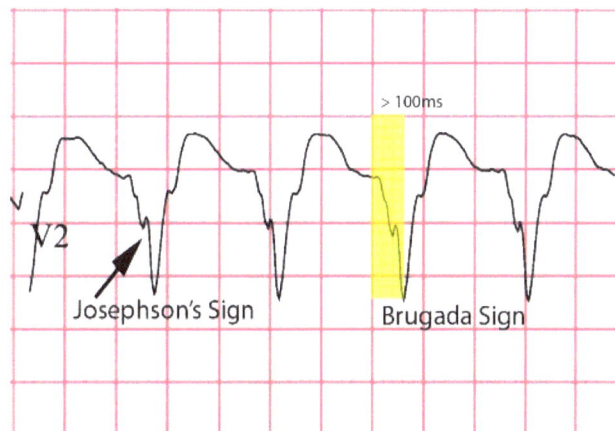

EKG Case 33

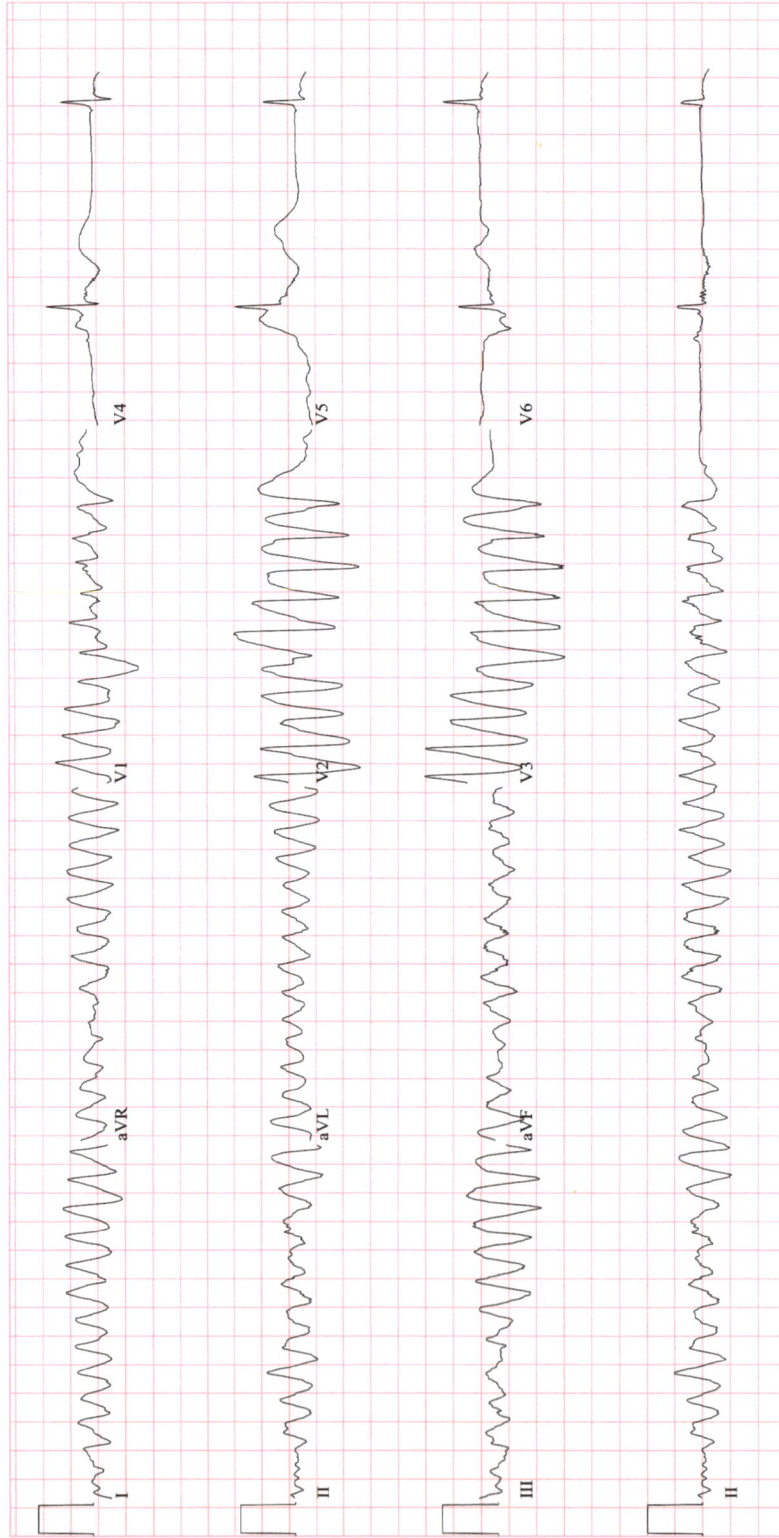

A 55-year-old male with a history of hypothyroidism, CHF, and ischemic heart disease is brought to the ER with lethargy and intermittent syncope. Blood chemistry reveals potassium of 1.6 mEq/L. An EKG is shown. What does it reveal?

DIAGNOSIS: Torsades de Pointes (TdP)

The EKG shows paroxysmal polymorphic ventricular tachycardia (PVT) with characteristics of Torsades de Pointes (TdP), which reverts spontaneously to low voltage QRS with marked QT prolongation.

- Polymorphic ventricular tachycardia is a form of ventricular tachycardia in which the morphology of QRS complexes varies from beat to beat, delineating the absence of a fixed electrical circuit. Torsades de pointes has a characteristic morphology in which the QRS complexes "twist" around the isoelectric line. It happens in the context of QT prolongation.

- For TdP to be diagnosed, the patient has to have evidence of both PVT *and* QT prolongation.

- A prolonged QT reflects prolonged myocyte repolarization due to ion channel malfunction, medication effects, ischemia, or congenital channelopathies.

- This prolonged repolarization period gives rise to early after depolarization (EADs). EADs may manifest on the EKG as tall U waves; if these reach threshold amplitude, they may manifest as premature ventricular contractions (PVCs).

- TdP is initiated when a PVC occurs during the preceding T wave, known as "R on T" phenomenon (not visible on this EKG strip).

- The onset of TdP is often preceded by a sequence of long-short R-R intervals, so called "pause dependent" TdP.

- Depending on their cause, most individual episodes of torsades de pointes revert to normal sinus rhythm within a few seconds, but may also persist and possibly degenerate into ventricular fibrillation, which can lead to sudden death in the absence of prompt defibrillation.

EKG Case 34

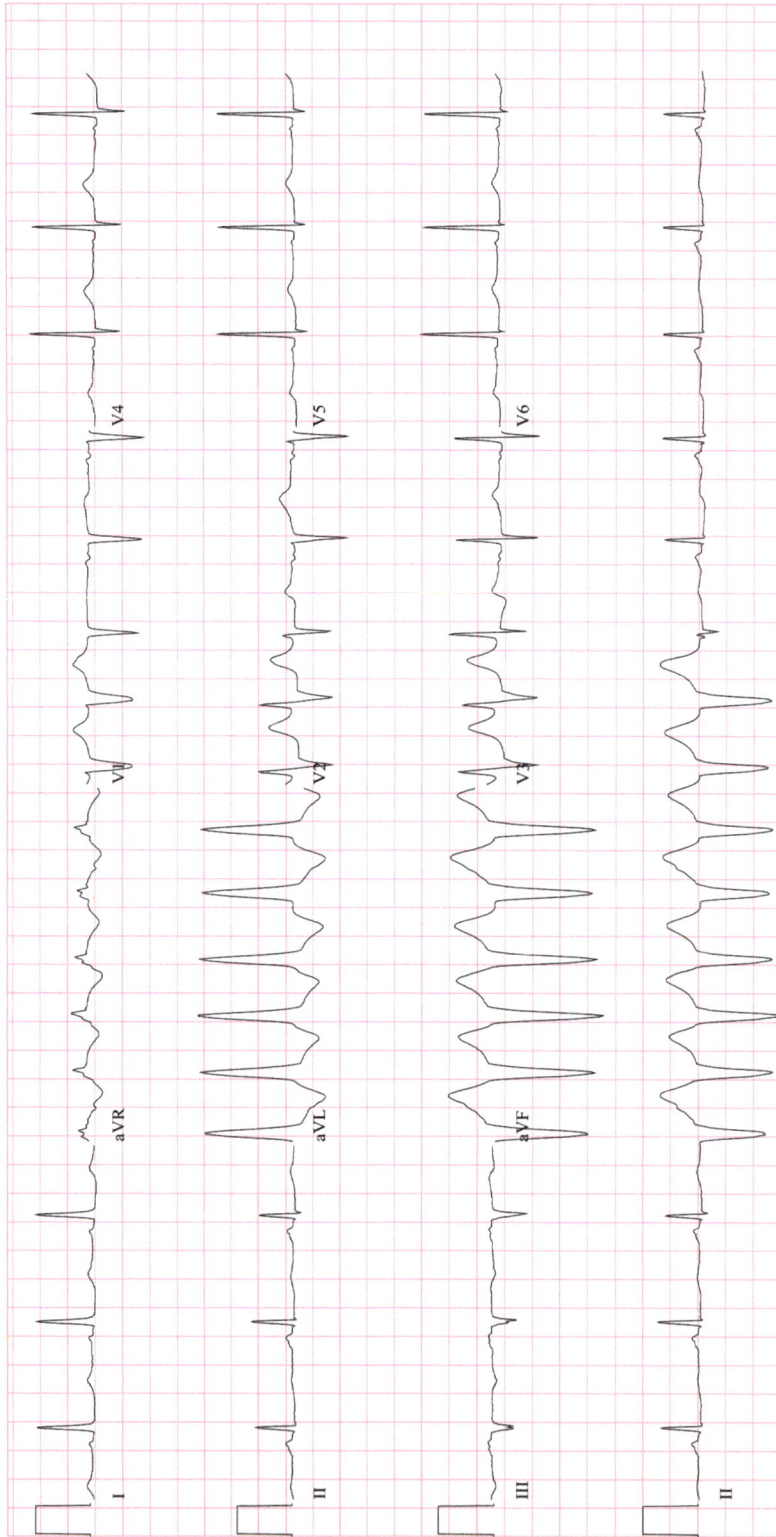

An EKG is recorded from a patient during hemodialysis when he reported palpitations. What does the EKG show?

DIAGNOSIS: Non-Sustained Ventricular Tachycardia (NSVT), Fusion Beat

- The EKG starts with normal sinus rhythm at 85bpm, but after 3rd normal QRS complex follows a run of eight non-sustained beats of wide QRS complexes (> 160ms) - The rhythm is known as non-sustained ventricular tachycardia and is defined by three or more consecutive ventricular complexes terminating spontaneously in < 30 seconds. The 9th beat exhibits fusion, which occurs when a supraventricular and a ventricular impulse coincide to produce a hybrid complex. Fusion beats are of intermediate width and morphology to the normally-conducted supraventricular beats and the ventricular complexes. The last five complexes are normally-conducted sinus beats.

- In the absence of prior cardiac arrest or sustained VT, NSVT is not an indication for ICD placement.

EKG Case 35

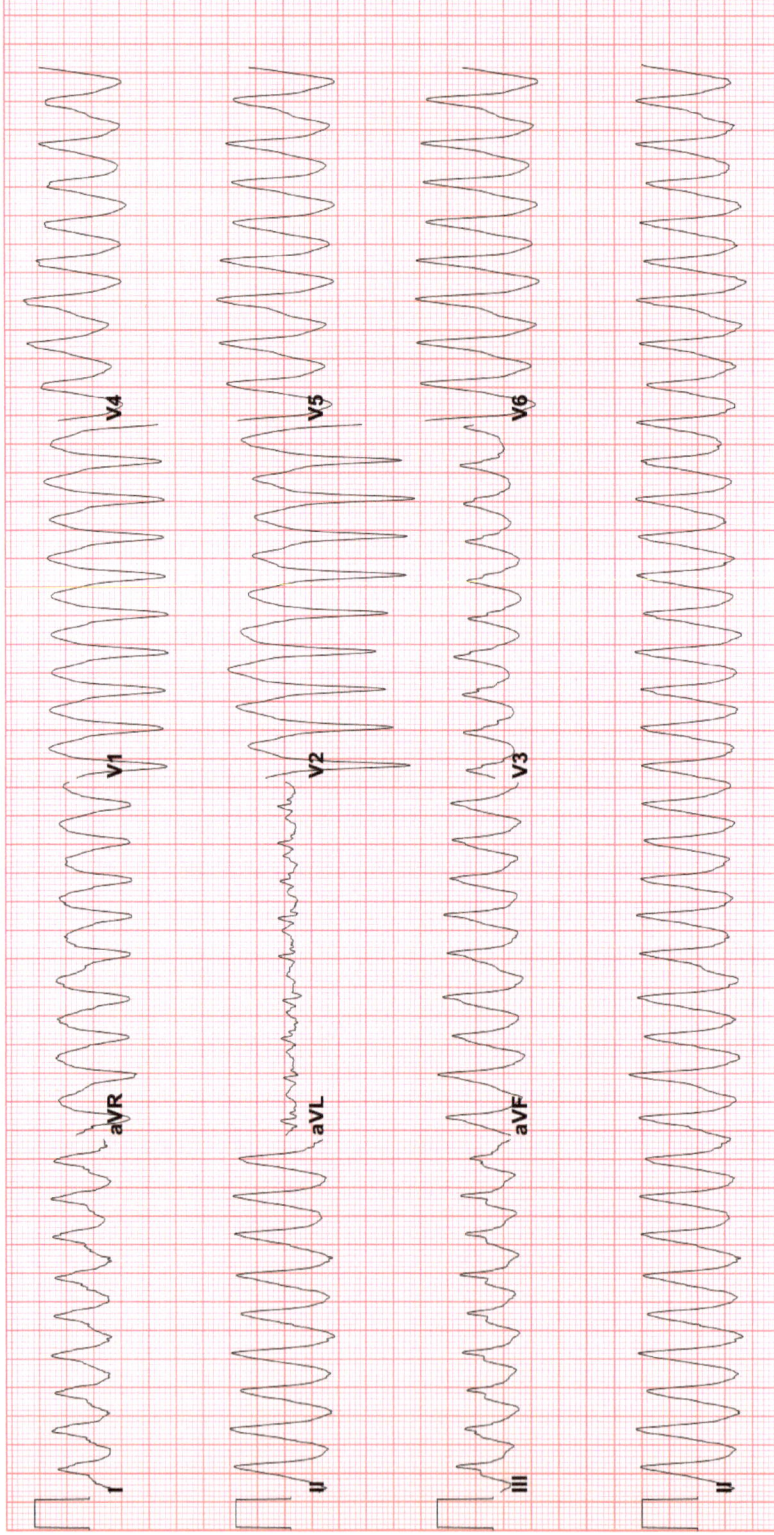

A 55-year-old male with an unremarkable past medical history complains of intermittent but rapid palpitations especially after heavy exertion. An EKG is obtained. What does it reveal?

DIAGNOSIS: Right Ventricular Outflow Tract (RVOT) Tachycardia (Idiopathic VT)

- This EKG shows wide complex tachycardia consistent with monomorphic VT of LBBB and inferior axis morphology.

- Right ventricular outflow tract (RVOT) tachycardia is a form of monomorphic VT originating from the outflow tract of the right ventricle or occasionally from the tricuspid annulus. It occurs in structurally normal hearts (idiopathic VT) and accounts for 10% of all VTs.

- RVOT could also be confused with life-threatening VT in the context of arrhythmogenic right ventricular cardiomyopathy (ARVC). A cardiac MRI may help differentiate between the two diagnoses.

- EKG diagnostic features of RVOT VT include, heart rate > 100 bpm, QRS duration > 120 ms LBBB morphology, rightward / inferior axis (around +90 degrees), and atrioventricular dissociation (if it can be seen on surface EKG).

This patient had a cardiac stress test which did not reveal underlying ischemia, and a cardiac MRI which did not show ARVC or other structural cardiac abnormalities. EP mapping revealed frequent ventricular ectopy originating from the anterior superior portion of the right ventricular outflow tract free wall, which was successfully ablated.

EKG Case 36

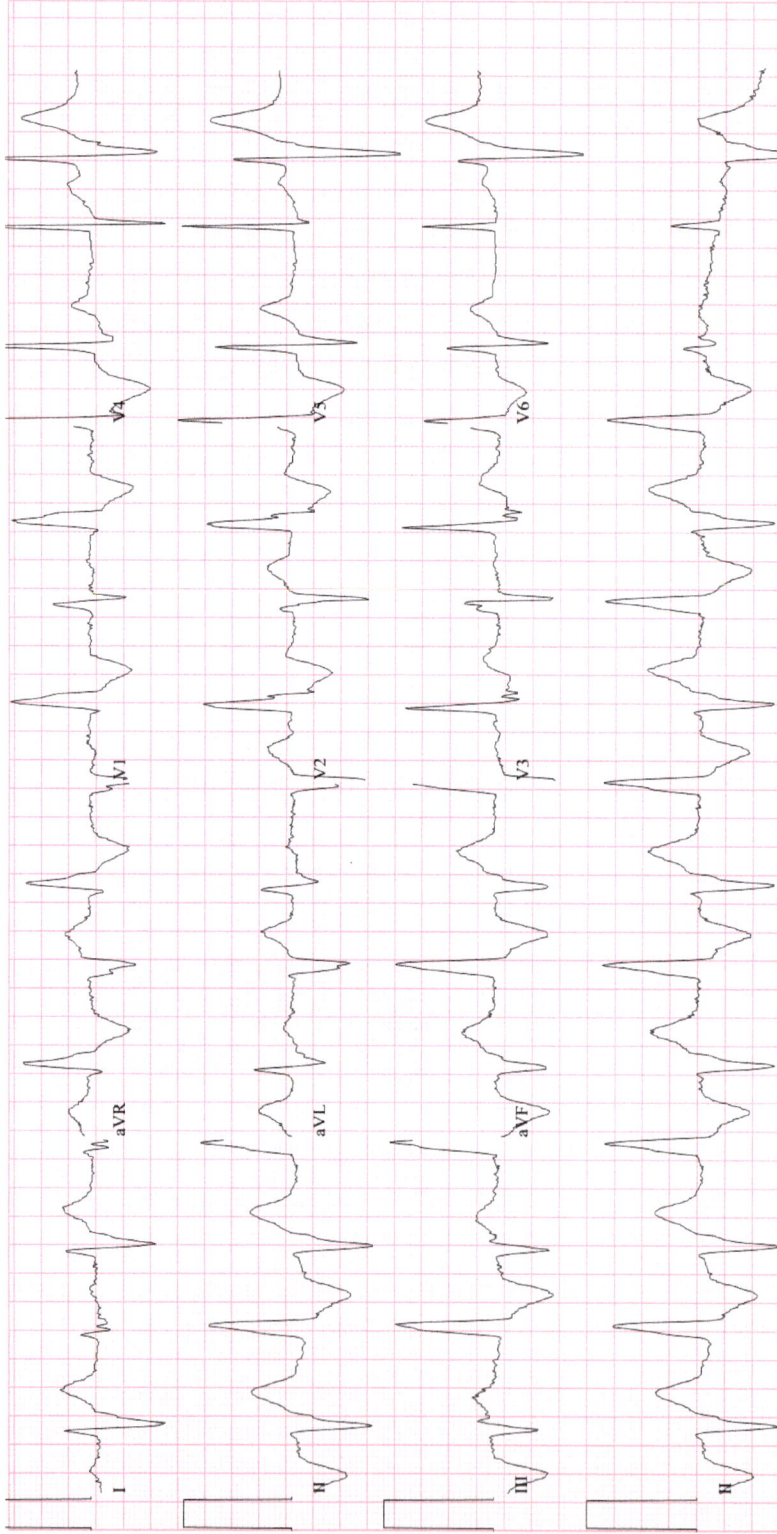

A 50-year-old male with a history of atrial fibrillation on digoxin presents with palpitations for the past three hours. An EKG is obtained. What does it show?

DIAGNOSIS: Slow Bi-directional Ventricular Tachycardia

- This EKG shows an example of bi-directional ventricular tachycardia with alternating wide QRS complexes (> 120ms) of different morphologies. Underlying fibrillatory waves could be seen in lead II with complete AV block.

- The bidirectional tachycardia is defined as a ventricular arrhythmia with an alternating 180° QRS axis on a beat-to-beat basis.

- This rhythm is most commonly seen in the context of severe digoxin toxicity. It may also be the presenting rhythm in patients with familial catecholaminergic polymorphic ventricular tachycardia (CPVT).

CPVT is characterized by episodic syncope occurring during exercise or acute emotional excitement, or stress in individuals without structural cardiac abnormalities. Mutation in four genes – *RYR2, CASQ2, TRDN*, and *CALM1* – have been implicated in CPVT. The most important diagnostic test is exercise stress testing, which can reproducibly evoke the clinical ventricular tachycardia during acute adrenergic activation. The use of beta-blockers is a cornerstone of CPVT therapy. When there is evidence of incomplete protection (recurrence of syncope or complex arrhythmias during exercise) beta blockers, flecainide should be added. Beta-blockers and flecainide are also indicated for affected individuals who have experienced a previous aborted sudden death. An implantable cardioverter defibrillator (ICD) may be necessary to protect patients with cardiac arrest while on beta-blocker therapy or for those unable to take beta-blockers.

EKG Case 37

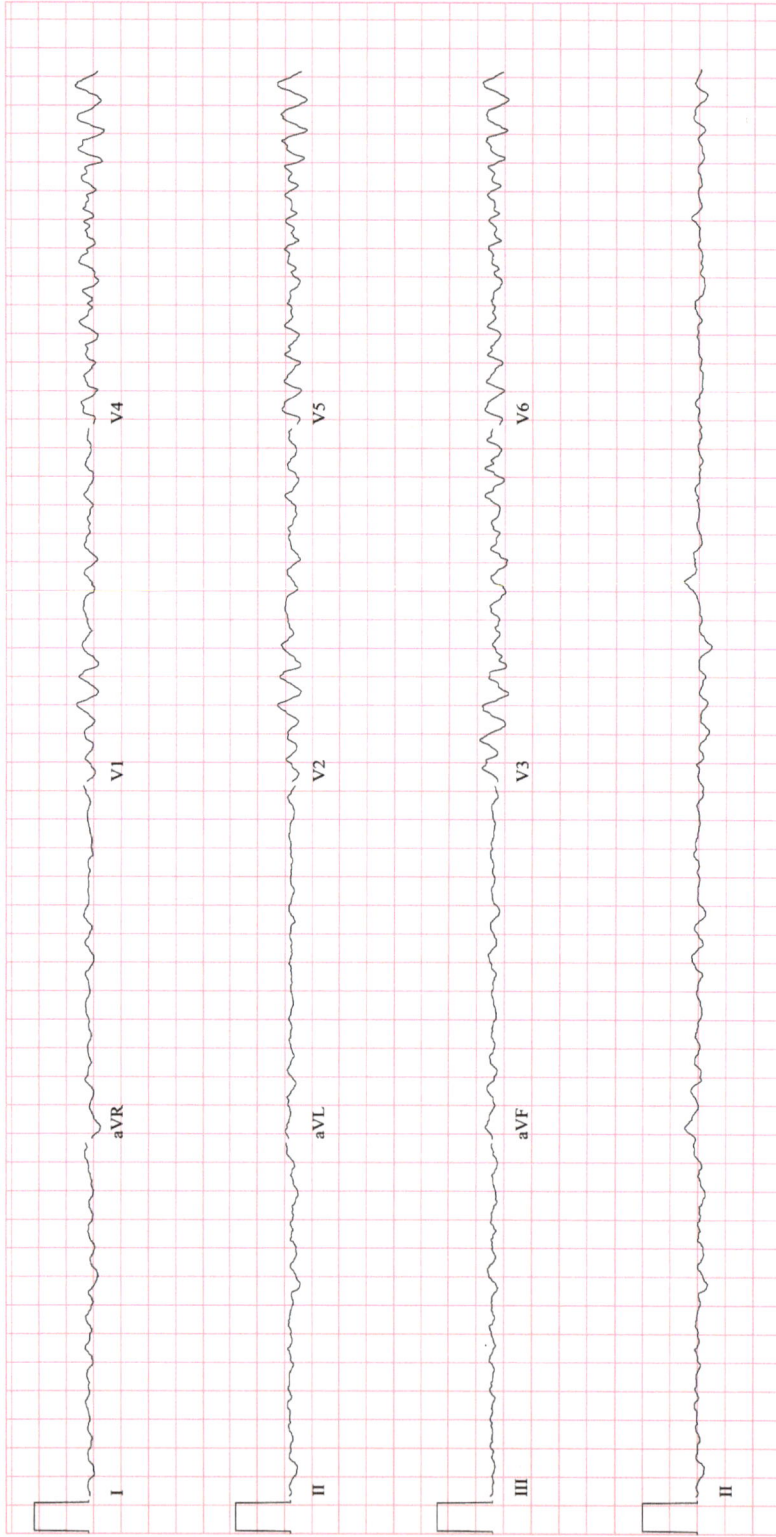

I   aVR   V1   V4

II   aVL   V2   V5

III   aVF   V3   V6

II

A 60-year-old male is brought to the ER with severe chest pain. As EKG is being recorded when he suddenly collapses. What does the EKG show?

DIAGNOSIS: Ventricular Fibrillation (VF)

This EKG shows chaotic, irregular, and disorganized ventricular complexes without discrete or discernable QRS complexes - the rhythm is compatible with ventricular fibrillation.

- Ventricular fibrillation (VF) is the most frequent mechanism of sudden cardiac death.

- In VF, rapid and irregular electrical activity renders the ventricles unable to contract in a synchronized manner, resulting in immediate loss of cardiac output. Unless advanced life support is rapidly instituted, this rhythm is invariably fatal.

- Prolonged ventricular fibrillation is associated with decreasing waveform amplitude, from coarse VF initially to fine VF later on and ultimately to asystole.

- Prompt non-synchronized defibrillation is needed to abort sudden cardiac death.

EKG Findings Include:

- Chaotic irregular deflections of varying amplitude.

- No identifiable P waves, QRS complexes, or T waves.

- Rate of 150 to 500 bpm.

- Amplitude decreases with duration (coarse VF to fine VF).

EKG Case 38

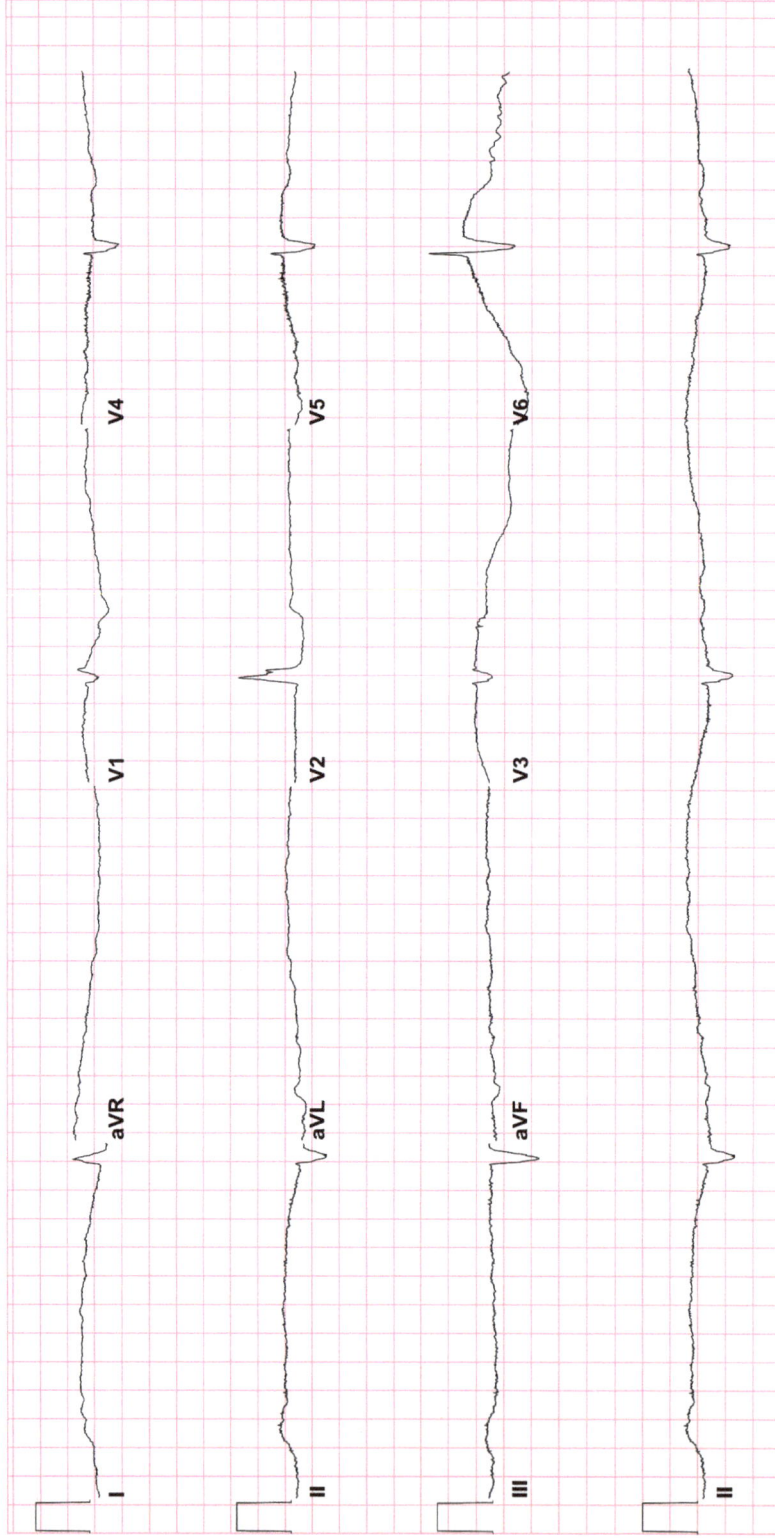

An EKG is obtained by medical student on an 85-year-old male with metastatic prostate cancer who is found confused and in agonal breathing. What does the EKG show?

DIAGNOSIS: Agonal Rhythm

- This is an end-of-life rhythm. Agonal rhythm is often the last ordered semblance of organized electrical activity in the heart prior to death.

- Heart rate is less than 20 bpm, with a wide, bizarre QRS complex and no discernable P waves.

- The rate is often so slow that it is difficult to determine whether the rhythm is regular or irregular on a short rhythm segment.

EKG Case 39

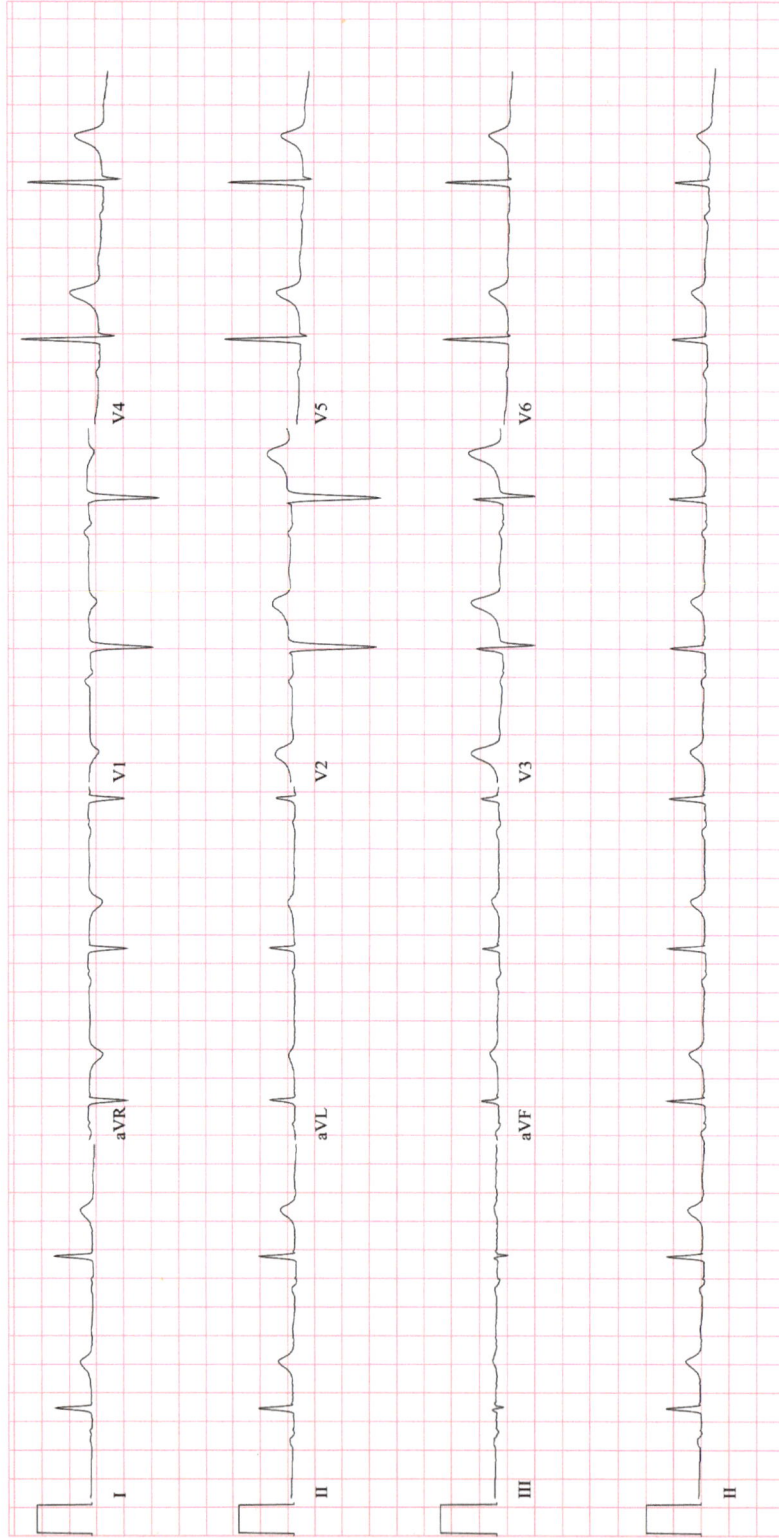

A 53-year-old female presents to the office for yearly physical exam. The EKG performed is read as abnormal by the automated system. What does the EKG show?

DIAGNOSIS: First Degree A-V Block

This EKG shows sinus rhythm with a heart rate of 55 bpm and a prolonged PR interval (which is measured from the start of the P wave to the start of the QRS complex). PR interval in the above patient is approximately 230 ms.

- First degree AV block defined by PR interval > 200 ms (five small squares).

- "Marked" first degree block if PR interval > 300 ms.

- In first degree atrioventricular block (first-degree heart block) there is delayed conduction of the electrical impulse from the atrium to the ventricles through the AV node. The prolongation of the PR interval is constant for each cardiac cycle.

- Conditions that may cause first degree AV block are increased vagal tone (during sleep, athletes), hypokalemia, ischemic heart disease, myocarditis (rheumatic heart disease, Lyme's disease), AV nodal blocking drugs including beta blockers, calcium channel blockers, amiodarone, digoxin, etc.

- First degree A-V block does not usually cause any specific symptoms and does not result in any hemodynamic compromise. No specific intervention is recommended. First degree AV block is not an indication for pacemaker insertion.

EKG Case 40

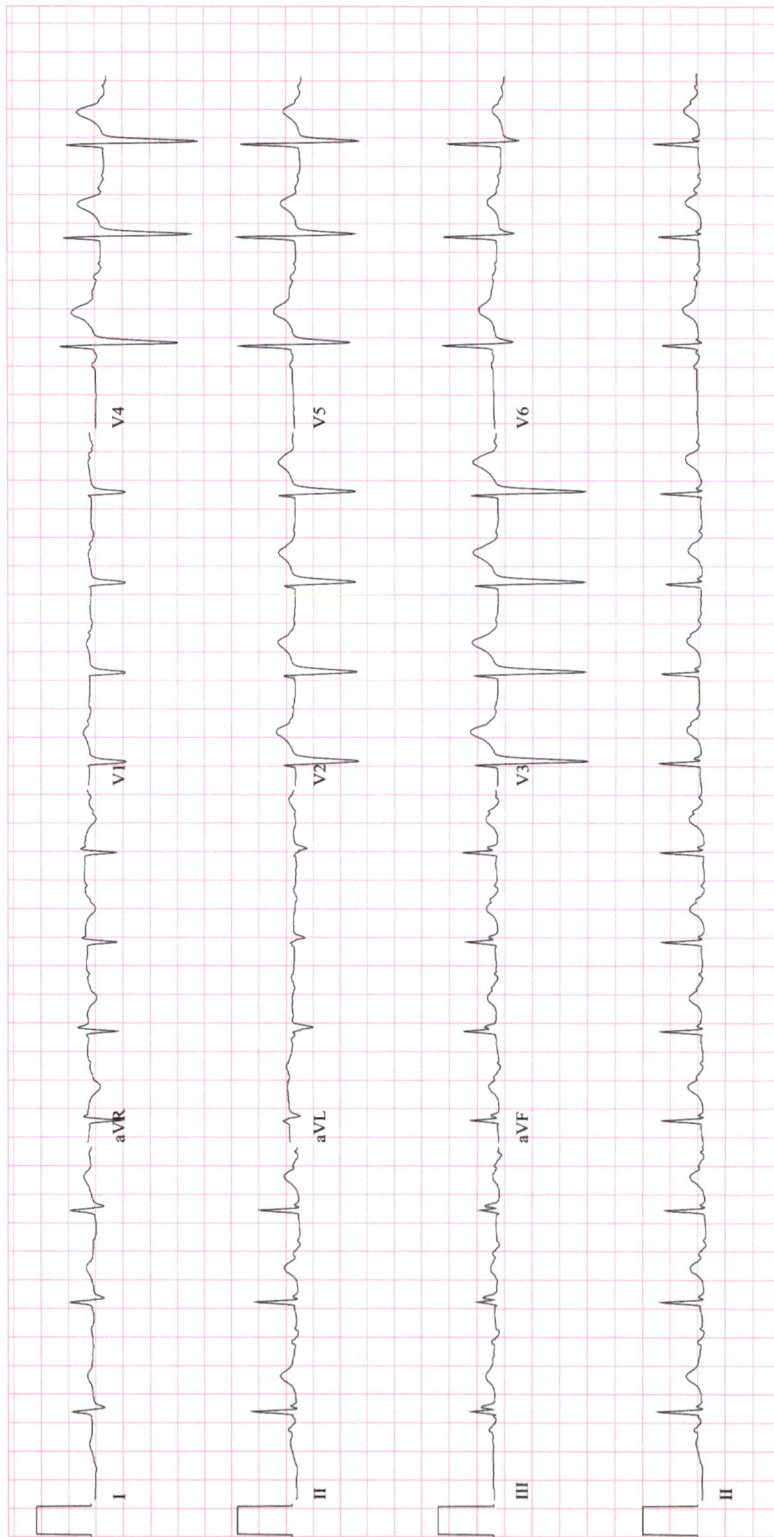

A 75-year-old male with a previous medical history of hypertension presents to the clinic with occasional palpitations which he describes as "skipped beats". An EKG is obtained. What does it show?

DIAGNOSIS: Second Degree A-V Block with Mobitz Type I Conduction. (Wenckebach Phenomenon)

This EKG shows normal sinus rhythm with progressive lengthening of PR interval (shown by arrows, below) after each successive P wave until the 12th P wave in the rhythm strip is not followed by a QRS complex. The subsequent PR interval after the dropped QRS complex is back to normal and the cycle repeats again.

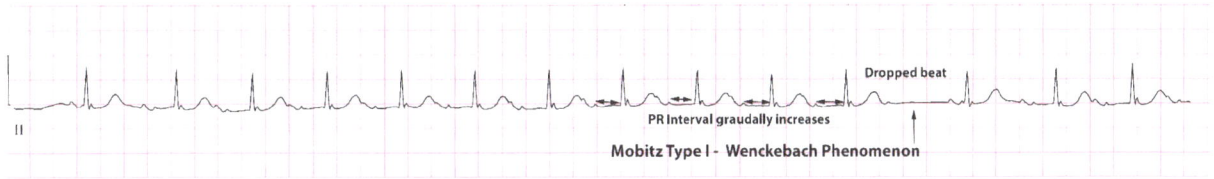

II

Dropped beat

PR Interval graudally increases

Mobitz Type I - Wenckebach Phenomenon

EKG features include:

- Progressive prolongation of the PR interval culminating in a non-conducted P wave.

- The PR interval is longest immediately before the dropped beat.

- The PR interval is shortest immediately after the dropped beat.

- The P-P interval remains relatively constant.

- The RR interval progressively shortens with each beat of the cycle.

- The Wenckebach pattern tends to repeat in P:QRS groups with ratios of 3:2, 4:3, or 5:4.

The impaired conduction through the AV node is often due to a reversible conduction abnormality within the AV node. It is benign and may occur with increased vagal tone (e.g. during sleep), AV node blocking drugs, inferior wall MI, myocarditis, and following cardiac surgery.

Wenckebach phenomenon does not require any intervention or pacing unless the patient has symptomatic bradycardia.

EKG Case 41

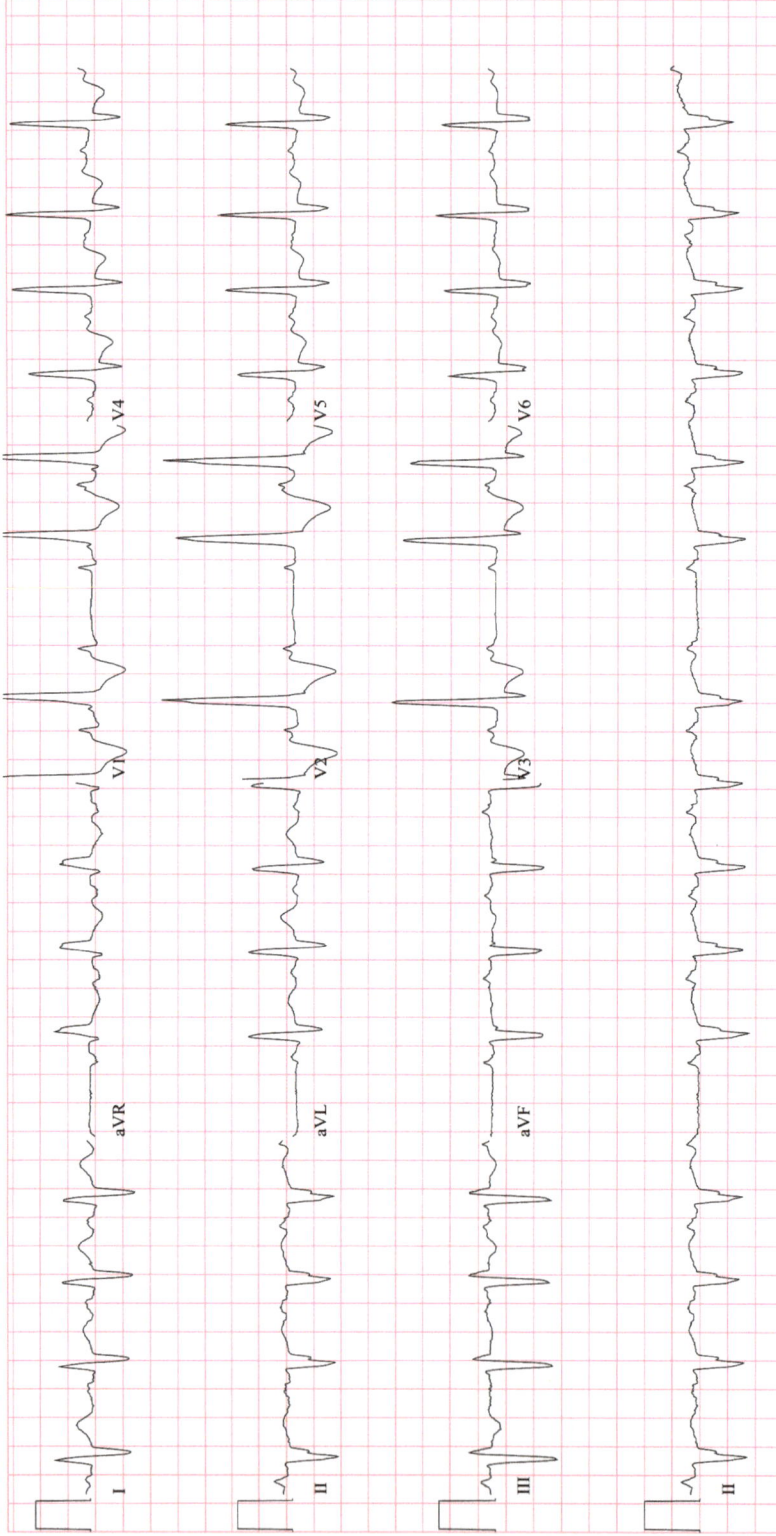

A 65-year-old man presenting with frequent episodes of palpitations and occasionally feeling faint. An EKG was obtained in the office. What does it show?

DIAGNOSIS: Second Degree AV Block, Mobitz type II Conduction.

This EKG shows normal sinus rhythm, Left bundle branch block, left axis deviation, and two intermittently non-conducted beats marked by x below. Please note that the PR and RR intervals on the conducted beats remain unchanged throughout the strip.

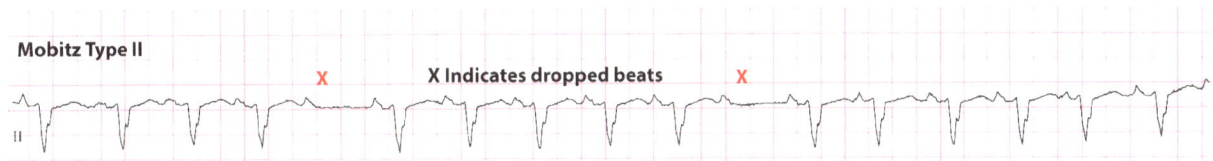

In Mobitz type II conduction:

- Intermittent non-conducted P waves without progressive prolongation of the PR interval (compare this to Mobitz I).

- The PR interval in the conducted beats remains constant.

- The P waves "march through" at a constant rate.

- The RR interval surrounding the dropped beat(s) is an exact multiple of the preceding RR interval (e.g, double the preceding RR interval for a single dropped beat, triple for two dropped beats, etc.).

- There is usually evidence of His-Purkinje disease on the EKG (RBBB/LAFP on the present EKG).

Mechanism

- Mobitz II is usually due to failure of conduction at the level of the His-Purkinje system (i.e, below the AV node).

- While Mobitz I is usually due to a functional suppression of AV conduction (e.g, due to drugs, reversible ischemia), Mobitz II is more likely to be due to structural damage to the conducting system (e.g, infarction, fibrosis, necrosis).

- In around 75% of cases, the conduction block is located distal to the Bundle of His, producing broad QRS complexes. In the remaining 25% of cases, the conduction block is located within the His Bundle itself, producing narrow QRS complexes.

- Unlike Mobitz I, which is produced by progressive fatigue of the AV nodal cells, Mobitz II is an "all or none" phenomenon whereby the His-Purkinje cells suddenly and unexpectedly fail to conduct a supraventricular impulse.

- There may be no pattern to the conduction block, or alternatively there may be a fixed relationship between the P waves and QRS complexes, e.g, 2:1 block, 3:1 block.

- Mobitz II mandates immediate admission for cardiac monitoring, backup temporary pacing, and ultimately insertion of a permanent pacemaker.

EKG Case 42

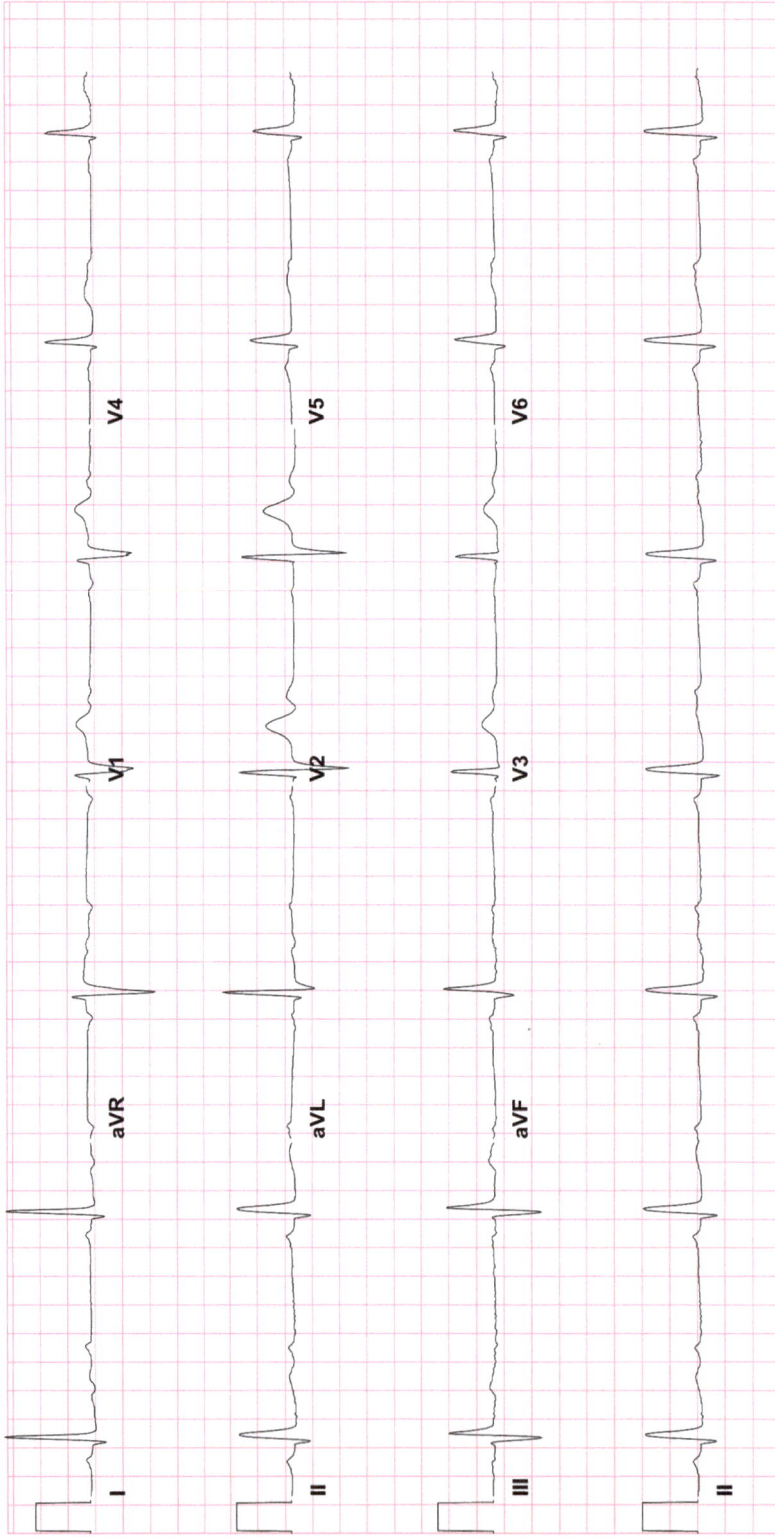

A 57-year-old male admitted to the hospital showed abnormalities on continuous cardiac monitoring while the patient was asleep. EKG was obtained immediately and Cardiology consulted for recommendations. What does the EKG show?

DIAGNOSIS: Second Degree AV Block with Fixed Ratio 2:1 Block

The EKG shows sinus bradycardia with every second P wave being blocked likely at the level of the AV node, hence every second P wave is not followed by a QRS complex. The EKG also shows Q waves in inferior leads (II, III, and aVF) indicating prior inferior wall MI.

Second degree AV block can also occur with other fixed ratios of P waves: QRS complexes. (e.g, 2:1, 3:1, 4:1). When two or more consecutive P waves are not conducted, it is termed "high degree AV block".

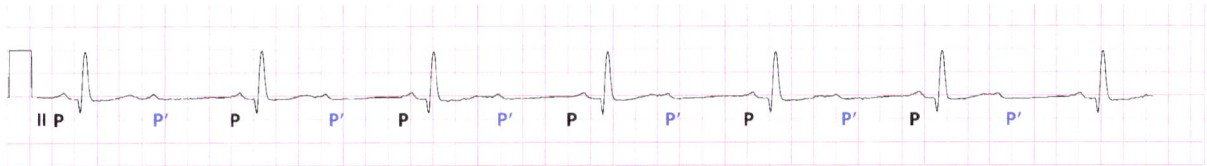

Figure: Second degree AV block with fixed ratio 2:1 block, P waves are conducted to the ventricles but P' are not.

- It is important to distinguish whether 2:1 AV block is either due to second degree Mobitz type I AV nodal block (Wenckebach), or second degree Mobitz type II AV nodal block, since the former is usually benign while the latter requires permanent pacing.

- A quick way to distinguish between the two is to look at the QRS complex.

- In Mobitz type I, conduction of the QRS complex is usually narrow, as the block is located at the level of the AV node and improves with administration of atropine or an increase in adrenergic tone.

- In Mobitz type II, conduction of the QRS duration is prolonged, as it usually occurs in the setting of preexisting His-Purkinje disease. This type of conduction worsens or does not improve with atropine or adrenergic stimulation.

- However, this strategy has its own pitfalls, as in 25% of Mobitz type II the block is located at the Bundle of His, producing narrow QRS complexes. Moreover, Mobitz type I may be associated with preexisting bundle branch block or interventricular conduction delay, resulting in a wide QRS complex.

- The best method to ascertain the type of block is to observe the patient's cardiac rhythm and monitor the PR interval. Frequently periods of 2:1 or 3:1 block will be interspersed with more characteristic Wenckebach (Mobitz type I) or Mobitz II sequences, which can indicate the actual type of block in that patient.

EKG Case 43

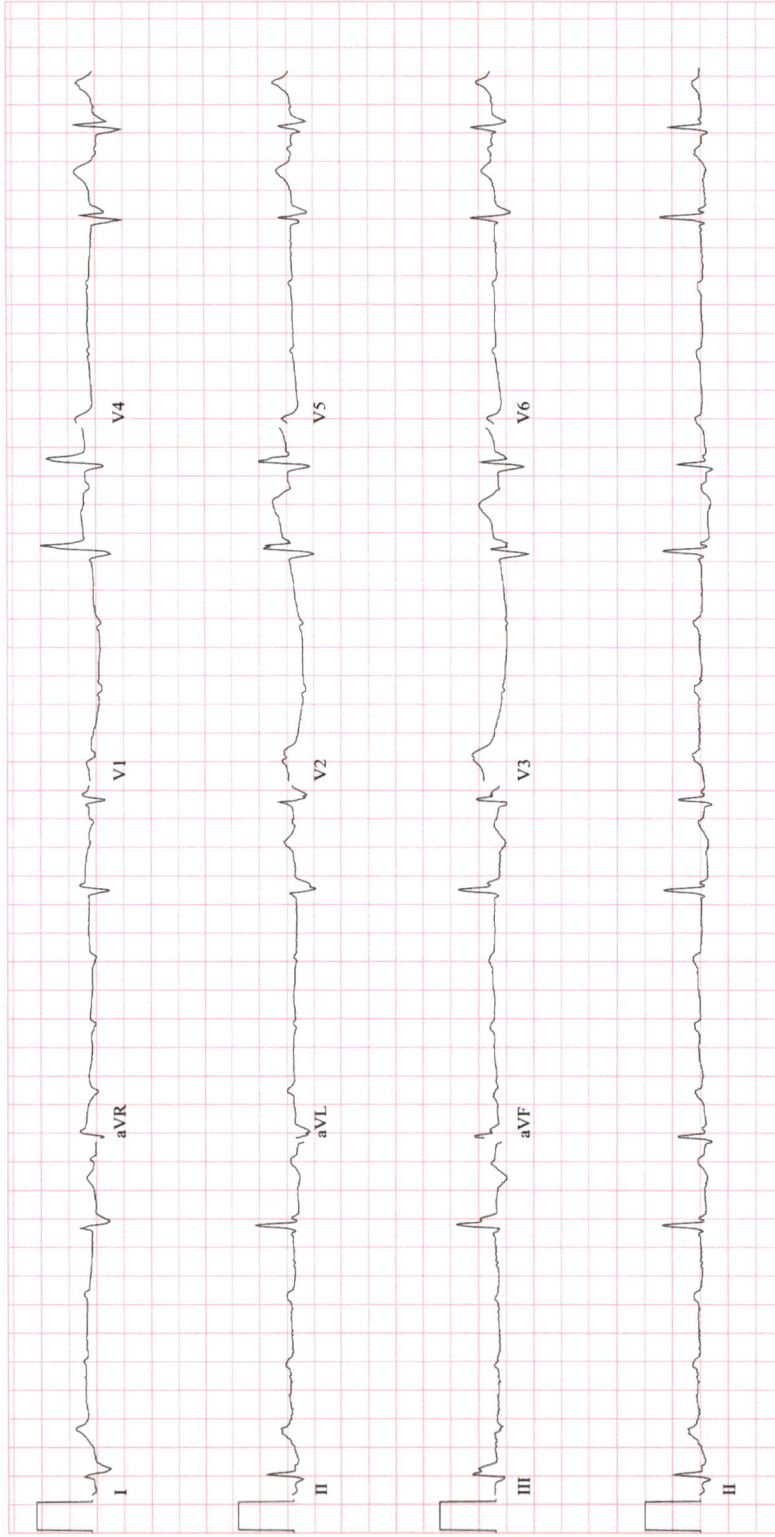

A 55-year-old man, with an unremarkable past medical history presents to the hospital with a femur fracture from a fall. He reports frequent falls and dizziness. Patient is hemodynamically stable. An EKG is obtained in the ER for pre-op clearance. What does it show and will you clear him for surgery?

DIAGNOSIS: High Grade AV Block

This EKG shows high grade AV block with consecutive non-conducted sinus beats and intermittent sinus conduction beats. The junctional escape beats and the conducted sinus beats are in a pattern of bigeminy. Atrial rate of 150 bpm with ventricular rate of 54 bpm. EKG also shows right bundle branch block.

High grade AV block is the type of second degree heart block defined by a P:QRS ratio of 3:1 or higher, producing an extremely slow ventricular rate. Unlike 3rd degree heart block, there is still some relationship between the P waves and the QRS complexes at least on a few beats. High grade AV block may result from progression of either Mobitz I or Mobitz II AV block.

Due to the emergent nature of the surgery, the patient was cleared for surgery after a temporary pacemaker was placed. Post-op, the patient needs to be assessed for implantation of a permanent pacemaker.

EKG Case 44

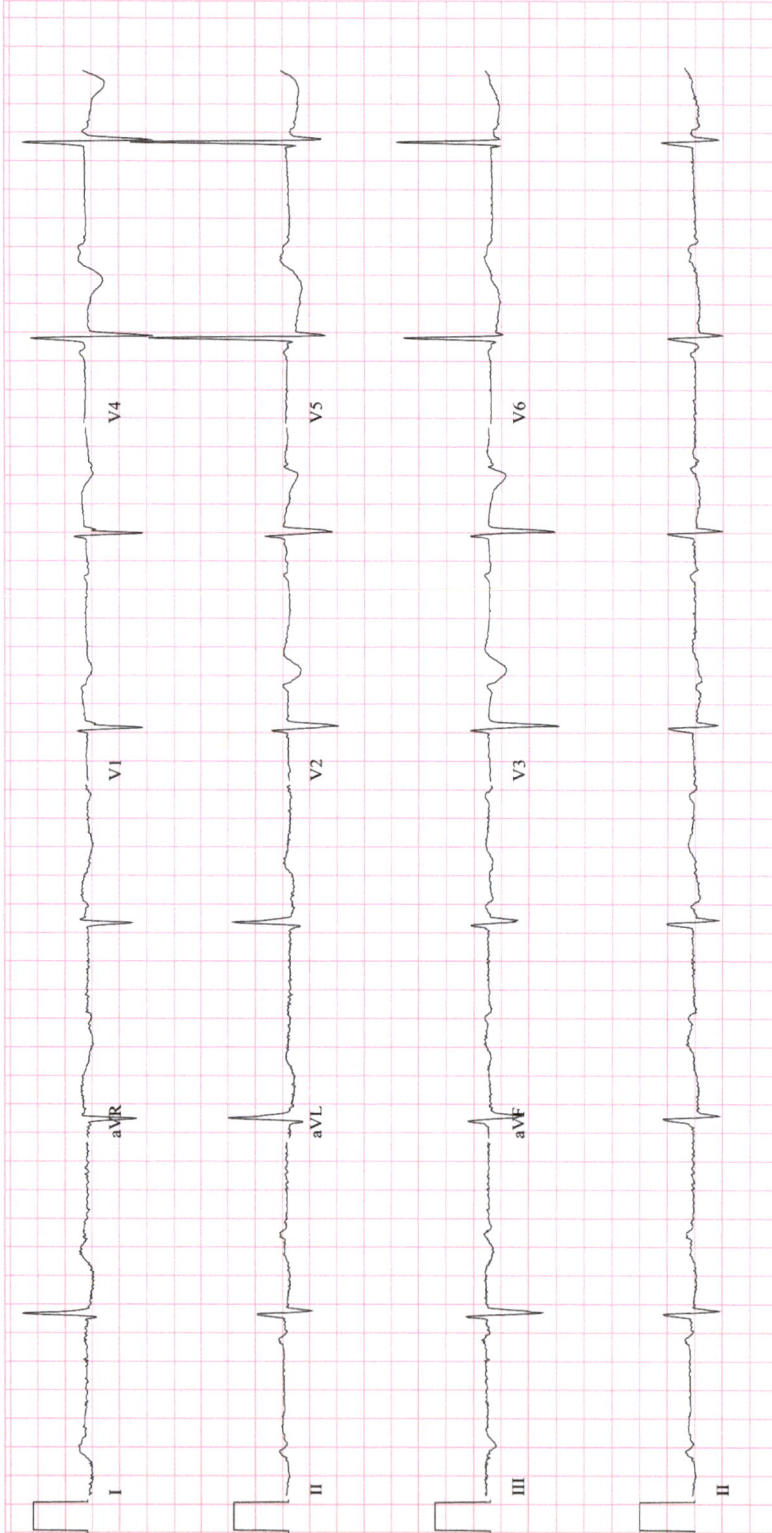

An 85-year-old man is brought to the ER after a witnessed syncopal episode. A 12-lead EKG was done immediately on arrival to the ER. What does it show?

DIAGNOSIS: Third Degree AV Block (Complete Heart Block)

The above EKG shows sinus bradycardia with third degree AV block with a junctional escape rhythm (note the narrow QRS complexes).The P-P and R-R intervals are constant. Atrial rate is approximately 79 bpm and ventricular rate is 45 bpm.

- In third degree AV block, no supraventricular impulses are conducted to the ventricles. The atria and ventricles beat independently of each other and ventricular excitation is maintained by a junctional or ventricular escape rhythm.

- Causes for third degree AV block are ischemic heart disease, AV nodal blocking drugs, fibrosis and calcification of the conduction system (Lev's and Lenegre's disease), and Lyme's disease, among other causes.

- Third degree AV block patients may require admission for cardiac monitoring, backup temporary pacing if hemodynamically unstable or if the level of block is below the AV node, and permanent pacemaker implantation if the cause of third degree AV block is irreversible.

EKG Features Include:

- In complete heart block the atrial rate (P wave) is faster than the ventricular rate (QRS wave) and bears no association with the QRS complexes.

- The QRS complex arises from a nodal origin (narrow QRS) or His-Purkinje-ventricular origin (wide QRS) Third degree AV block can exist with any atrial rhythm, hence P waves may be abnormal or absent (such as in atrial fibrillation with AV block).

EKG Case 45

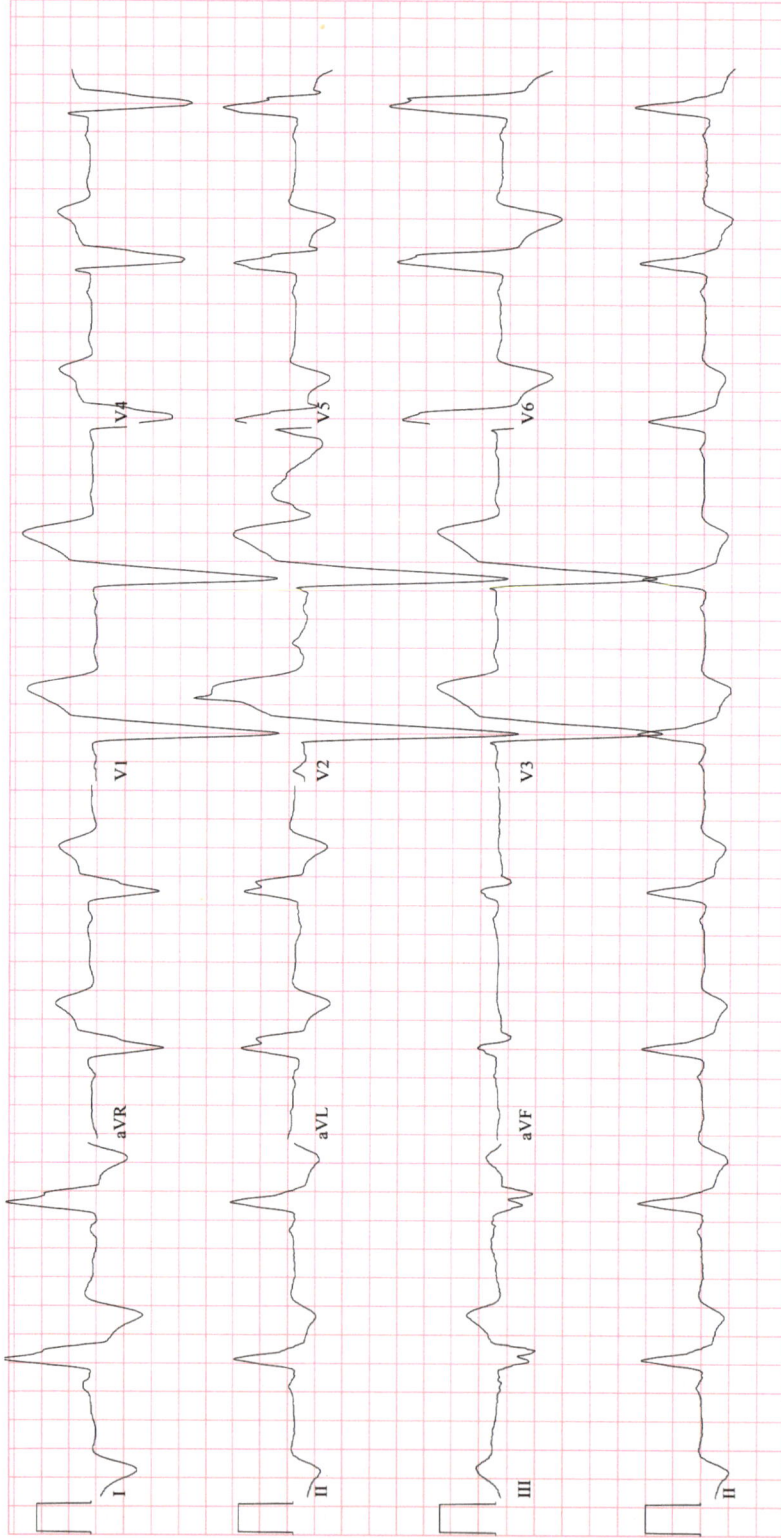

A 75-year-old male presents to the office with exertional shortness of breath. An EKG is obtained. What does it show?

DIAGNOSIS: Left Bundle Branch Block (LBBB) with Sinus Bradycardia

The EKG shows LBBB with sinus bradycardia at a rate of 55 bpm. The QRS duration is 200 ms, the R waves in leads aVL, V5, and V6 are notched, and with a deep S wave in V1.

- Left bundle branch block results from failed or delayed conduction through the left bundle branch. As a result, the left ventricle must be activated indirectly through the impulse coming from the right bundle branch across the interventricular septum. This results in activation of the right ventricle before the left ventricle, which prolongs the duration of ventricular depolarization and broadens the QRS complexes (> 120 ms).

- Causes of LBBB are ischemic heart disease, anterior MI, dilated cardiomyopathy, primary degenerative disease of the conducting system, hyperkalemia, and digitalis toxicity.

- Left ventricular hypertrophy is one of the differential diagnosis of LBBB, as it may have a similar appearance to LBBB, with QRS widening and ST depression / T-wave inversion in the lateral leads.

- Diagnosis of incomplete LBBB is made when LBBB morphology is present but with a relatively narrow QRS complex (<120 ms).

- LBBB could possibly be associated with structural heart disease and requires further investigation, but LBBB itself would not explain dyspnea.

EKG Features Include:

- QRS duration ≥ 120 ms in adults.

- Broad, notched, or slurred R wave in leads aVL, V5, and V6.

- Deep S wave in V1.

- Absent Q waves in leads I, V5, and V6, with the exception of lead aVL.

- Delayed time to peak R wave (> 60 ms in leads V5 and V6 but normal in leads V1, V2, and V3).

- ST and T waves are polarized in the opposite direction of the main QRS deflection.

EKG Case 46

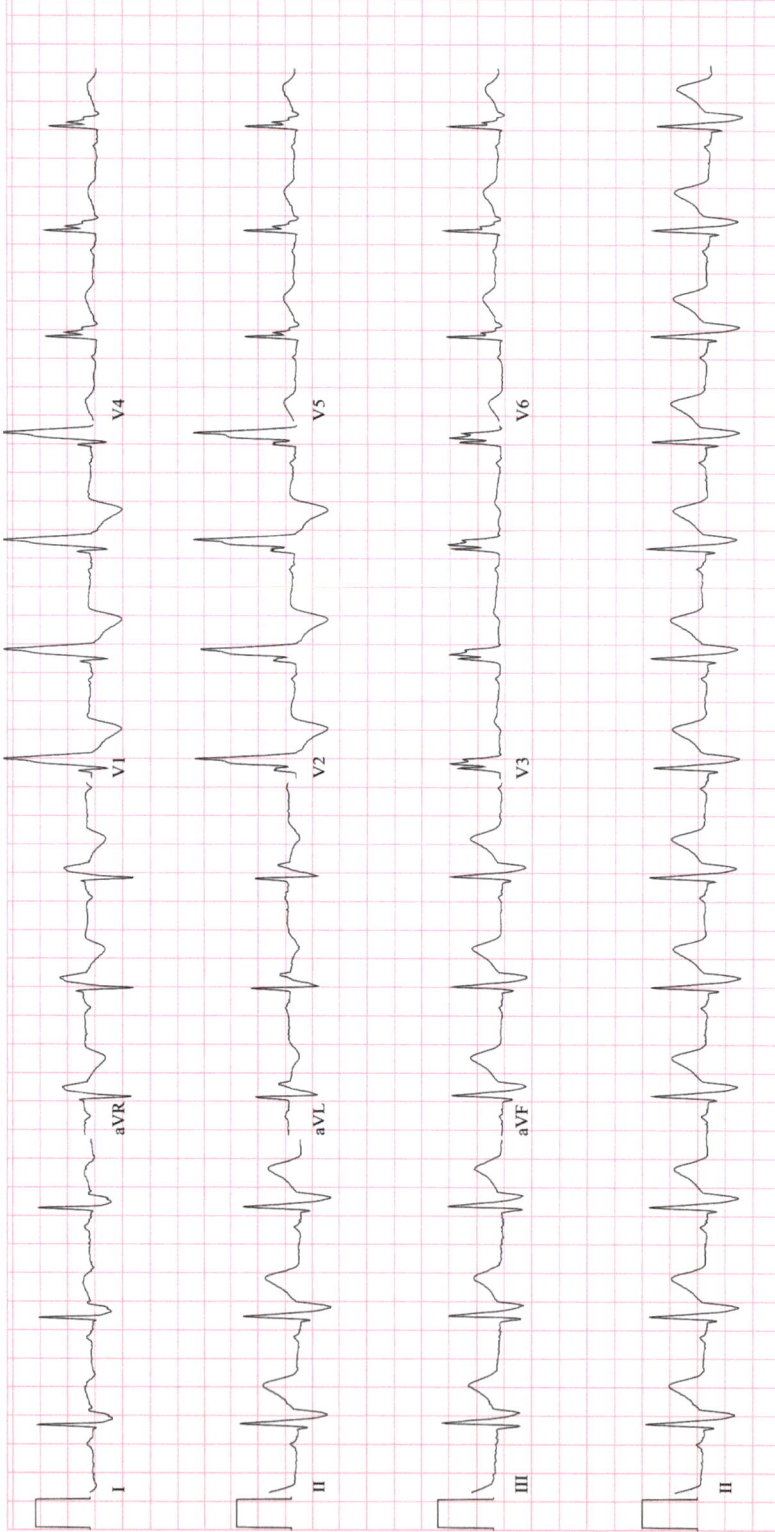

A 70-year-old male had an EKG performed for pre-op evaluation. What does the EKG show?

DIAGNOSIS: Right Bundle Branch Block

This EKG shows normal sinus rhythm at 79 bpm. The QRS duration is approximately 140 ms. An rSR' pattern is seen in V1-V3 as well as a broad slurred S wave in lead I. There are also ST segment depressions and T wave inversions in the right precordial leads (V1 and V2).

- In RBBB, the impulse travels normally down the left bundle and then depolarizes the ventricles from left to right through the interventricular septum. This leads to delayed right ventricular depolarization and gives rise to a wide QRS complex and to the typical rSR' pattern in lead V1 (rabbit ears with taller right ear).

- Causes of RBBB are RVH, Cor Pulmonale, Pulmonary embolus, ischemic heart disease, myocarditis, cardiomyopathy and degenerative disease of the conduction system.

- An rSR' pattern in the leads V1-V3 may also be caused by Brugada syndrome and one needs to be aware of this potentially fatal condition.

- Incomplete RBBB is diagnosed when morphology of RBBB is present with a QRS < 120 ms.

EKG Features Include:

- ST depression and T wave inversion in the right precordial leads (V1-V3).

- QRS duration ≥ 120 ms in adults.

- S wave of longer duration than R wave or greater than 40 ms in leads I and V6 in adults.

- Time to R wave peak normal in leads V5 and V6 but greater than 50 ms in lead V1.

EKG Case 47

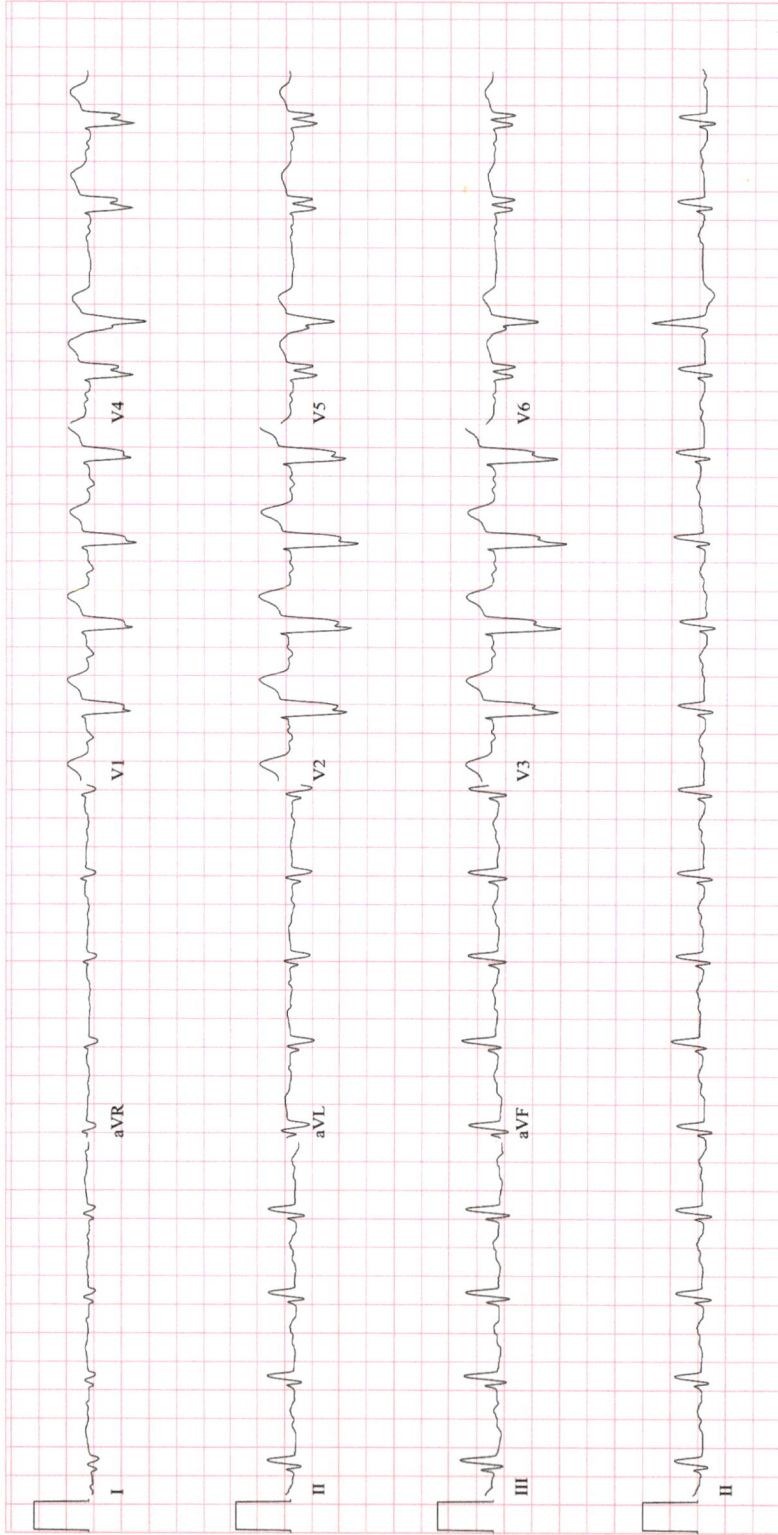

An EKG is recorded from a 75-year-old male with a history of hypertension who is admitted to the hospital for acute on chronic heart failure. What does the EKG show?

DIAGNOSIS: Interventricular Conduction Delay (IVCD), Also known as Nonspecific Intraventricular Conduction Delay (NICD)

This EKG shows sinus tachycardia at 100 bpm with wide QRS complexes of 135 ms. QRS morphology is not typical for either RBBB or LBBB. Rhythm is regular with the exception of 15th QRS complex which represents a premature ventricular contraction.

Assessment of QRS Widening[1]

If the QRS complex is wide (>120 ms) and the rhythm is supraventricular (i.e,, not wide due to ventricular tachycardia, ventricular pacing, or preexcitation), then there are three possibilities: a) RBBB; b) LBBB; or c) IVCD.

IVCD is a diagnosis of exclusion.

- Expected morphology for typical RBBB includes an rSR' complex in right-sided lead V1 and wide terminal S waves in left-sided leads I and V6 . Above EKG does not meet morphology of RBBB.

- Expected morphology for typical LBBB includes broad upright, monophasic QRS in left-sided leads I and V6, and a predominantly negative QRS in right-sided lead V1. Although QRS morphology above is consistent with LBBB in lead V1, it is clearly not consistent with it in either lead I or V6.

- By process of elimination, the conduction defect in the above EKG represents IVCD.

1   ECG Interpretation.": *Review #13 (BBB, Wide QRS, Is this LBBB vs RBBB vs IVCD)*. Web. 28 Jun. 2015. http://
     ecg-interpretation.blogspot.com/2011/01/ecg-interpretation-review-13-bbb-wide.html

EKG Case 48

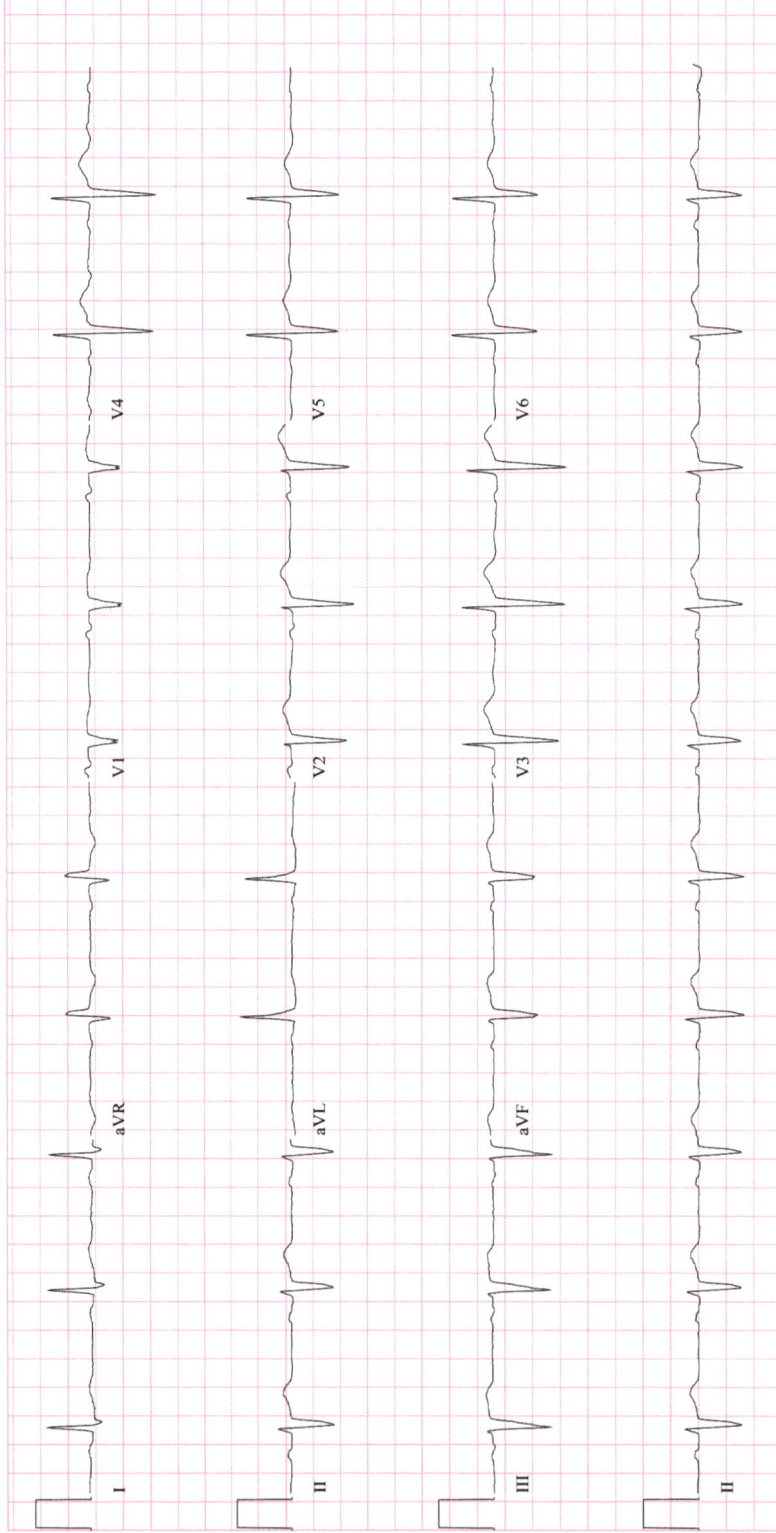

A 82-year-old female with a past medical history of coronary artery disease presents to your office for a routine medical checkup. An EKG is obtained. What does it show?

DIAGNOSIS: Left Anterior Fascicular Block (LAFB)

The EKG shows normal sinus rhythm with left anterior fascicular block. qR complex in leads I and AVL and rS complexes in leads II and III.

- The left anterior fascicle normally initiates conduction in the anterolateral left ventricular free wall, left anterior papillary muscle, and upper part of the septum. In left anterior fascicular block, the initial electrical impulse/vector is propagated through the left posterior fascicle which inserts into the infero-septal wall of the left ventricular endocardial surface. As a result, the initial electrical vector is directed downwards and rightward. This produces small R waves in the inferior leads and small Q waves in the left sided leads (I, aVL).

- The depolarization wave then spreads upwards and leftwards, producing positive voltages (tall R waves) in the left side leads and large negative voltages (deep S waves) in the inferior leads. This process takes approximately 20 ms longer than normal conduction through both fascicles, resulting in a minimal widening of QRS complexes.

- LAFB in the absence of organic heart disease and other associated electrical blocks is a benign condition that is observed more frequently with aging. LAFB, however can be associated with other pathological conditions such as coronary artery disease, Chaga's disease, infiltrative and inflammatory diseases, congenital heart diseases (including tricuspid atresia, endocardial cushion defects, single ventricle, spontaneous and surgical closure of a VSD, and other disorders), and as part of a primary sclerotic degenerative disorder. LAFB is not an uncommon finding after aortic valve surgery.

- Differential diagnoses of LAFB are left ventricular hypertrophy, hypertrophic obstructive cardiomyopathy, inferior or inferolateral wall myocardial infarction, chronic obstructive pulmonary disease, Wolff-Parkinson-White syndrome, congenital heart disease including corrected transposition, tricuspid atresia, single ventricle, endocardial cushion malformations, and Ebstein's disease.

EKG Features Include:

- Left axis deviation (usually between -45 and -90 degrees).
- Small Q waves with tall R waves (qR complexes) in leads I and aVL.
- Small R waves with deep S waves (rS complexes) in leads II, III and aVF.
- QRS duration normal or slightly prolonged (80 -110 ms).
- Delayed time to R wave peak in aVL (greater than 45 ms).
- Increased QRS voltage in the limb leads.

EKG Case 49

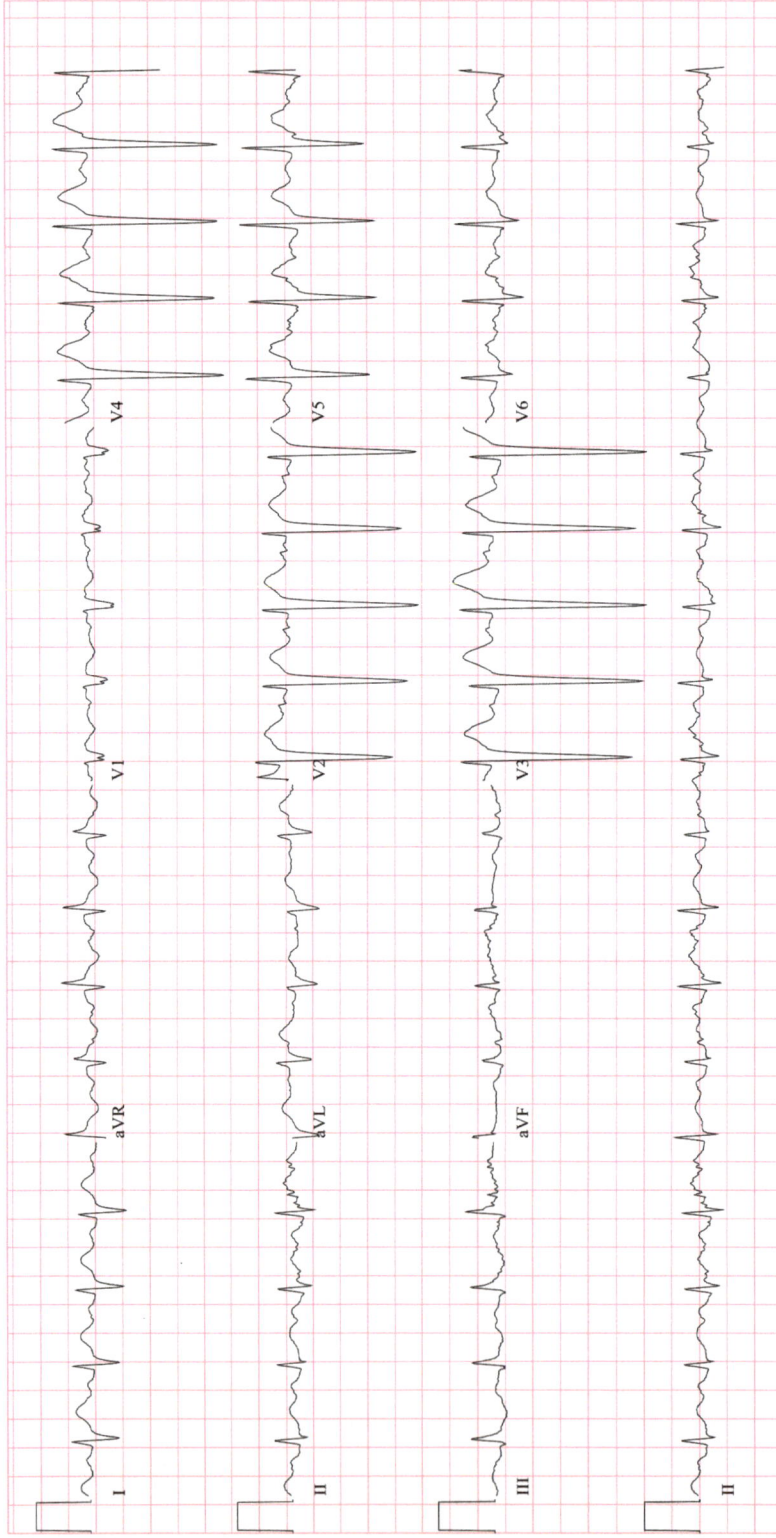

A 70-year-old man presents to the emergency room with chest pain, fever, and new onset cough. Chest x-ray shows right lower lobe pneumonia. An EKG is also obtained as part of the workup. What does it show?

DIAGNOSIS: Left Posterior Fascicular Block (and sinus tachycardia)

This EKG shows sinus tachycardia at 100 bpm with right axis deviation and left posterior fascicular block.

- Left Posterior Fascicular Block (LPFB) is less common than Left Anterior Fascicular Block (LAFB) in isolation. It is however commonly seen with RBBB in the setting of bifascicular or trifascicular block.

- The broad bundle of fibers that make up the left posterior fascicle is more resistant to damage when compared with the thin single tract that makes up the left anterior fascicle.

- In LPFB, the impulses are conducted through the left anterior fascicle through the upper and lateral wall of the left ventricle. The initial electrical vector is directed upwards and leftwards, causing small R waves in the lateral leads (I, aVL) and small Q waves in the inferior leads. The next wave of depolarization spreads along the free left ventricular wall downwards and rightwards, producing positive voltages (tall R waves) in the inferior leads and negative voltages (deep S waves) in the lateral leads (I, aVL).

- This process takes up to 20 ms longer than normal simultaneous conduction via both anterior and posterior fascicles, resulting in a slight widening of the QRS.

- Isolated LPFB is uncommon and one of the causes of LPFB is ischemic heart disease.

- Situations that need to be distinguished from LPFB are right ventricular hypertrophy (due to valvular heart disease or cor pulmonale) and high lateral or anterolateral myocardial infarction.

EKG Features Include:

- Right axis deviation (> +110 degrees).

- Small R waves with deep S waves (rS complexes) in leads I and aVL.

- Small Q waves with tall R waves (qR complexes) in leads II, III, and aVF.

- QRS duration normal or slightly prolonged (80 -110ms).

- Delayed time to peak R wave in aVF.

- Increased QRS voltage in the limb leads.

- No evidence of any other cause for right axis deviation, such as RVH.

EKG Case 50

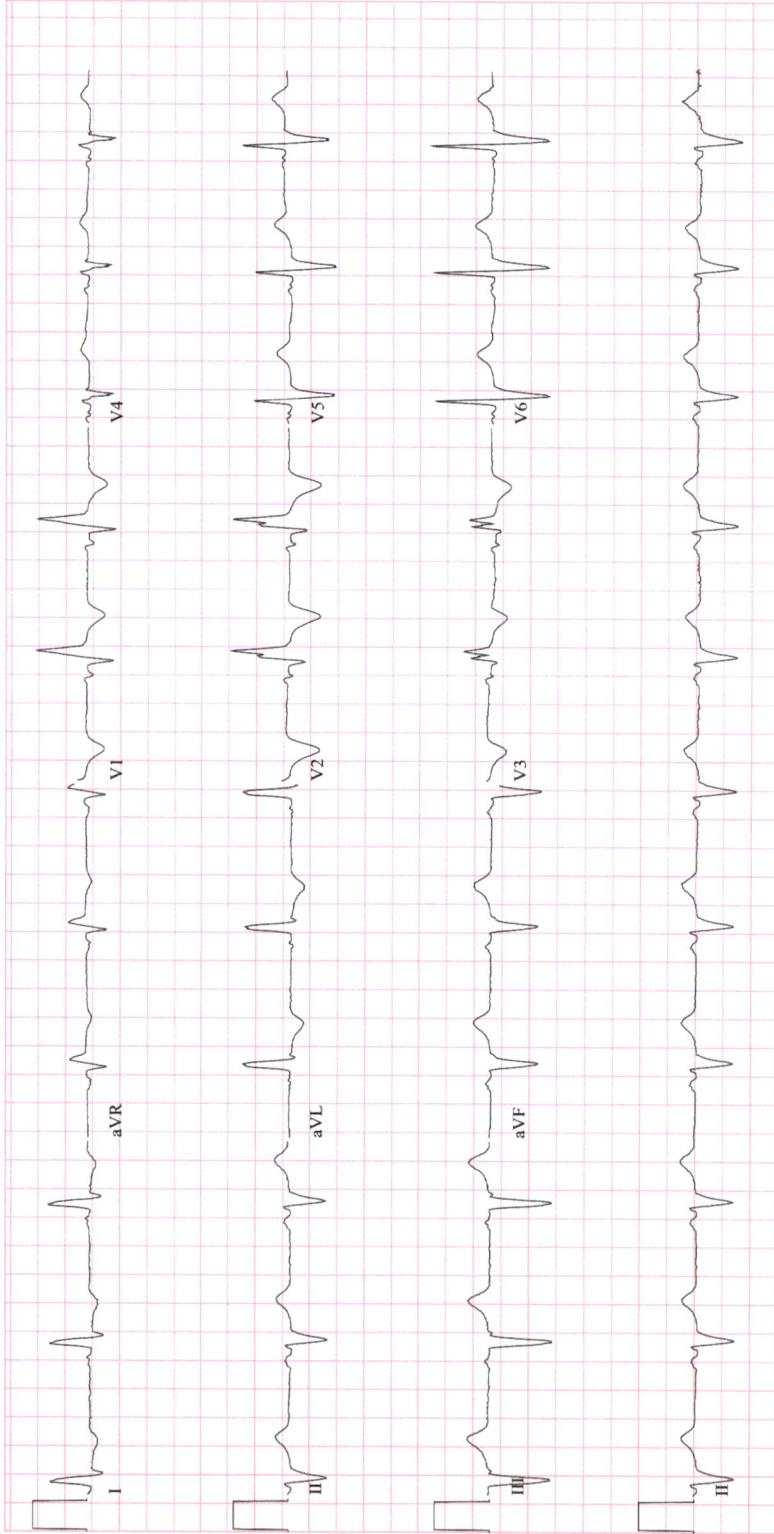

A 60-year-old male with a previous medical history of coronary artery disease and myocardial infarction presents to the ER with exertional chest discomfort. An EKG is obtained. What does it show?

DIAGNOSIS: Bifascicular Block

The EKG shows sinus rhythm with RBBB and left anterior fascicular block (bifascicular block).

- Bifascicular block is defined as RBBB, plus one of either LAFB or LPFB.
- The single remaining fascicle is the one through which conduction to the ventricles occurs.
- RBBB+LAFB is the more common pattern of blockade.
- Bifascicular block signifies extensive conduction system disease, although the risk of progression to complete heart block is low.
- Common causes of bifascicular block are ischemic heart disease, anterior myocardial infarction, primary degenerative disease of the conduction system, and congenital heart disease.
- Patients with chronic bifascicular block and unexplained syncope should be considered for permanent pacemaker implantation.
- Electrocardiogram will show features of RBBB and left or right axis deviation based on the fascicle involved.

EKG Case 51

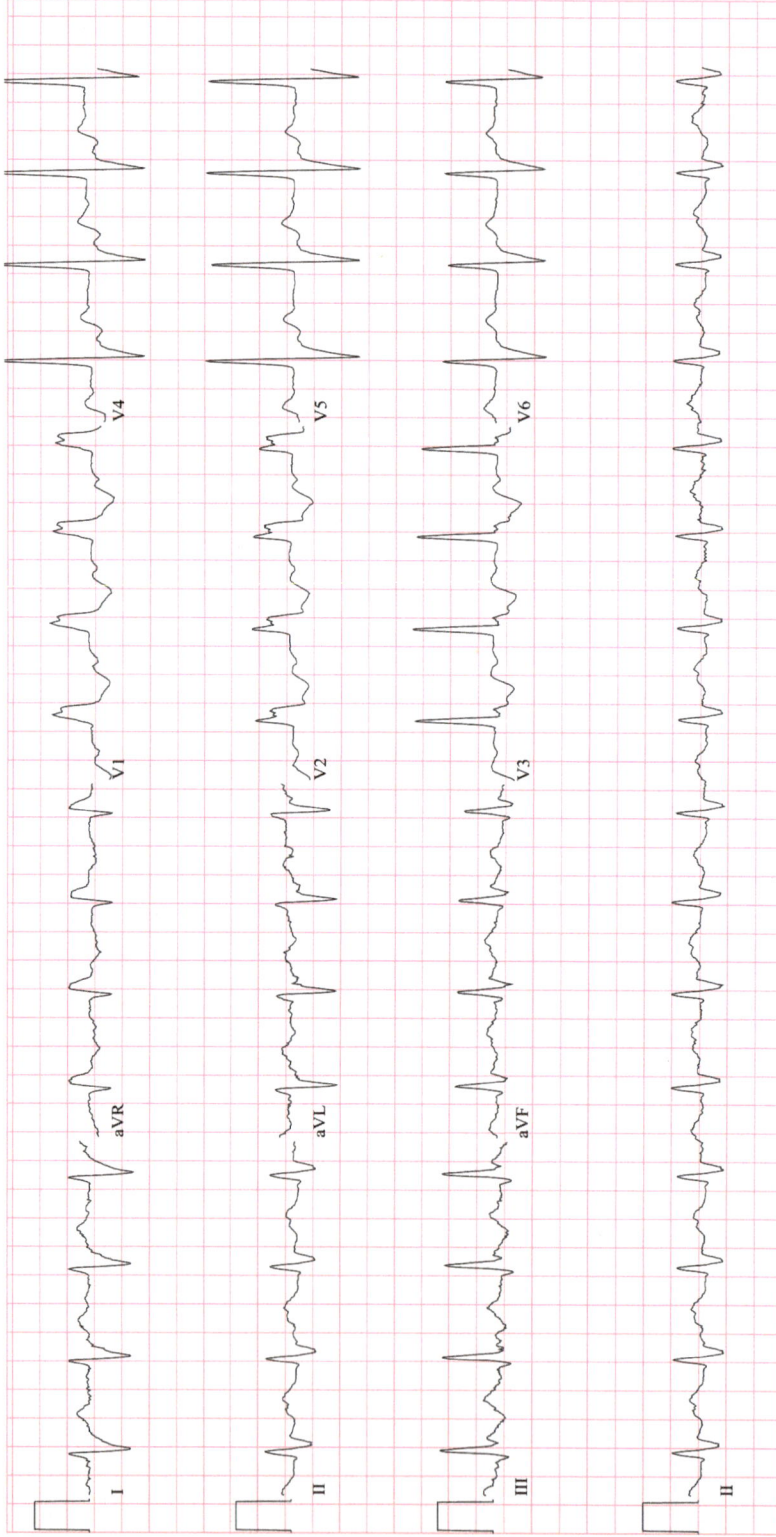

A 78-year-old man presents to the ER with a syncopal episode. An electrocardiogram was obtained on arrival. What does it show?

DIAGNOSIS: Trifascicular Block: First Degree AV Block, Right Bundle Branch Block, and Left Posterior Fascicular Block

This EKG shows right bundle branch block, first degree AV block, and left posterior fascicular block, also known as trifascicular block.

- First degree AV block, RBBB, and LPFB have been described in previous cases.

- Trifascicular block is a misnomer because not all fascicles are blocked, but rather all three have delayed conduction, thus the prolonged PR interval.

- In the presence of syncope, trifascicular block (like bifascicular block) is an indication for permanent pacemaker implantation.

EKG Case 52

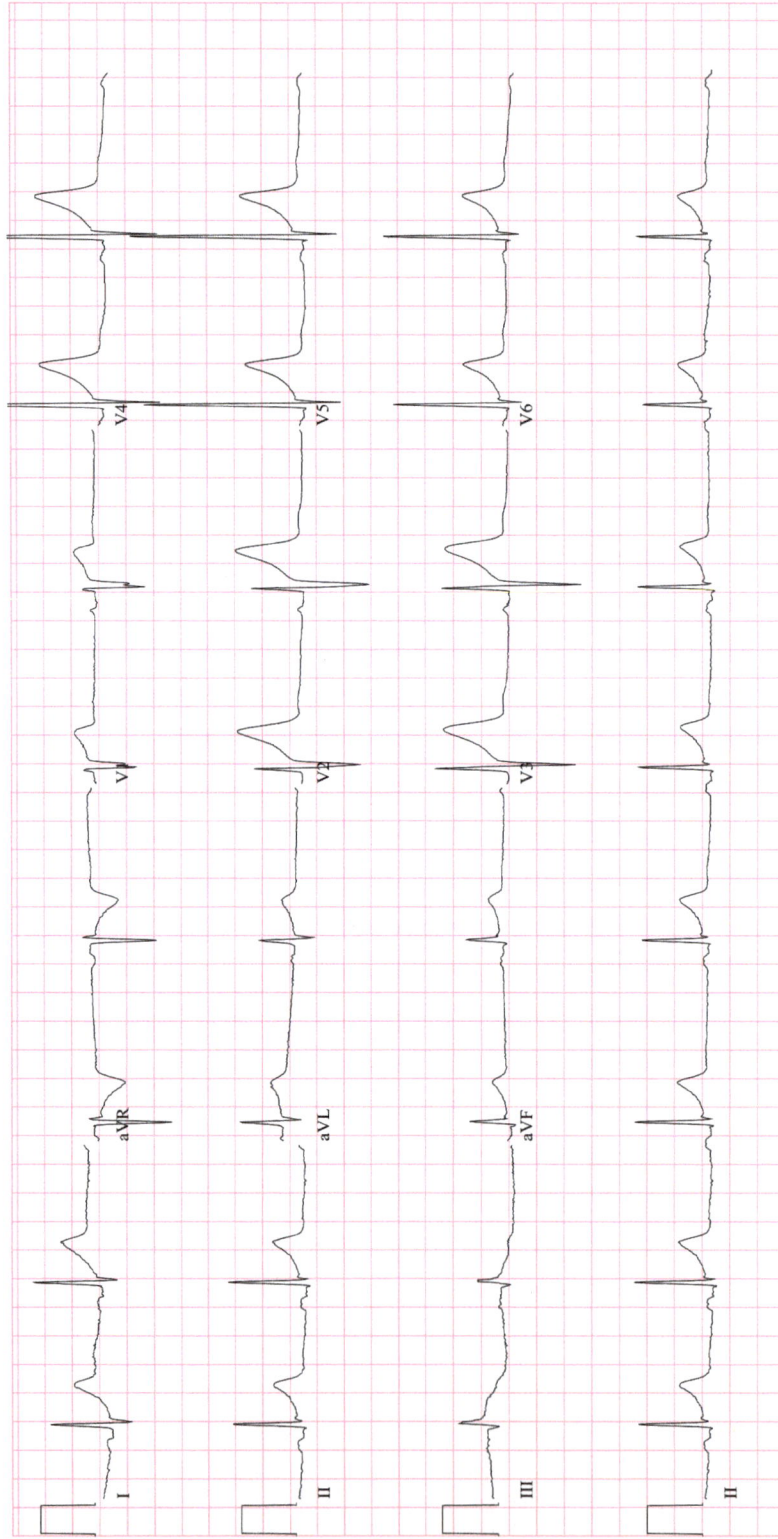

A 40-year-old male presents to the ER with central typical chest pain. He has no risk factors for coronary artery disease. Labs including cardiac troponin are normal. An EKG is obtained. What does it show?

DIAGNOSIS: Early Benign Repolarization (EBP), High Uptake, J Point Elevation Pattern

This EKG shows normal sinus rhythm at 60 bpm with generalized concave ST elevation in the precordial (V2 - V6) and limb leads (II, III, aVF). J point notching in evident in inferior leads II, III and aVF.

Early repolarization (ER) pattern is a common EKG variant, characterized by J point elevation manifesting either as terminal QRS slurring (the transition from the QRS segment to the ST segment) or notching (a positive deflection inscribed on terminal QRS complex) associated with concave upward ST-segment elevation and prominent T waves in at least two contiguous leads.[1]

- Common in fit young people.

- Generally disappears in middle age, rare in the elderly.

- Elevated J point, often with notching: the so-called "fish hook" pattern.

- Predominantly in anterior chest leads, but can occur elsewhere.

- Associated with large, symmetrical, concordant T waves.

- Absence of reciprocal changes or pathological Q waves.

- Possibly related to high sympathetic tone on heart – can normalize with exercise or beta-blockade.

ER has generally been considered a normal EKG variant with good long-term prognosis. However, this long-held concept has been challenged, and recently published population-based studies have reported an association with ventricular fibrillation and sudden death.[2] ER has also emerged as a marker of increased long-term mortality (cardiac and arrhythmic) in the general population. Interestingly, Watanabe et al.[3] recently reported that patients with short QR syndrome (SQTS) have a higher prevalence of early repolarization pattern in the EKG and that the presence of early repolarization is strongly associated with arrhythmic events. Thus, ER is probably not as benign as traditionally believed.[4]

1   Derval, Nicolas, Ashok Shah, and Pierre Jaïs. "Definition of Early Repolarization A Tug of War." *Circulation* 124, no. 20 (2011): 2185-2186.

2   Derval, Nicolas, Christopher S. Simpson, David H. Birnie, Jeffrey S. Healey, Vijay Chauhan, Jean Champagne, Martin Gardner et al. "Prevalence and characteristics of early repolarization in the CASPER registry: cardiac arrest survivors with preserved ejection fraction registry." *Journal of the American College of Cardiology* 58, no. 7 (2011): 722-728.

3   Watanabe, Hiroshi, Takeru Makiyama, Taku Koyama, Prince J. Kannankeril, Shinji Seto, Kazuki Okamura, Hirotaka Oda et al. "High prevalence of early repolarization in short QT syndrome." Heart rhythm 7, no. 5 (2010): 647-652.

4   Sinner, Moritz F., Wibke Reinhard, Martina Müller, Britt-Maria Beckmann, Eimo Martens, Siegfried Perz, Arne Pfeufer et al. "Association of early repolarization pattern on ECG with risk of cardiac and all-cause mortality: a population-based prospective cohort study (MONICA/KORA)." *PLoS medicine* 7, no. 7 (2010): 879.

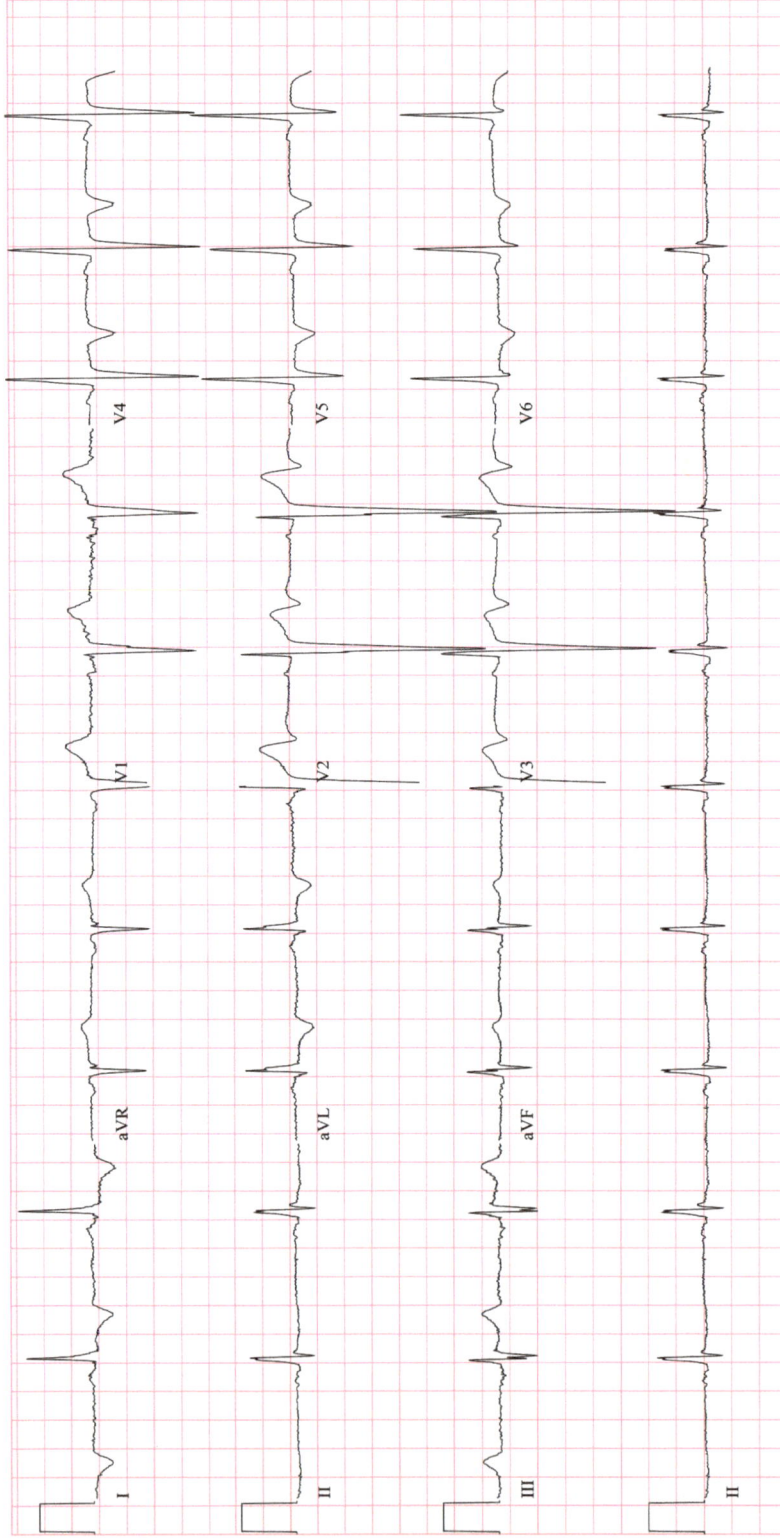

A 45-year-old man with an unremarkable past medical history presents to the ER with symptoms of dyspepsia and indigestion. He has experienced epigastric pain radiating to his chest in the last week, but currently is symptom free. An EKG is obtained. What does it show?

DIAGNOSIS: Wellens' Syndrome Type A

This EKG shows normal sinus rhythm with biphasic T waves in in V2-V3 with extended T waves inversions in V4 - V6, I, and aVL.

- Wellens' syndrome was first described in the early 1980s by de Zwaan, Wellens, and colleagues[1], who identified a subset of patients with unstable angina who had specific precordial T wave changes and subsequently developed a large anterior wall myocardial infarction (MI).

- Wellens' syndrome is a pattern of deeply inverted or biphasic T waves in V2- V3, which is highly specific for a critical stenosis of the left anterior descending artery (LAD). Patients may be pain free at the time the EKG is recorded and have normal or minimally elevated cardiac enzymes. Patients are, however, at extremely high risk for extensive anterior wall MI within the next few days to weeks. Due to the critical LAD stenosis, these patients usually require invasive therapy, do poorly with medical management, and may suffer MI or cardiac arrest if inappropriately stress tested.

Diagnostic Criteria

- Rhinehart et al.[2] describe the following diagnostic criteria for Wellens' syndrome:

- Deeply inverted or biphasic T waves in V2-V3 (may extend to V1-6).

- Isoelectric or minimally-elevated ST segment (< 1mm).

- No precordial Q waves.

- Preserved precordial R wave progression.

- Recent history of angina.

- EKG pattern present in pain-free state.

- Normal or slightly elevated serum cardiac markers.

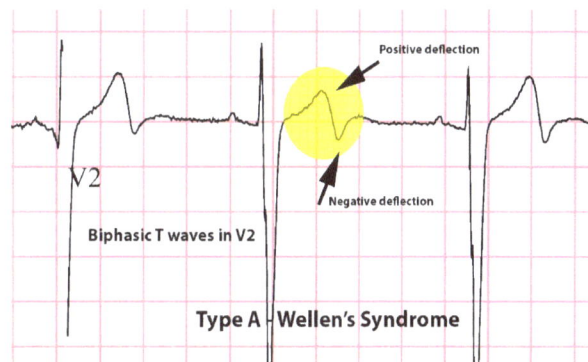

Biphasic T waves in V2

Positive deflection

Negative deflection

Type A - Wellen's Syndrome

There are two patterns of T wave abnormality in Wellens' syndrome:

- Type A = Biphasic, with initial positivity and terminal negativity (25% of cases), as in this case.

- Type B = Deeply and symmetrically inverted (75% of cases).

---

1   De Zwaan, Chris, Frits WHM Bär, and Hein JJ Wellens. "Characteristic electrocardiographic pattern indicating a critical stenosis high in left anterior descending coronary artery in patients admitted because of impending myocardial infarction." In *Professor Hein JJ Wellens*, pp. 245-252. Springer Netherlands, 2000.

2   Rhinehardt, Joseph, William J. Brady, Andrew D. Perron, and Amal Mattu. "Electrocardiographic manifestations of Wellens' syndrome." The American journal of emergency medicine20, no. 7 (2002): 638-643.

EKG Case 54

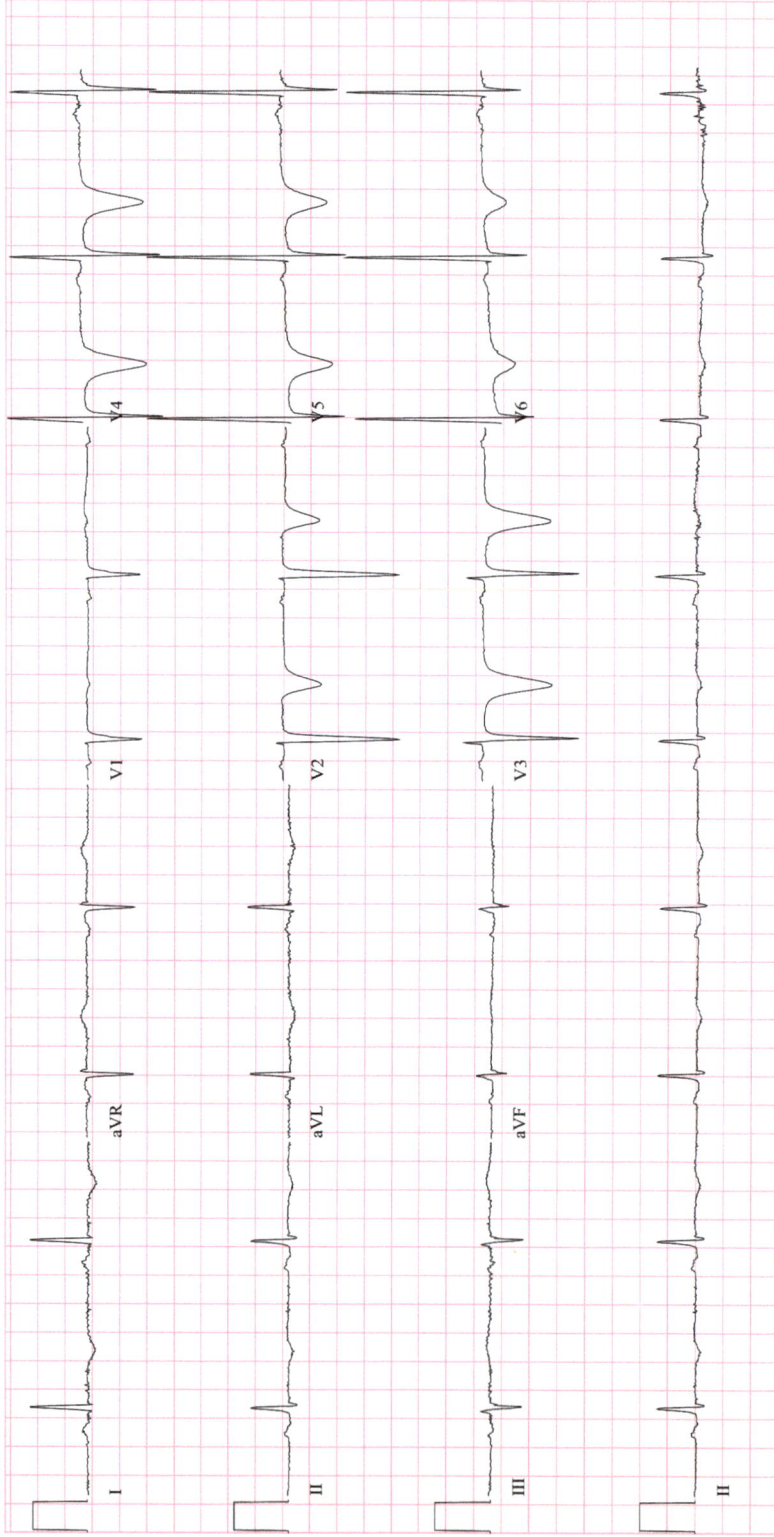

A 75-year-old male with a history of diabetes mellitus and hypertension presents to the ER with shortness of breath for the past three days. An EKG is recorded. What does it show?

DIAGNOSIS: Wellens' Syndrome Type B

The EKG shows normal sinus rhythm with deep T waves inversions in anterior (V2-V4) and lateral (V5-V6, I, and aVL) leads.

As discussed in previous case, Wellens' syndrome represents critical LAD disease.

EKG features of Wellens' syndrome are:

- Type A pattern: Positive to negative biphasic T waves in leads V2 and V3 (previous case).
- Type B pattern: Deep symmetrically inverted T waves in leads V2 and V3 (As above) with no pathological precordial Q waves and no loss of R wave progression. Patient with recent history of chest pain.

Note:

- Typical Wellens' EKG features are usually noted on pain free EKG.
- T wave changes may extend into the lateral precordial leads.
- Patients may have normal cardiac enzymes.
- Exercise stress testing may precipitate acute infarction and should be avoided.

This patient underwent percutaneous transluminal coronary angioplasty and stent placement in proximal left anterior descending, the mid left anterior descending, and the mid right coronary arteries.

EKG Case 55

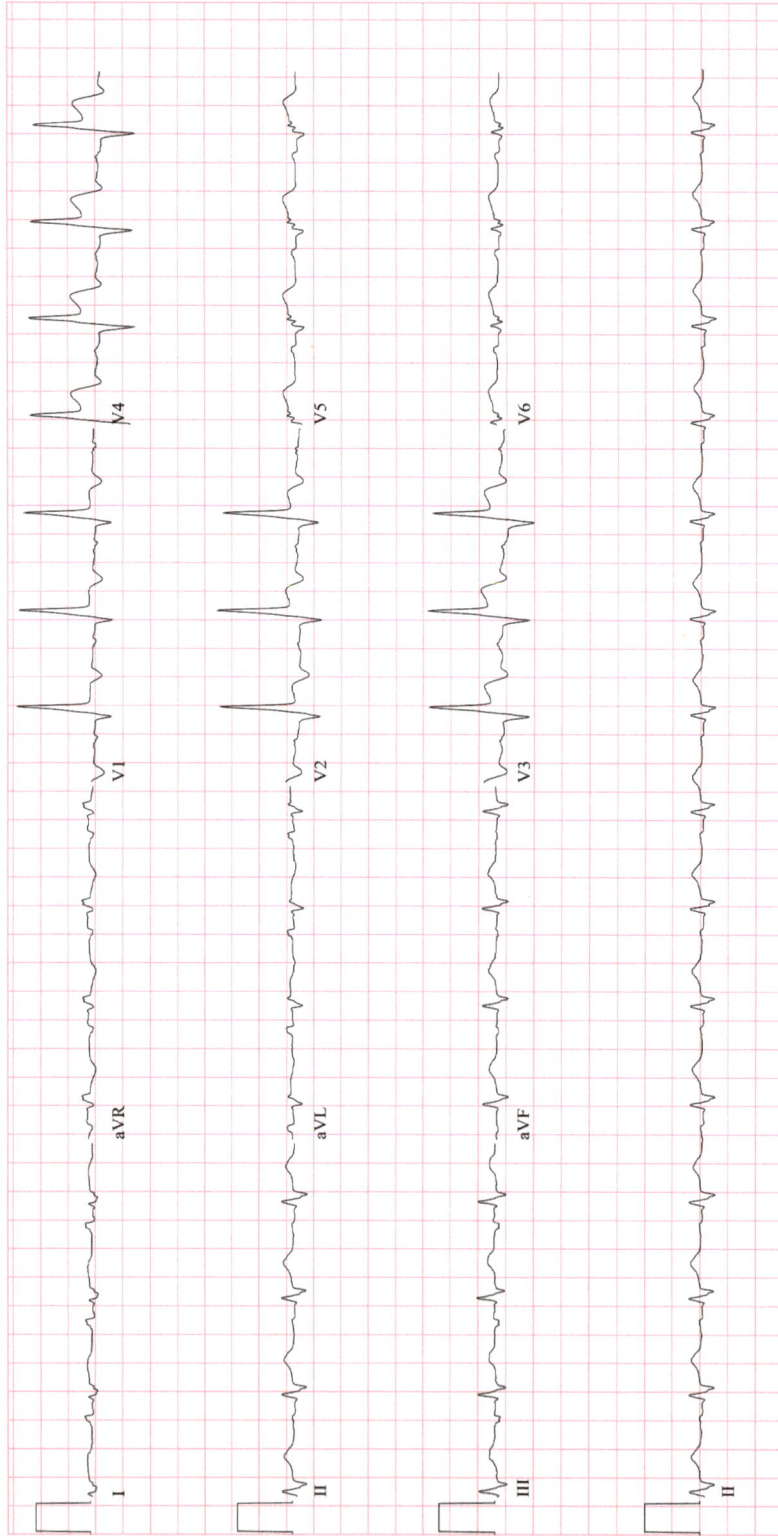

A 56-year-old man with a history of poorly controlled insulin-dependent diabetes mellitus, hypertension, hyperlipidemia, and who smokes two packs of cigarettes per day presents with crushing chest pain and shortness of breath. An EKG is obtained by the paramedics en route to the hospital. What does it show?

DIAGNOSIS: Acute Extensive Anterior, Septal, and Lateral wall ST Elevation Myocardial Infarction (STEMI)

This EKG shows normal sinus rhythm with acute anteroseptal STEMI with maximal STE in V1-V4. Proximal LAD occlusion signs in this EKG are, STE in V1 and new onset RBBB. STE in aVR and aVL suggests left main coronary artery (LMCA) occlusion. Similarly, there is subtle ST elevation in lateral leads I, V5, and V6. This EKG pattern is suggestive of extensive coronary artery disease as evident by cardiac catheterization (below).

- Proximal LAD occlusion is suggested by: ST-segment elevation in V1 (> 2.5 mm) or new right bundle branch block with Q wave or both (sensitivity 12%, specificity 100%, positive predictive value 100%, negative predictive value 61%).

- Proximal LAD / LMCA occlusion has a significantly worse prognosis due to larger infarct size and subsequently more severe hemodynamic compromise.

- An emergent cardiac catheterization revealed significant coronary artery occlusions with Left Main: 90%, Proximal LAD: 100%, Proximal Circumflex 70%, Distal Circumflex: 90%, Proximal RCA: 99 %, and Mid RCA: 80 %. Patient underwent urgent coronary artery bypass grafting.

EKG Case 56

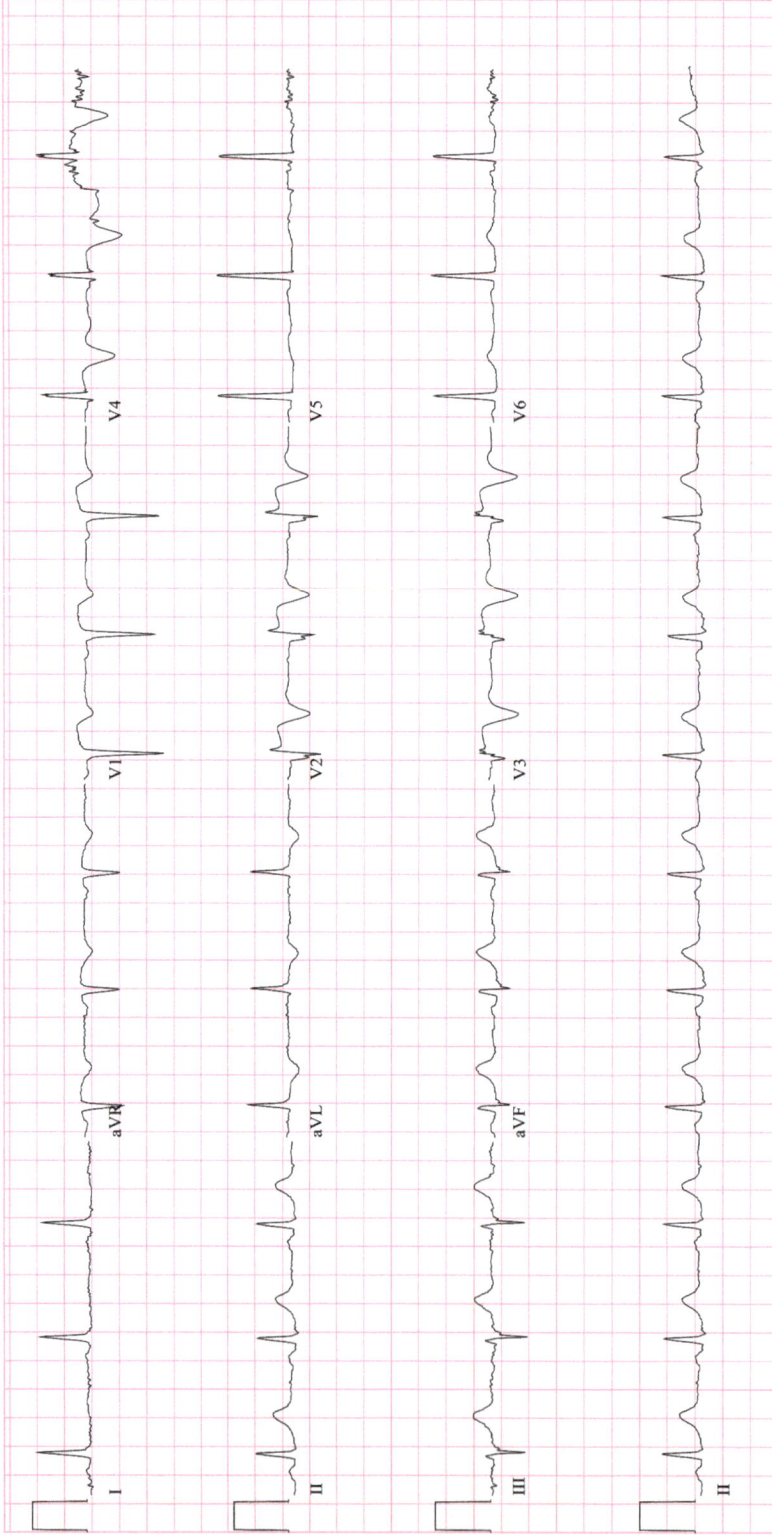

A 45-year-old male with a history of hypertension presents to the ER with complaints of chest pain. An EKG is recorded. What does it show?

DIAGNOSIS: Anteroseptal Myocardial Infarction

The EKG shows normal sinus rhythm with ST segment elevation in leads V1- V3 with biphasic T waves extending to V4. Development of Q waves in V1- V3. The EKG also shows reciprocal changes with T wave inversion in lateral lead aVL and subtle ST segment depression in leads III and aVF.

- There is an anteroseptal STEMI with maximal ST elevation in V1-V2 (extending out to V3).

- Marked ST elevation (> 2.5 mm) in V1 and STE in aVR. These features suggest occlusion proximal to 1st septal perforators (S1).

- The patient underwent cardiac catheterization which revealed multivessel occlusions with Left main 20%, Proximal LAD 100%, Dominant RCA 20%, stenosis, and right to left collaterals. Successful PCI of proximal LAD with a drug eluting stent was performed.

EKG Case 57

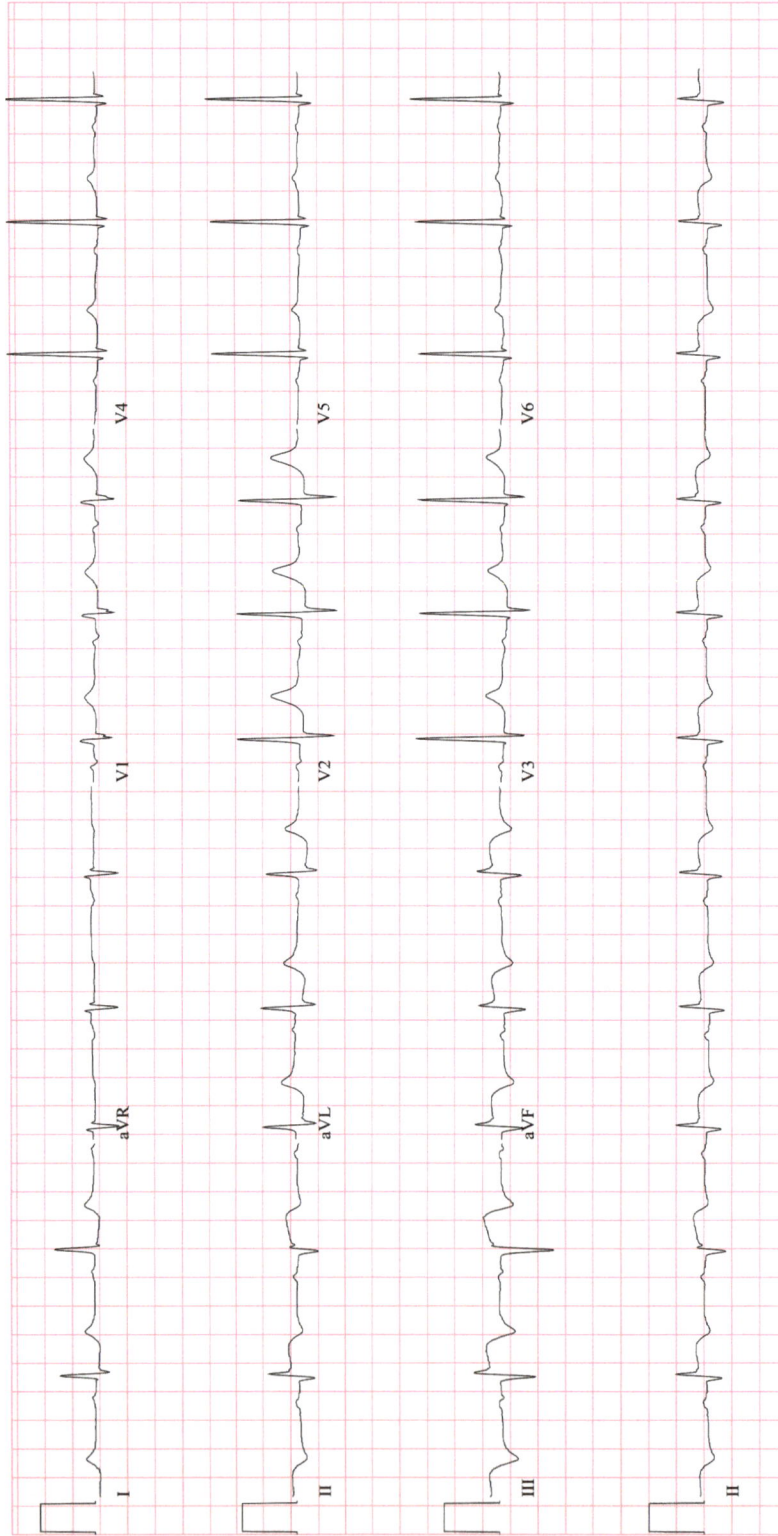

I aVR V1 V4
II aVL V2 V5
III aVF V3 V6
II

A 64-year-old female presents to the hospital with substernal chest pain and shortness of breath for the past five hours. An EKG is obtained. What does it show?

DIAGNOSIS: Acute ST Elevation Inferior Wall Myocardial Infarction Due to Distal RCA Occlusion.

This EKG shows normal sinus rhythm with ST elevation in leads II, III, and aVF, and development of Q waves in II, III, and aVF. Reciprocal ST depression in aVL and lead I. Findings suggestive of acute inferior wall myocardial infarction due to RCA occlusion.[1]

- Inferior Wall MI can result from occlusion of any of the three coronary arteries. The vast majority (~80%) of inferior STEMIs are due to occlusion of the dominant right coronary artery (RCA). Less commonly (around 18% of the time), the culprit vessel is a dominant left circumflex artery (LCx). Occasionally, inferior STEMI may result from occlusion of a "type III" or "wraparound" left anterior descending artery (LAD). This produces the unusual pattern of concomitant inferior and anterior ST elevation (see Case 58).

- While both RCA and left circumflex occlusion may cause infarction of the inferior wall, the precise area of infarction in each case is slightly different, as indicated by subtle differences on the EKG.

- **RCA occlusion:** The RCA territory covers the medial part of the inferior wall, including the inferior septum. The injury current in RCA occlusion is directed inferiorly and rightward, producing ST elevation in lead III > lead II (as lead III is more rightward facing). **Distal RCA occlusion** (as in this case) is suggested by ST elevation in lead III > lead II and presence of reciprocal ST depression in lead I. **Proximal RCA occlusion** causes additional ST segment elevation in V1, V4R, or both, and is associated with right ventricular infarction (see Case 60).

- **LCx occlusion:** The LCx territory covers the lateral part of the inferior wall and the left postero-basal area. The injury current in LCx occlusion is directed inferiorly and leftward, producing ST elevation in the lateral leads I and V5- V6 and ST elevation in inferior leads, II and III. However, ST elevation in lead II is usually equal to lead III and there is an absence of reciprocal ST depression in lead I.

1   Zimetbaum, Peter J., and Mark E. Josephson. "Use of the electrocardiogram in acute myocardial infarction." *New England Journal of Medicine* 348, no. 10 (2003): 933-940.

EKG Case 58

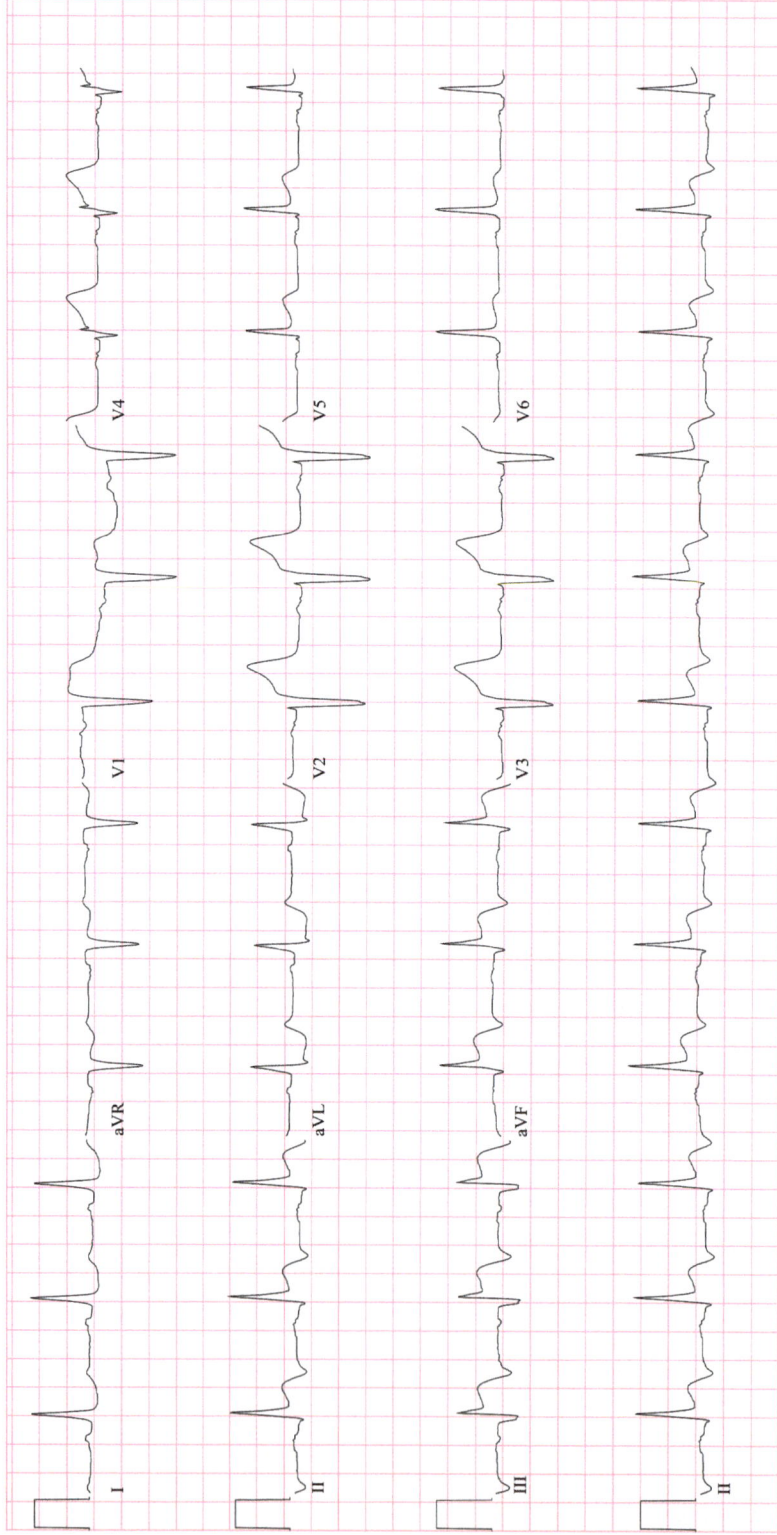

A 70-year-old male with a history of uncontrolled diabetes mellitus, hypertension, and hyperlipidemia presents with severe retrosternal chest pain that has persisted for the past seven hours. On arrival to the ER, the patient is diaphoretic and hypotensive. An EKG is obtained. What does it show?

DIAGNOSIS: Acute Inferior and Anterior Wall ST Elevation Myocardial Infarction

This EKG shows normal sinus rhythm with ST elevation in leads II, III, aVF, V1- V4; ST segment depression in leads I and aVL.

- Acute occlusion of the left anterior descending coronary artery (LAD) generally results in ST segment elevations in precordial leads and reciprocal ST segment depression in inferior leads. When ST segment elevation occurs in inferior leads, the culprit artery is either the right coronary artery (RCA) or left circumflex coronary artery (LCX).

- Simultaneous anterior and inferior myocardial infarction has been described due to occlusion of "wrapped LAD", i.e, a large LAD that supplies the anterior LV wall and wraps around the LV apex to supply blood to the inferior LV wall.

- Patient underwent percutaneous transluminal coronary angiogram and was found to have extensive LAD and LCX occlusion as 95% stenosis of the mid LAD, 60% stenosis of the proximal segment of the LAD, 60% stenosis of the proximal segment of the first diagonal branch of the LAD, 80% stenosis of the proximal segment of the LCX, and a 90% stenosis of the proximal segment of the OM2 branch of the LCX, requiring balloon angioplasty and deployment of bare metal stents.

EKG Case 59

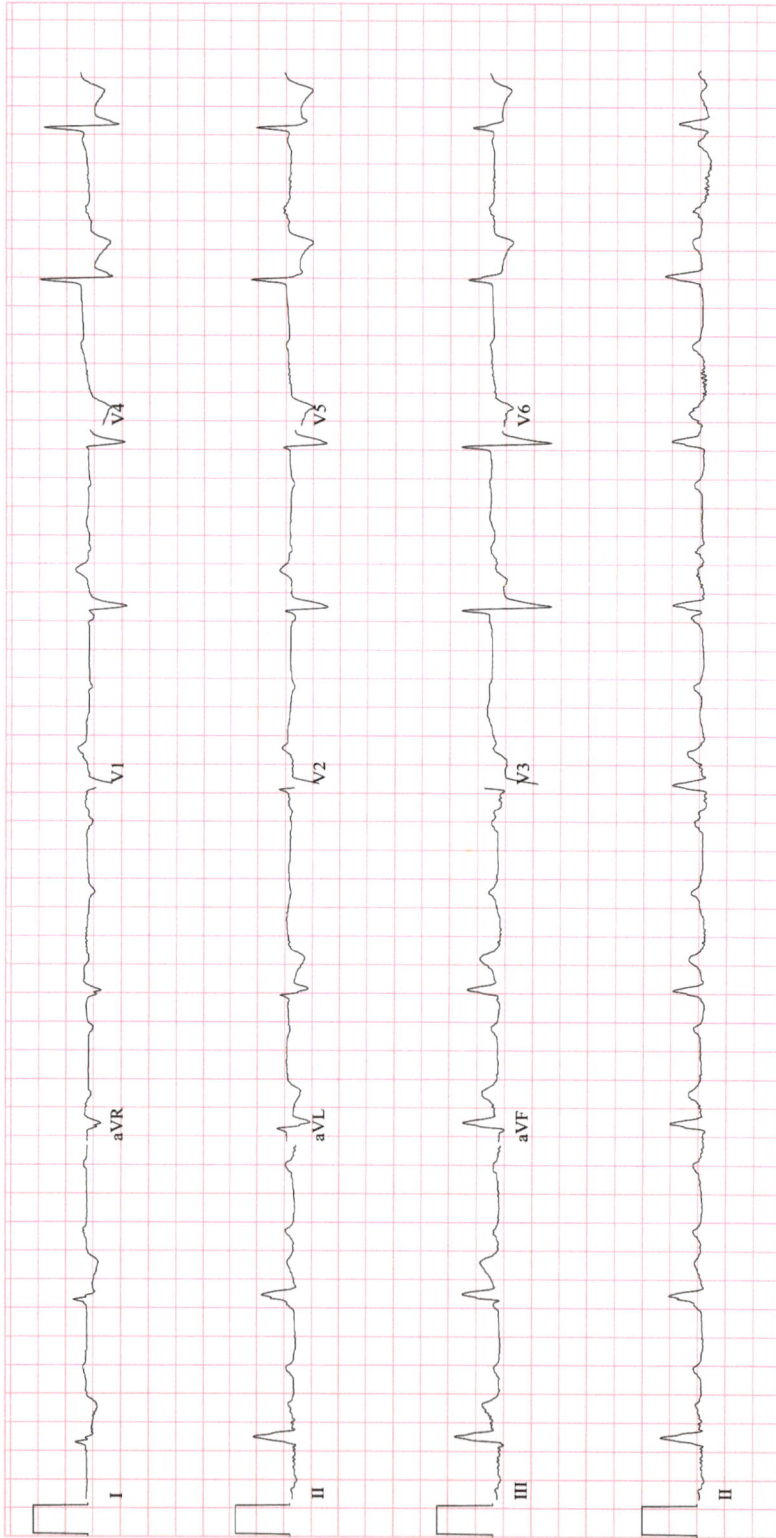

A 45-year-old diabetic male is brought to the ER after a syncopal episode. He is diaphoretic and hypotensive. An EKG is obtained. What does it show?

DIAGNOSIS: AV Block in Inferior ST Elevation Myocardial Infarction (STEMI)

This EKG shows 3rd degree AV block with ST elevation in leads III and aVF with reciprocal ST depression in lateral leads V4 - V6, I, and aVL, indicating acute inferior wall myocardial infarction.

- Up to 20% of patients with inferior STEMI will develop either second or third degree heart block.

- Presumed mechanisms for this includes (a) ischemia of the AV node due to impaired blood flow via the AV nodal artery. This artery arises from the RCA 80% of the time, hence its involvement in inferior STEMI due to RCA occlusion. (b) Bezold-Jarisch reflex = increased vagal tone secondary to ischemia.

- The conduction block may develop either as a step-wise progression from 1st degree heart block via Wenckebach to complete heart block (in 50% of cases), or as abrupt onset of second or third-degree heart block (in the remaining 50%).

- Patients may also manifest signs of sinus node dysfunction, such as sinus bradycardia, sinus pauses, sinoatrial exit block, and sinus arrest. Similarly to AV node dysfunction, this may result from increased vagal tone or ischemia of the SA node (which is supplied by the RCA in 60% of people).

- Bradyarrhythmias and AV block in the context of inferior STEMI are usually transient (lasting hours to days), respond well to atropine, and usually do not require permanent pacing.

EKG Case 60

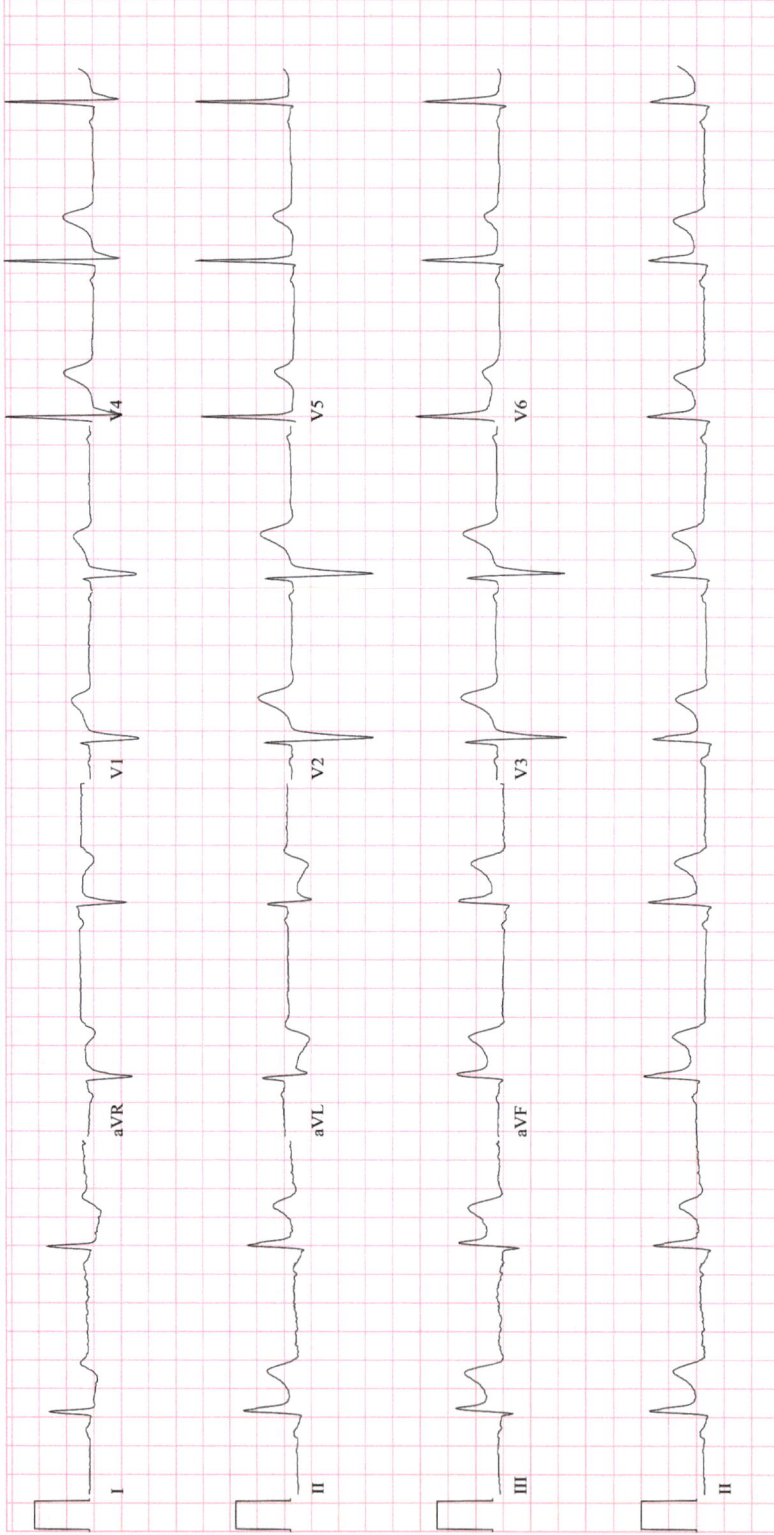

A 42-year-old man with a history of hypertension and diabetes mellitus presents to the hospital with retrosternal chest pain and dizziness. An EKG is obtained. What does it show?

DIAGNOSIS: Acute Inferior Wall MI with Right Ventricular Infarction

Right ventricular myocardial infarction is always associated with occlusion of the proximal segment of the right coronary artery. The most sensitive electrocardiographic sign of right ventricular infarction is ST segment elevation of more than 1 mm in lead V4R with an upright T wave in that lead (see right sided EKG of this patient below). The presence of ST segment elevation in lead V1 (subtle in this case) in association with ST segment elevation in leads II, III, and aVF (with greater elevation in lead III than in lead II) is highly correlated with the presence of right ventricular infarction[1]. Right ventricular infarction is confirmed by the presence of ST elevation in the right-sided leads (V3R - V6R).

- Right ventricular infarction complicates up to 40% of inferior STEMIs. Isolated RV infarction is extremely uncommon.

- Patients with RV infarction are very preload sensitive (due to poor RV contractility) and can develop severe hypotension in response to nitrates or other preload-reducing agents.

- Hypotension in right ventricular infarction is treated with fluid loading. Vasodilators such as nitrates are contraindicated in these cases as nitrates can cause syncope. Also avoid diuretics despite elevated JVP as it can lead to cardiogenic shock.

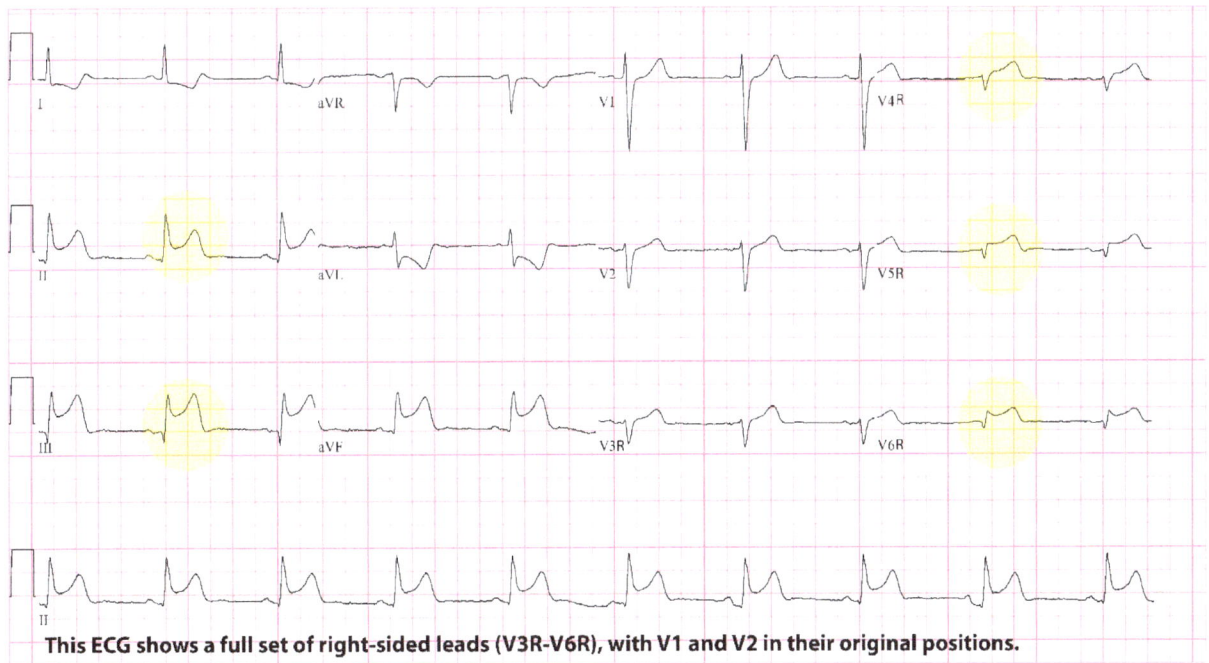

This ECG shows a full set of right-sided leads (V3R-V6R), with V1 and V2 in their original positions.

---

1   Zimetbaum, Peter J., and Mark E. Josephson. "Use of the electrocardiogram in acute myocardial infarction." *New England Journal of Medicine* 348, no. 10 (2003): 933-940.

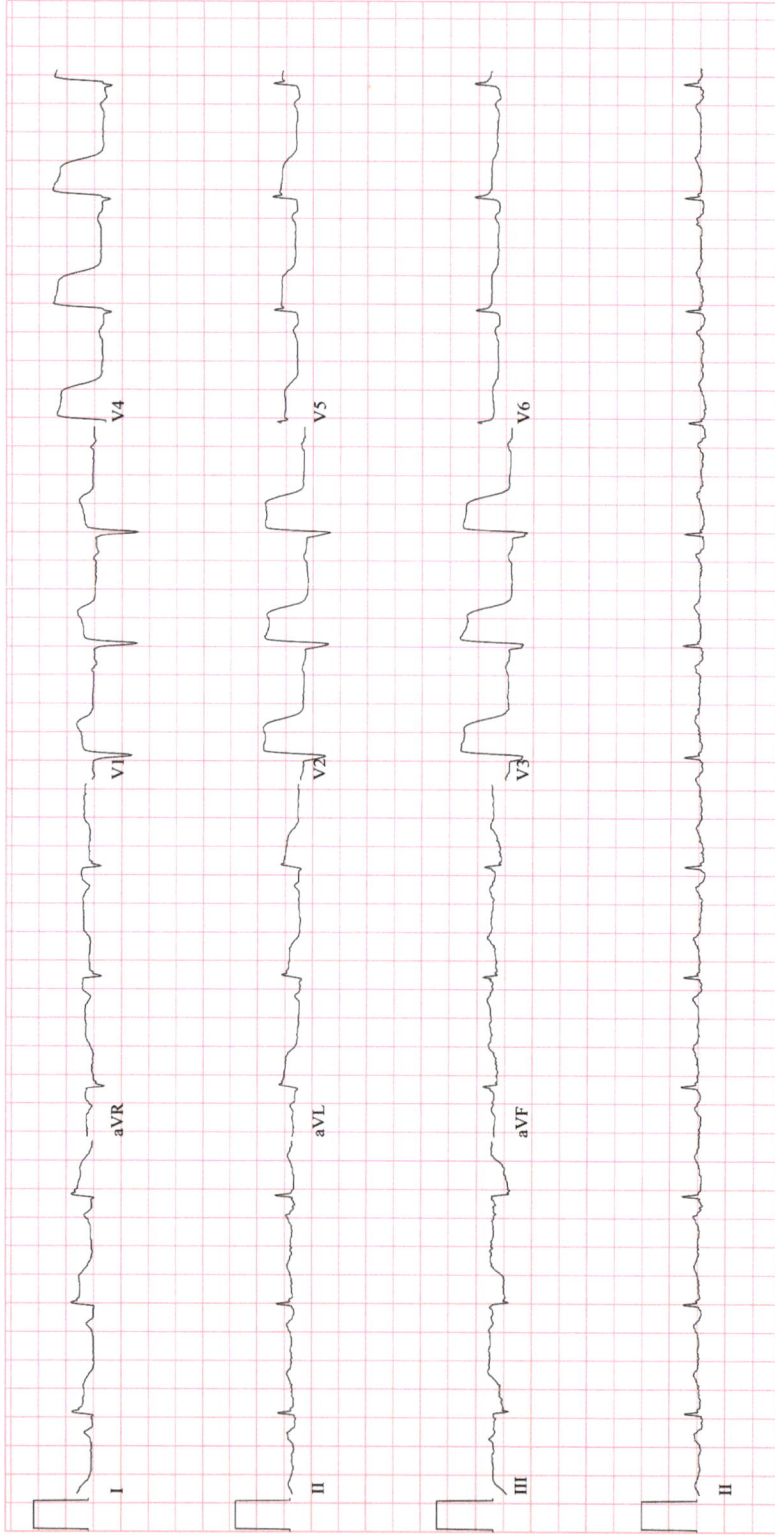

EKG Case 61

A 65-year-old woman with family history significant because of sudden cardiac death of father at age 50 presents to the ER with crushing chest pain for the past seven hours. An EKG is obtained. What does it show?

DIAGNOSIS: Anterolateral ST Elevation Myocardial

- This EKG shows normal sinus rhythm at 75 bpm with ST elevation in the anterior (V2-4) and lateral leads (I, aVL, V5 - V6). There is a loss of general R wave progression across the precordial leads. There is reciprocal ST depression in the inferior leads (III and aVF). This pattern indicates an extensive infarction involving the anterior and lateral walls of the left ventricle.

- Anterolateral myocardial infarctions frequently are caused by occlusion of the proximal left anterior descending coronary artery, or combined occlusions of the LAD together with the right coronary artery or left circumflex artery. It can also be due to an occlusion of the left main artery.

EKG Case 62

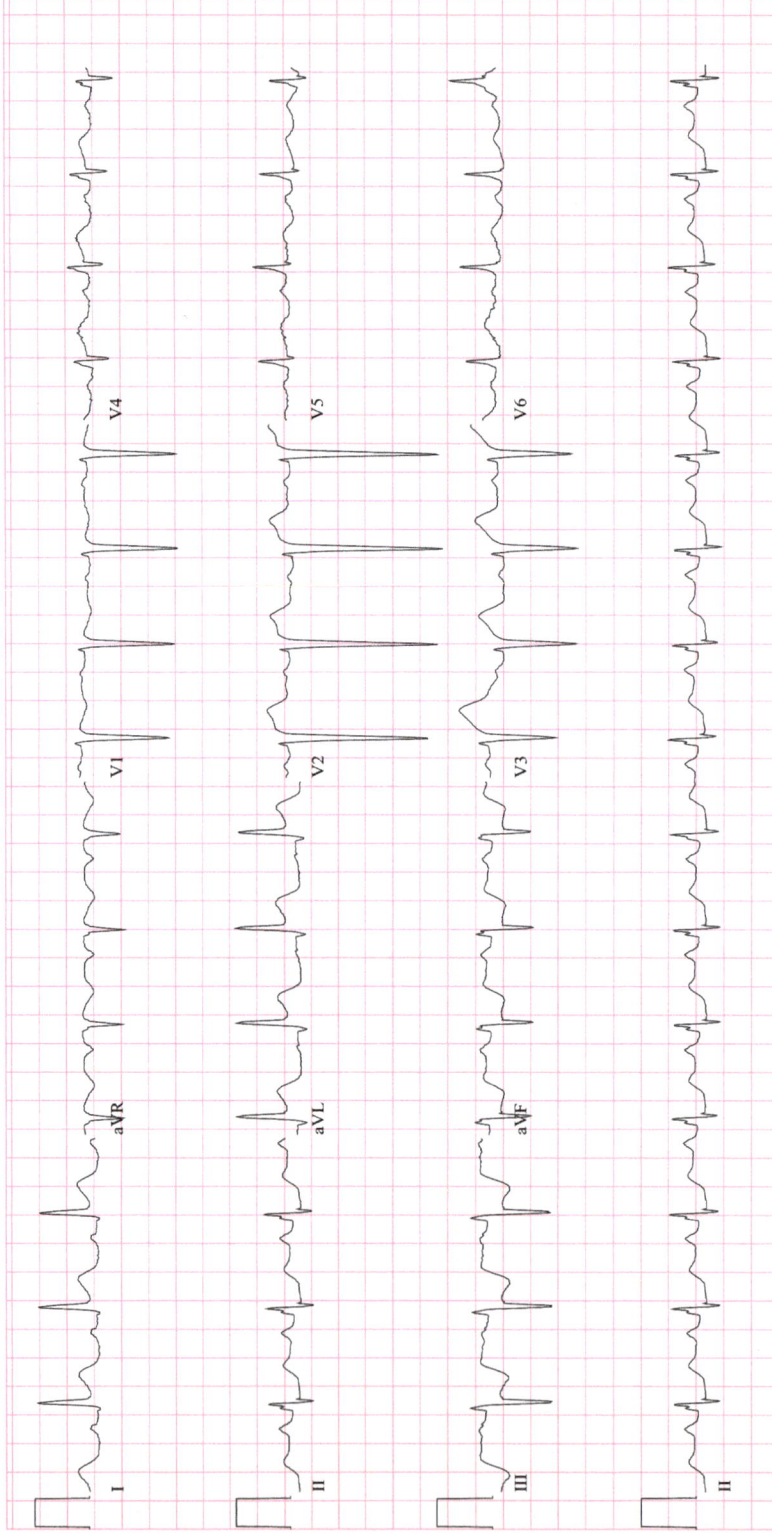

A 67-year-old male with a history of coronary artery disease, hypertension, and diabetes mellitus presents with crushing chest pain. In the ER, an EKG is obtained. What does it show?

DIAGNOSIS: High Lateral STEMI

This EKG shows normal sinus rhythm, leftward axis with marked ST elevation in leads I and aVL with reciprocal ST segment depression in inferior leads (II, III, and aVF). This pattern is consistent with an acute infarction localized to the superior portion of the lateral wall of the left ventricle (high lateral STEMI). This EKG also shows left ventricular hypertrophy by voltage criteria.

- ST elevation primarily localized to leads I and aVL is referred to as a high lateral STEMI.

- It is usually associated with reciprocal ST depression and T wave inversion in the inferior leads.

- Culprit vessels include: (a) occlusion of the first diagonal branch (D1) of the left anterior descending artery (LAD) which may produce isolated ST elevation in I and aVL; and (b) Occlusion of the circumflex artery which may cause ST elevation in I, aVL along with leads V5 - V6.

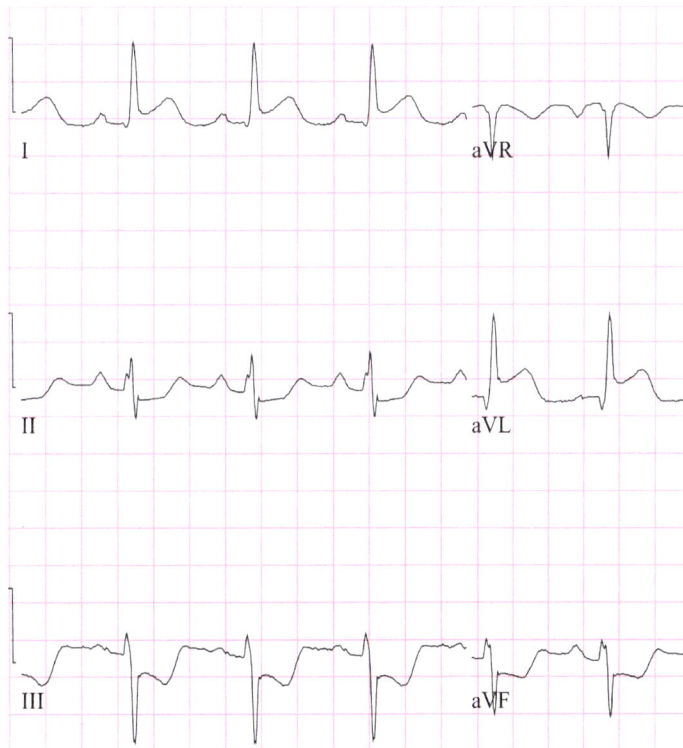

EKG Case 63

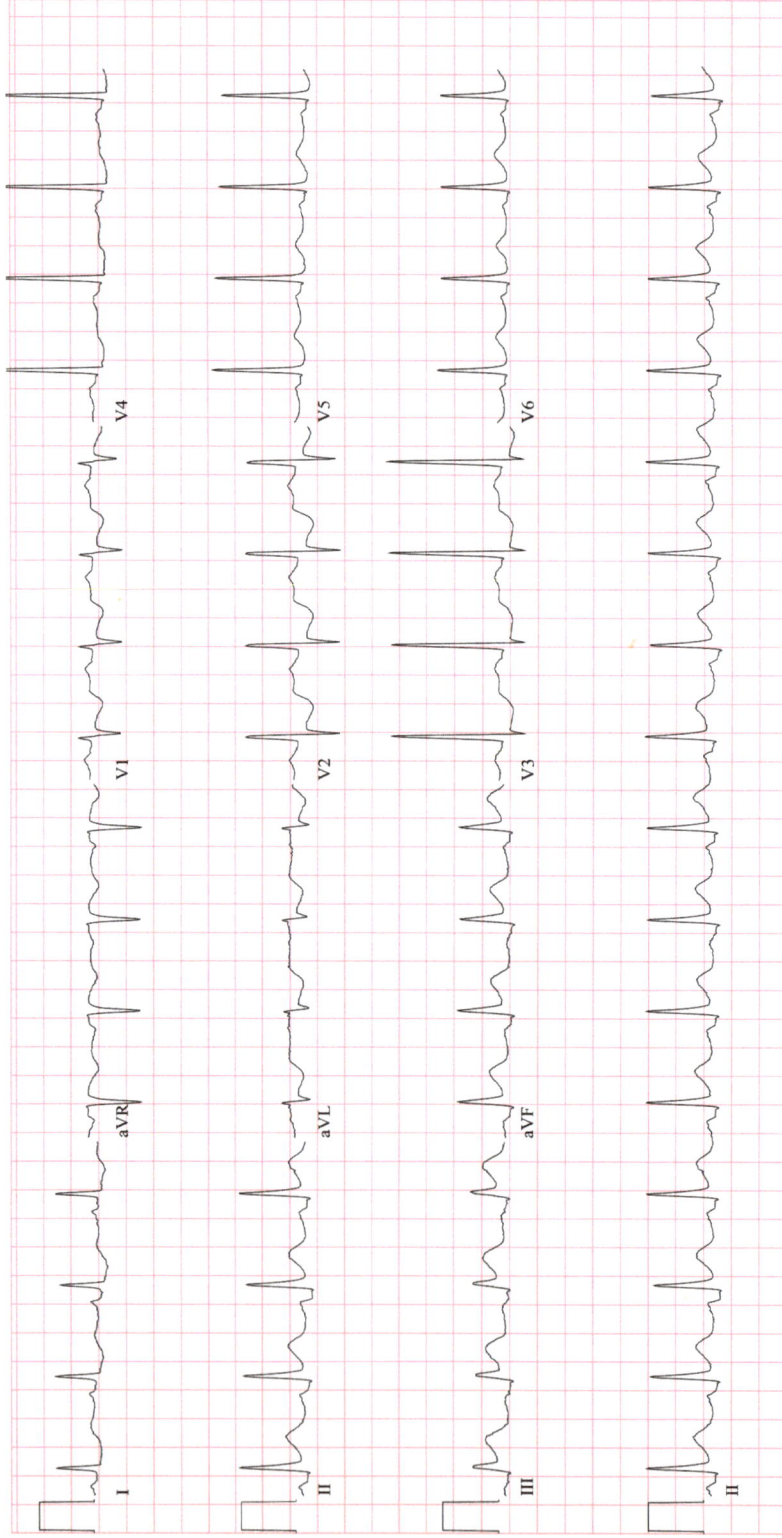

A 62-year-old female with a past history of hypertension, type II Diabetes Mellitus, and hyperlipidemia presents to the hospital with nausea, vomiting, and epigastric pain. Her blood pressure is 80/50. What does the EKG show and what will you do?

DIAGNOSIS: Acute ST Elevation Inferior and Posterior Wall Myocardial Infarction

- The EKG shows tall dominant R waves in leads V1 - V4 with ST segment depression and upright T waves. These reciprocal changes in anterior leads i.e, R waves instead of Q waves, V1 or V2 R/S >1, ST depression, and upright T waves are indicative of posterior wall ST elevation myocardial Infarction accompanying inferior wall MI.

- Differential diagnosis for tall R waves are limited, including posterior wall MI, right ventricular hypertrophy, RBBB, and WPW with left sided accessory pathway.

- Also note, ST elevation in leads II, III, and aVF showing inferior wall MI.

- Use of posterior leads V7 to V9 significantly increase the detection of posterior injury patterns compared with the standard 12-lead EKG. Lead V7 is placed at the level of lead V6 at the posterior axillary line, lead V8 on the left side of the back at the tip of the scapula, and lead V9 is placed at left spinal border. ST segment elevation of > 1 mm in the posterior leads is suggestive of PMI.

- Posterior infarction accompanies 15 - 20% of STEMIs. In 70% of cases, the right coronary artery is involved and in the rest of cases, the circumflex artery is involved.

- This patient's abdominal pain is secondary to acute myocardial infarction. The patient is in a state of cardiogenic shock, and she should be immediately treated with IV fluids, antiplatelets agents like aspirin or clopidogrel and IV heparin. Emergent percutaneous coronary intervention (PCI) to restore myocardial blood flow is required.

EKG Case 64

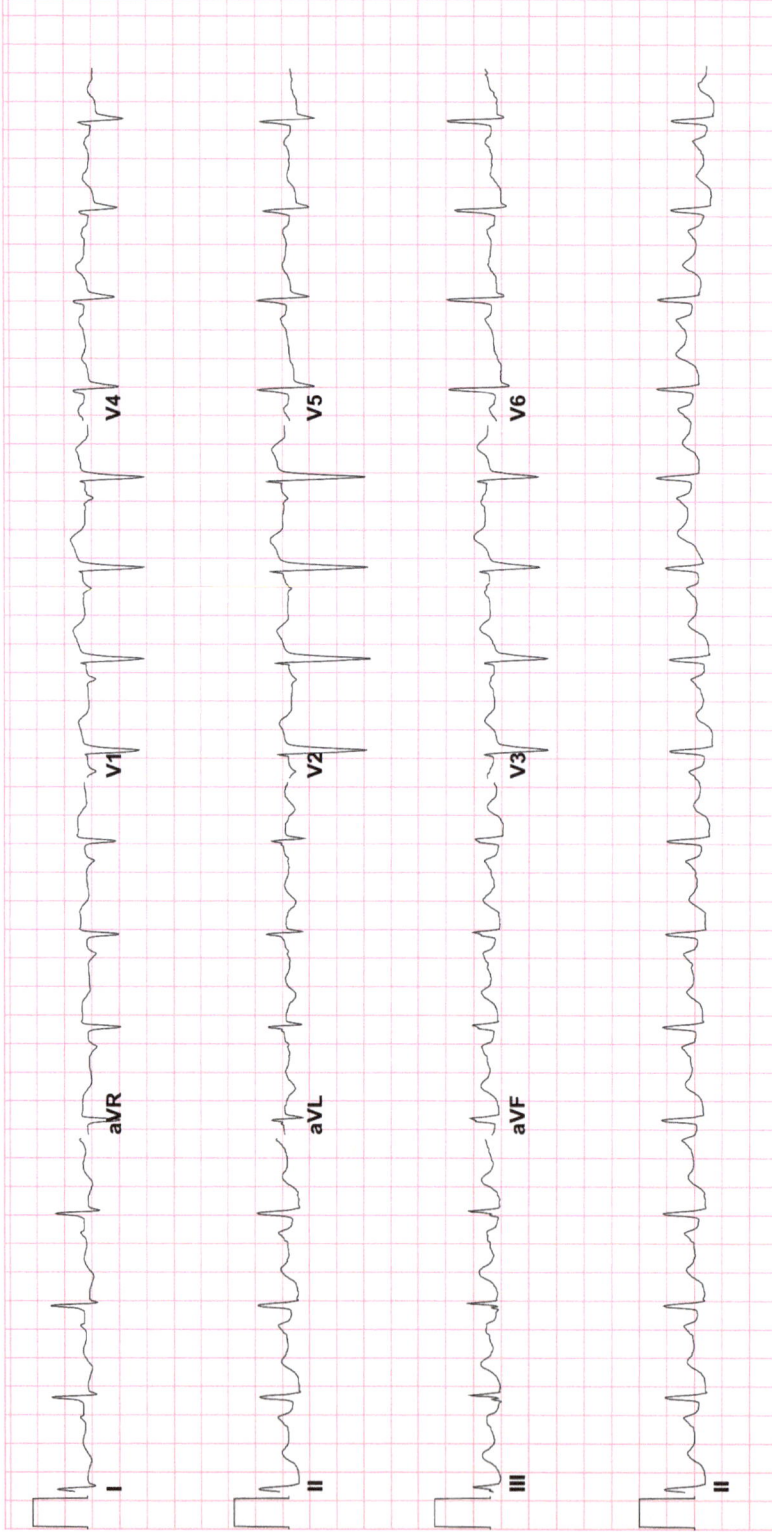

A 70-year-old female presents to the hospital with chief complaint of epigastric pain radiating to the chest and jaw. Pain has been ongoing for six weeks and patient had an unremarkable endocscopy. The pain is now "unbearable" and is associated with exertional dyspnea. An EKG is obtained. What does it show?

DIAGNOSIS: ST Segment Elevation in aVR (STE-aVR) - Left Main Coronary Artery (LMCA) Occlusion

This EKG demonstrates the classical pattern of left main coronary artery (LMCA) stenosis. Widespread horizontal ST depression, most prominent in leads I, II, aVF, and V4- V6, and ST elevation in aVR ≥ 1mm.

- Augmented vector right (aVR) lead is commonly "ignored" and designated as the "neglected lead"[1]. In the setting of acute coronary syndrome, severe left main coronary artery disease usually presents as widespread ST segment depression, whereas ST segment elevation (STE) in aVR (STE-aVR) is a less recognized finding. More importantly, STE-aVR can also be seen with left anterior descending (LAD) artery occlusion/sub-occlusion but is an uncommon electrocardiographic sign in this setting.[2]

Mechanism of STE in aVR

- Lead aVR is electrically opposite to the left-sided leads I, aVL, and V4 - V6; therefore, ST depression in these leads will produce reciprocal ST elevation in aVR.

- Lead aVR also directly records electrical activity from the right upper portion of the heart, including the right ventricular outflow tract and the basal portion of the interventricular septum. Infarction in this area could theoretically produce ST elevation in aVR.

ST elevation in aVR is therefore postulated to result from two possible mechanisms:

- Diffuse subendocardial ischemia, with ST depression in the lateral leads producing reciprocal change in aVR and infarction of the basal septum, i.e, an STEMI involving aVR.

- The basal septum is supplied by the first septal perforator artery (a very proximal branch of the LAD), so ischemia, infarction of the basal septum would imply involvement of the proximal LAD or LMCA.

An emergent coronary angiogram showed 95% distal LMCA occlusion and patent LAD. Patient underwent emergent coronary artery bypass grafting x2, consisting of left internal mammary artery to the left anterior descending artery and a reverse saphenous vein graft to the obtuse marginal.

---

1   Kossaify, Antoine. "ST Segment Elevation in aVR: Clinical Significance in Acute coronary syndrome." *Clinical medicine insights. Case reports* 6 (2013): 41.

2   de Winter RJ, Verouden NJ, Wellens HJ, Wilde AA. A New ECG Sign of Proximal LAD Occlusion. N Engl J Med. 2008;359:2071–3.

EKG Case 65

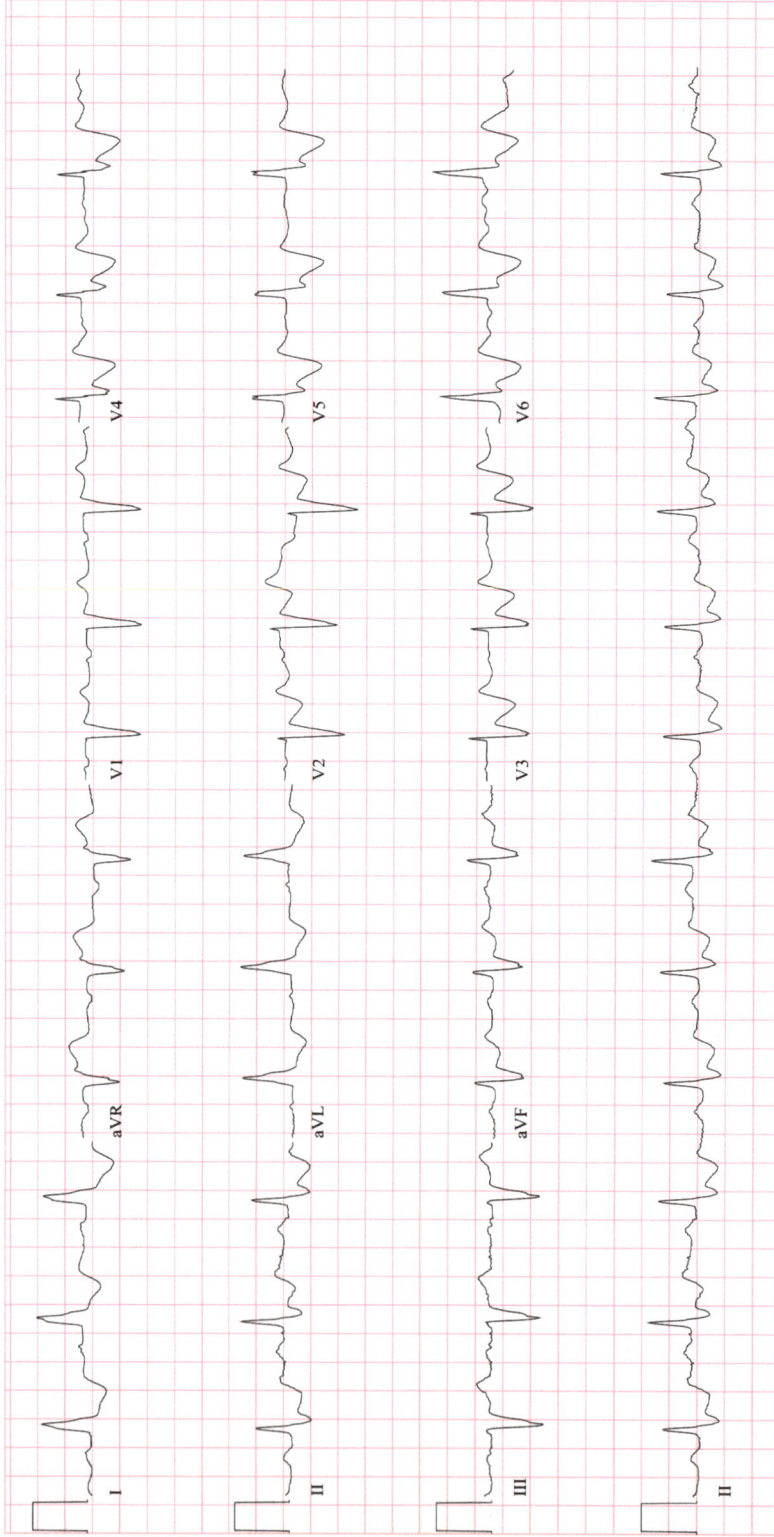

A 75-year-old woman with a history of metastatic breast cancer and hypertension presents to the hospital with chief complaint of chest pain and GI bleeding. Patient's lab revealed hemoglobin of 6g/dl and troponin of 4.5 ng/mL. An EKG is recorded. No previous EKGs are available for comparison. What does it show?

DIAGNOSIS: Acute Myocardial Infarction in LBBB (Sgarbossa Criteria)

This EKG shows normal sinus rhythm with first degree AV block, left bundle branch, and concordant ST depression in V2- V4 (anterior wall MI). T wave inversions could be seen in inferolateral leads.

Sgarbossa's criteria are a set of electrocardiographic findings generally used to identify acute myocardial infarction in the presence of a left bundle branch block (LBBB) or a ventricular paced rhythm. Acute myocardial infarction is often difficult to detect when LBBB is present on EKG.

Normally, in LBBB, we expect the J-point or ST segment to move in opposite direction of the QRS complex. In other words, in those leads where the QRS complex is normally a positive deflection, the J-point and ST-segment should be slightly below the isoelectric line, and in those leads where the QRS is negative (primarily V_1-V_3), the J-point and ST-segment should rise slightly above the isoelectric line. This is known as *discordance*, and a small amount of discordance is appropriate and expected in LBBB.

A large clinical trial of thrombolytic therapy for acute MI (GUSTO-1)[1] evaluated the electrocardiographic diagnosis of evolving acute MI in the presence of LBBB. Among 26,003 North American patients who had an acute myocardial infarction confirmed by enzyme studies, 131 (0.5%) had LBBB. A scoring system, now commonly called Sgarbossa criteria, was developed from the coefficients assigned by a logistic model for each independent criterion, on a scale of 0 to 5. Three parameters are included in Sgarbossa's criteria:

- ST elevation ≥1 mm in a lead with a positive QRS complex (ie: concordance): 5 points
- ST depression ≥1 mm in lead V1, V2, or V3: 3 points
- ST elevation ≥5 mm in a lead with a negative (discordant) QRS complex: 2 points

A total score of ≥ 3 has a specificity of 90% (sensitivity of 36%) for diagnosing acute myocardial infarction. During right ventricular pacing, the EKG also shows a left bundle branch block pattern and the above criteria can also be applied for the diagnosis of myocardial infarction, although they are less specific.

This patient was treated conservatively due to comorbidities and a follow-up EKG on day 10 of hospitalization showed resolution of concordant ST depression in leads V2 and V3.

---

1   Sgarbossa, Elena B., Sergio L. Pinski, Alejandro Barbagelata, Donald A. Underwood, Kathy B. Gates, Eric J. Topol, Robert M. Califf, and Galen S. Wagner. "Electrocardiographic diagnosis of evolving acute myocardial infarction in the presence of left bundle-branch block." New England Journal of Medicine 334, no. 8 (1996): 481-487.

EKG Case 66

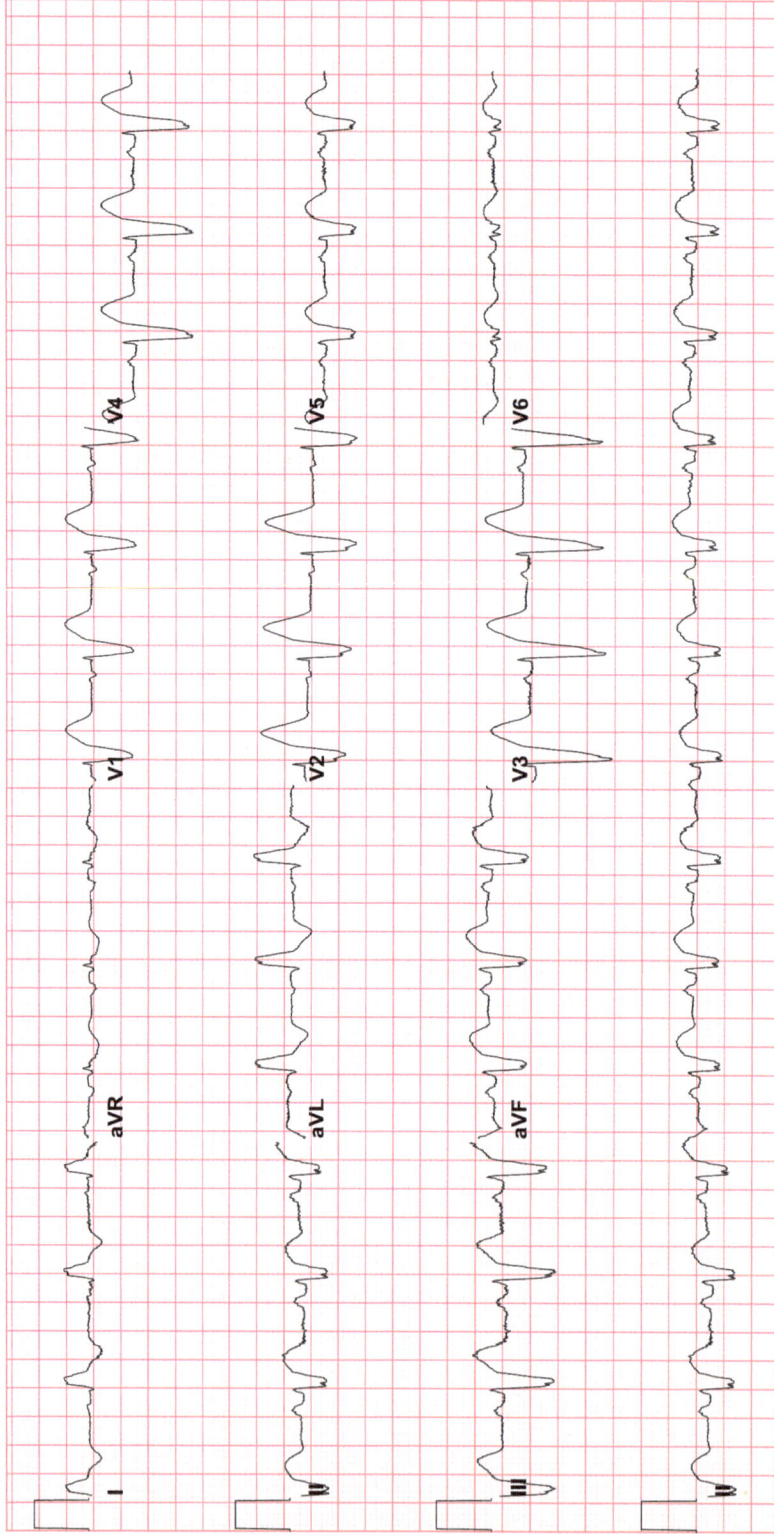

A 60-year-old male with history of hypertension presents to the hospital with the chief complaint of retrosternal chest pain. Cardiac troponin is elevated to 10.0 ng/ml. An EKG obtained 6 months ago shows LBBB. What does the present EKG show?

DIAGNOSIS: Acute Myocardial Infarction – Sgarbossa's Criteria

This EKG shows normal sinus rhythm, LBBB, and concordant ST elevation in V5 and V6 (leads with positive QRS complex).

As per our discussion in the previous EKG case, Sgarbossa's criteria are a set of electrocardiographic findings generally used to identify acute myocardial infarction in the presence of a left bundle branch block (LBBB) or a ventricular paced rhythm.

Sgarbossa's criteria is defined by:

- ST elevation ≥1 mm in a lead with a positive QRS complex (i.e, concordance): 5 points (**as above**).

- ST depression ≥1 mm in lead V1, V2, or V3: 3 points.

- ST elevation ≥5 mm in a lead with a negative (discordant) QRS complex: 2 points.

A total score of ≥ 3 has a specificity of 90% (sensitivity of 36%) for diagnosing acute myocardial infarction. During right ventricular pacing, the EKG also shows a left bundle branch block pattern and the above criteria also apply for the diagnosis of myocardial infarction, although they are less specific.

EKG Case 67

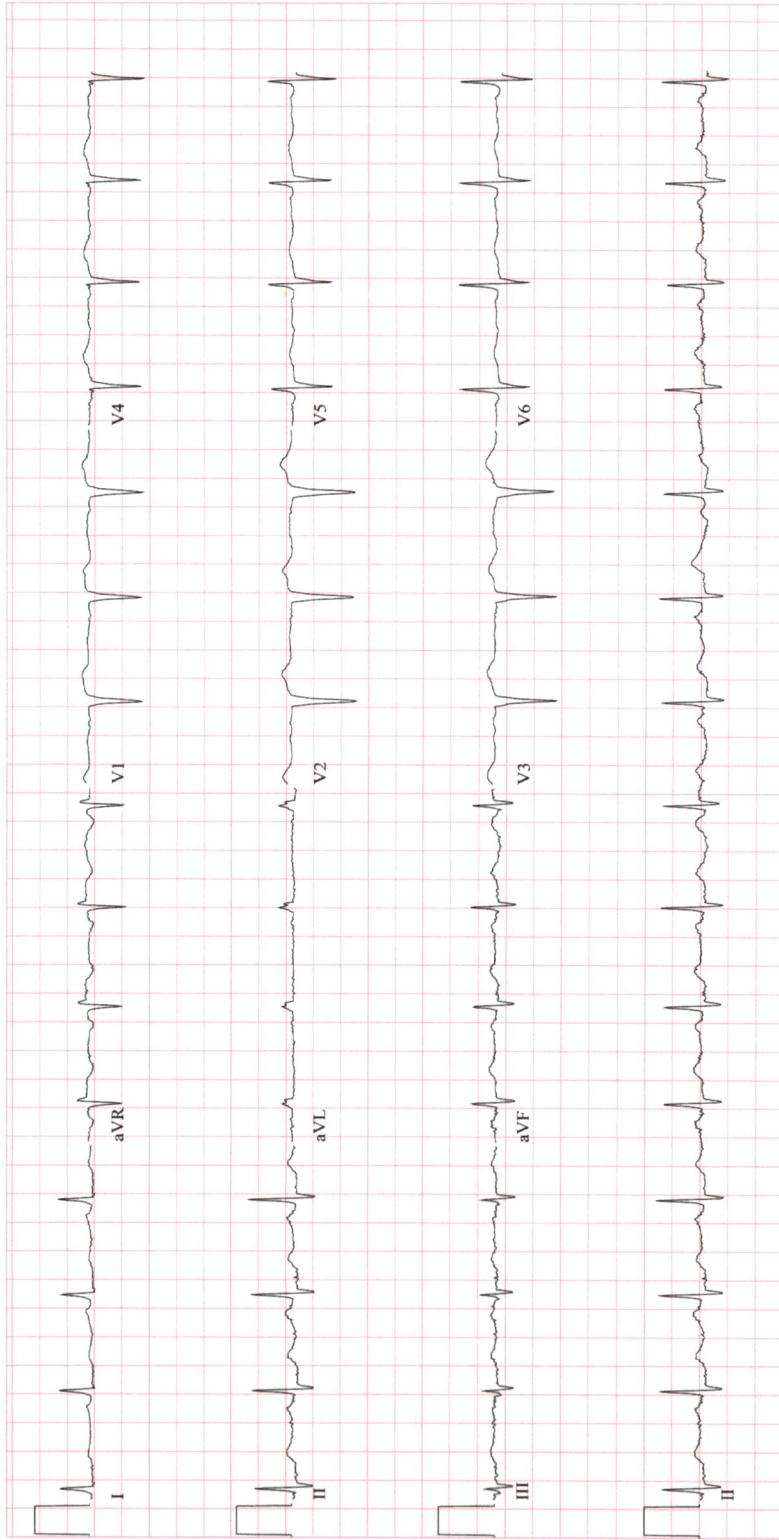

An EKG is obtained from an asymptomatic 75-year-old male with a history of coronary artery disease. What does the EKG show?

DIAGNOSIS: Anteroseptal Myocardial Infarction and Poor R Waves Progression

This EKG shows normal sinus rhythm at 75 bpm and pathologic Q waves in anteroseptal leads V1- V4 with poor progression of R waves.

Q waves are considered pathological if:

- > 40 ms (1 mm) wide

- > 2 mm deep

- > 25% of depth of QRS complex

- Seen in leads V1- V4

- Pathological Q waves usually indicate current or prior myocardial infarction.

Poor R wave progression refers to the absence of the normal increase in size of the R wave in the precordial leads as one progresses from lead V1 to V6. In lead V1, the R wave should be small. The R wave becomes larger throughout the precordial leads to the point where the R wave is larger than the S wave in lead V4.

The causes of poor R wave progression include:

- Prior anteroseptal, anterior, or anterolateral myocardial infarction.

- Lead misplacement (frequently in obese women), e.g, transposition of V1 and V3.

- Left bundle branch block or left anterior fascicular block.

- Left ventricular hypertrophy.

- Dilated cardiomyopathy.

- Dextrocardia.

- Tension pneumothorax with mediastinal shift.

- May be a normal variant.

EKG Case 68

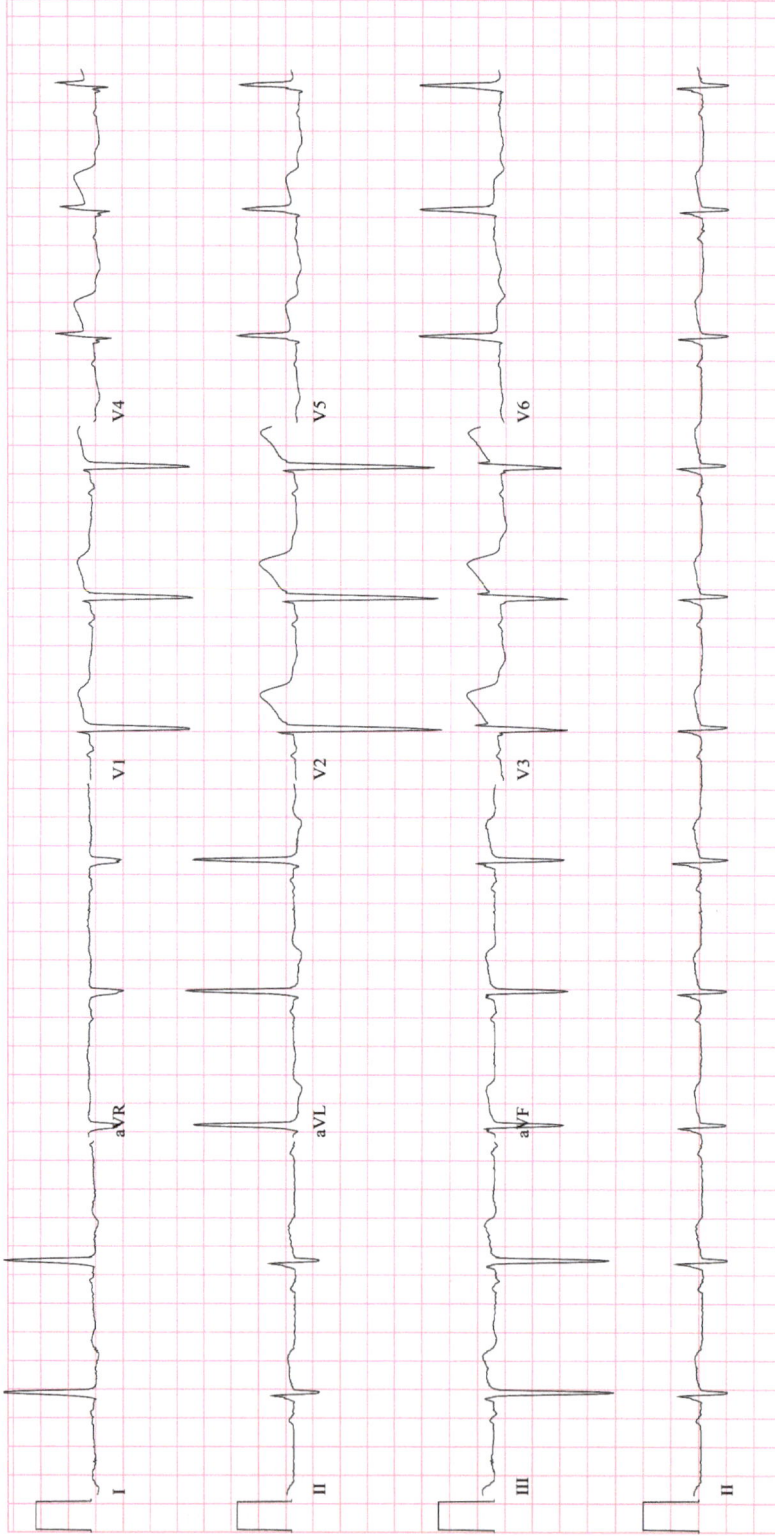

A 54-year-old male presents to the clinic for follow-up after a recent anterior myocardial infarction eight weeks ago. His only complaint today is exertional dyspnea. An EKG is obtained. What does it show and what should be done next?

DIAGNOSIS: Left Ventricular Aneurysm

Persistent ST elevation in the chest leads often indicates formation of a ventricular aneurysm. This EKG shows the presence of deep Q waves in V1- V4 (previous transmural myocardial infarction) with persistent ST segment elevation in leads V2- V5, eight weeks after known anterior myocardial infarction. This is highly suggestive of left ventricular aneurysm.

- ST elevation can be of convex or concave morphology with usual biphasic, non-hyperacute T waves.

- Myocardial scar tissue is arrhythmogenic and can lead to ventricular arrhythmias and sudden cardiac death.

- Ventricular aneurysm can also lead to congestive heart failure, and mural thrombosis and subsequent thromboembolism.

- An echocardiogram or cardiac MRI should be performed to confirm the diagnosis and assess myocardial viability.

- Treatment encompasses managing heart failure, anticoagulation to prevent thromboembolism, and surgical evaluation for possible aneurysmectomy.

EKG Case 69

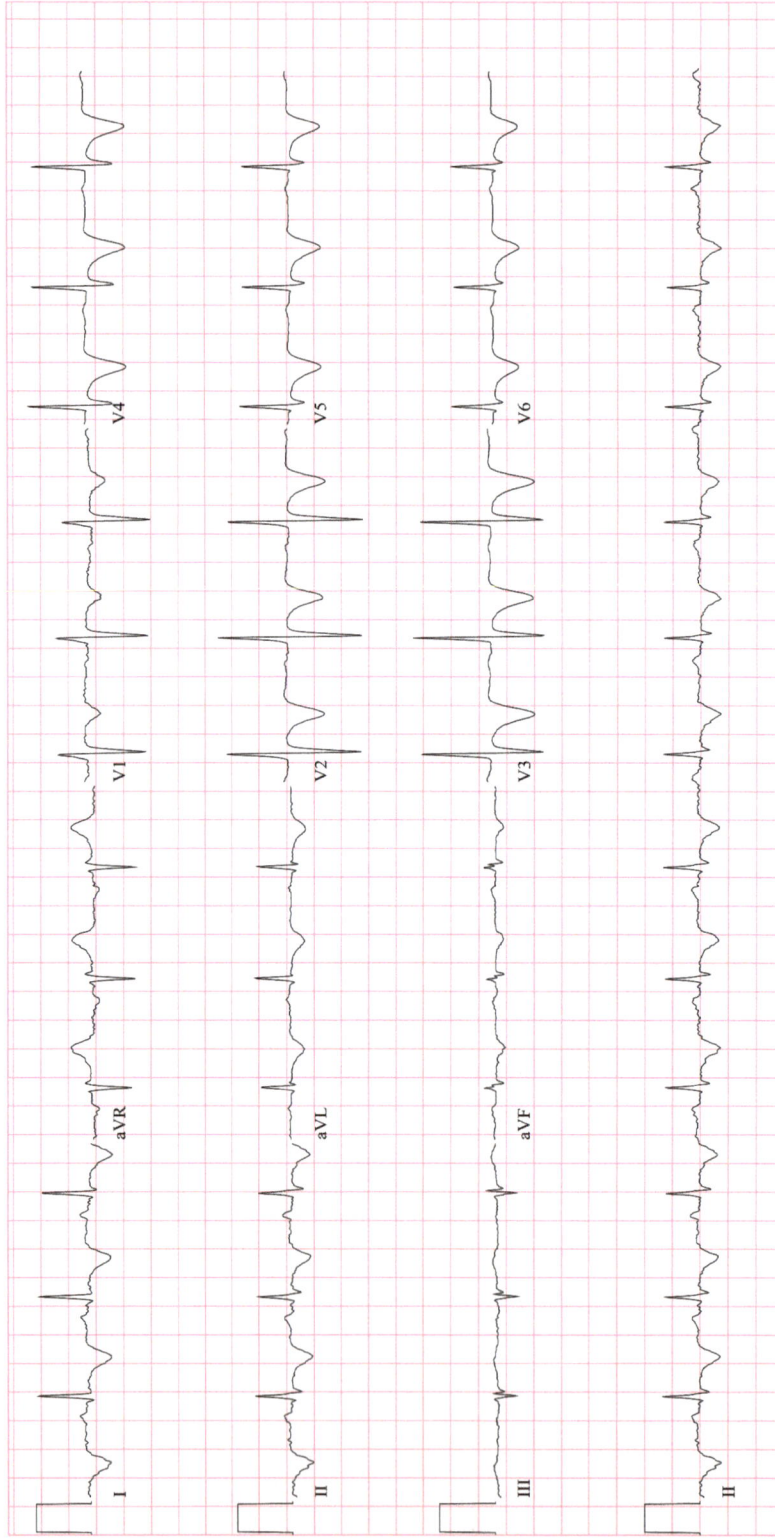

A 22-year-old male presents to the ER with retrosternal chest pain with dyspnea and diaphoresis for the past three weeks. He underwent cardiac stress test followed by coronary angiogram last week which revealed mild non-obstructive coronary artery disease. The patient continues to have chest pain. Urine drug screen is positive for cocaine use. Troponins are negative. What EKG changes could be seen?

DIAGNOSIS: Cocaine Associated Chest Pain (CACP) and Ischemic Changes on EKG

- EKG shows normal sinus rhythm at 80 bpm with diffuse T wave inversions in almost all leads. QTc is prolonged at 480 ms.

- Patients presenting with CACP are typically young, male, cigarette smokers with few other cardiac risk factors. CACP is often substernal and pressure-like and may be associated with dyspnea and diaphoresis.

- In absence of underlying atherosclerotic coronary artery disease, the EKG findings of prolonged QTc and T waves inversions are reversible as they disappear with abstinence from cocaine use. [1] [2]

- Clinicians should have a high index of suspicion for cocaine use in young patients presenting with chest pain, and should pursue a history of cocaine use with direct questioning in all patients, and with urine toxicology in select patients.

- For cocaine-using patients with chest pain, cessation of cocaine is the primary therapeutic goal. For patients who discontinue cocaine, the incidence of recurrent chest pain is reduced and MI and death are rare. Cardiac risk factors should be modified, especially cigarette smoking.

- Current treatment options for the management of cocaine-associated chest pain and MI include initial treatment with aspirin and benzodiazepines. Intravenous nitroglycerin, nitroprusside, or phentolamine may also be used for persistent hypertension. The practice of avoiding the use of beta blockers in patients with cocaine-associated cardiovascular complications began in 1985 when researchers theorized that b-adrenergic blockade, specifically with propranolol during cocaine use, leads to unopposed a-adrenergic stimulation[3]. They speculated that increased concentrations of norepinephrine induced by cocaine activate a1 adrenoreceptors causing arterial constriction, while beta inhibition hinders compensatory b2-mediated vasodilation. A 2012 update to the guidelines for UA/NSTEMI supports the use of nonselective agents such as labetalol (alpha and beta adrenergic blocker) as reasonable for patients after cocaine use with hypertension or sinus tachycardia, provided that the patient received a vasodilator agent. More recent data show that many clinicians now use beta-blockers in this setting.[4]

1   PATEL, MRUGESH, and UMANG SHAH. "Cocaine-Induced QTc Prolongation."*Consultant* 53, no. 5 (2013): 372.

2   Schwartz, Bryan G., Shereif Rezkalla, and Robert A. Kloner. "Cardiovascular effects of cocaine." *Circulation* 122, no. 24 (2010): 2558-2569.

3   Ramoska, Edward, and Alfred D. Sacchetti. "Propranolol-induced hypertension in treatment of cocaine intoxication." *Annals of emergency medicine* 14, no. 11 (1985): 1112-1113.

4   Gupta, Navdeep, Jeffrey B. Washam, Stavros E. Mountantonakis, Shuang Li, Matthew T. Roe, James A. de Lemos, and Rohit Arora. "Characteristics, management, and outcomes of cocaine-positive patients with acute coronary syndrome (from the National Cardiovascular Data Registry)." *The American journal of cardiology* 113, no. 5 (2014): 749-756.

EKG Case 70

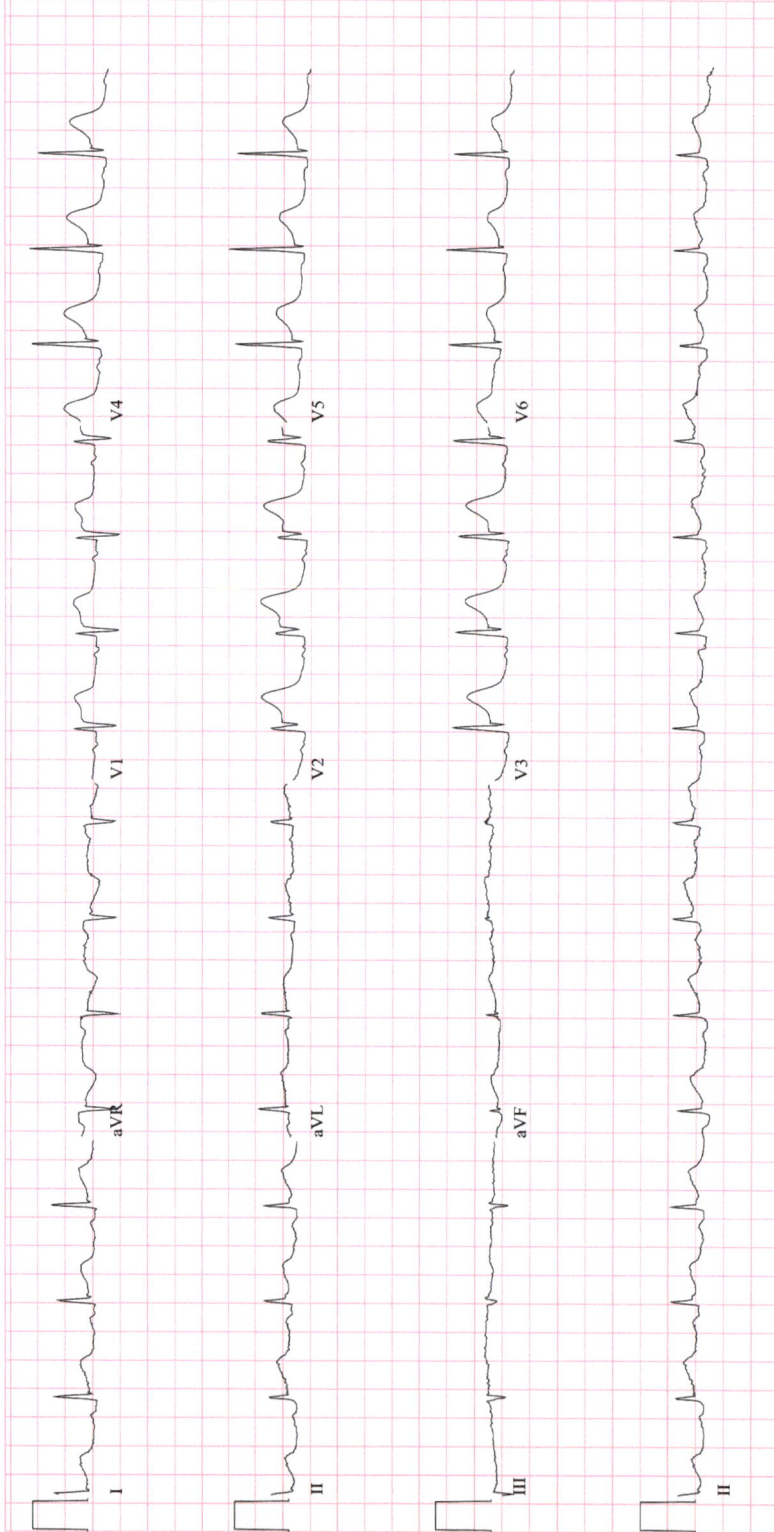

A 19-year-old male is brought to the ER with severe, sharp anterior chest pain which worsens with inspiration. Two weeks ago, he had flu-like symptoms which have now resolved. An EKG is obtained. What does it show?

DIAGNOSIS: Acute Pericarditis

- The EKG shows normal sinus rhythm with diffuse ST segment elevation in leads I, II, and V1-V6 with reciprocal ST depression in aVR. It also shows PR segment depression in the inferior leads.

- Inflammation of the pericardium (e.g, following viral infection) produces characteristic chest pain (anterior or retrosternal, pleuritic, worse when lying flat, relieved by sitting forward), tachycardia, and dyspnea. There may be an associated pericardial friction rub on auscultation or evidence of a pericardial effusion by echocardiography.

- Widespread ST segment changes occur due to involvement of the underlying epicardium (i.e, myopericarditis). Sinus tachycardia is also common in acute pericarditis due to pain and/or pericardial effusion.

Some of the causes of pericarditis include:

- Infectious – mainly viral (e.g, coxsackie virus); occasionally bacterial, fungal, TB.
- Immunological – SLE, rheumatic fever
- Uremia
- Post-myocardial infarction / Dressler's syndrome
- Trauma
- Following cardiac surgery (post-pericardiotomy syndrome)
- Paraneoplastic syndromes
- Drug-induced (e.g, isoniazid, cyclosporine)
- Post-radiotherapy

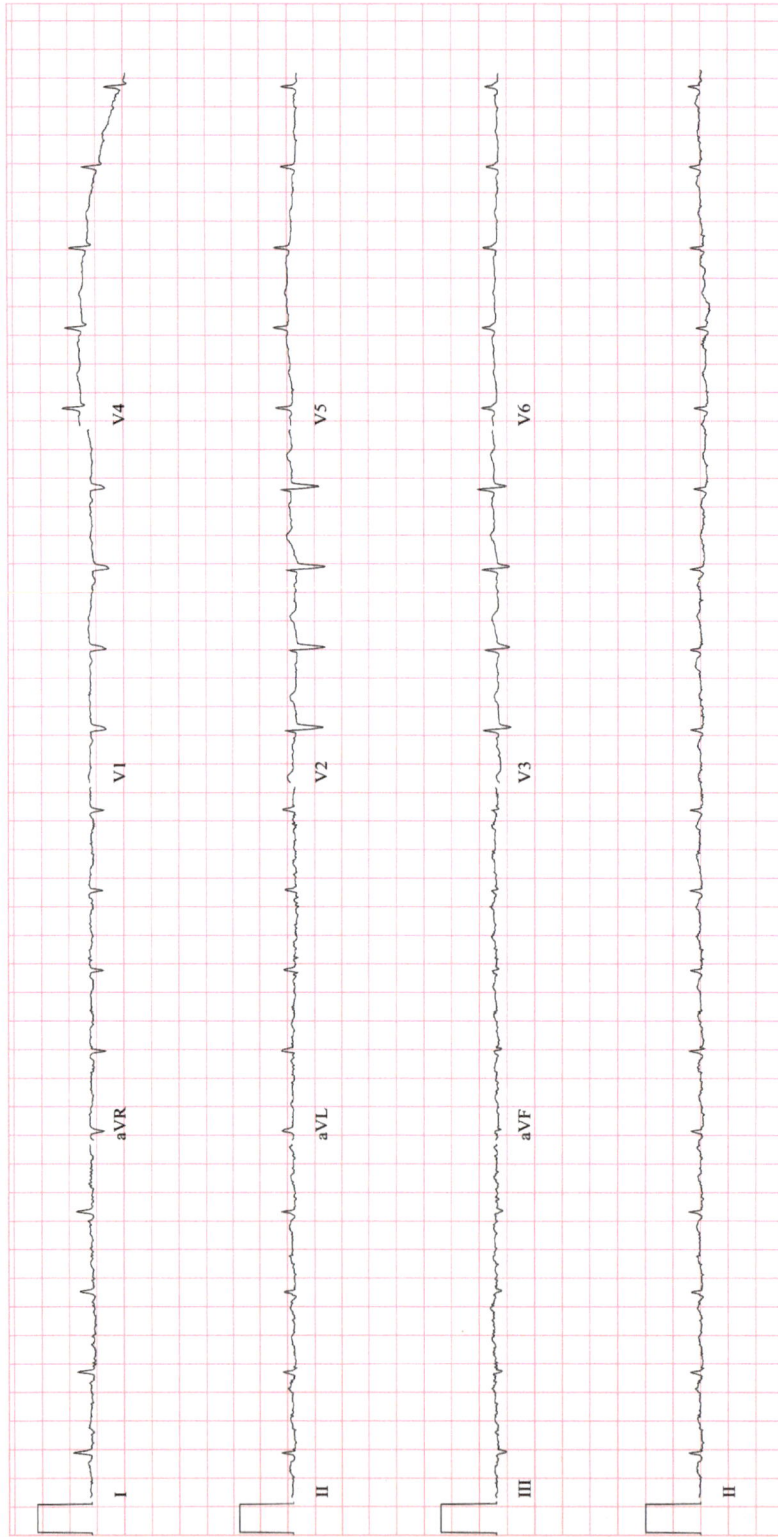

A 65-year-old obese woman with a history of constrictive pericarditis is admitted to the ICU with sepsis. An EKG is obtained. What does it show?

DIAGNOSIS: Low Voltage QRS Complex EKG

This EKG shows sinus tachycardia at about 115 bpm. The QRS voltages are low in the limb leads (5 mm or less) and relatively low in the precordial leads (10 mm or less). Non-specific ST-T changes are present.

The QRS is said to be low voltage when:

- The amplitudes of all the QRS complexes in the limb leads are < 5 mm; or
- The amplitudes of all the QRS complexes in the precordial leads are < 10 mm

Specific causes of low voltage EKG include:

- Pericardial effusion, especially with tamponade; usually has a triad of low voltage QRS complexes, sinus tachycardia, and electrical alternans.
- Pleural effusion.
- Obesity.
- Emphysema: low voltage and R wave progression are sometimes accompanied by rightward QRS and P wave deviation, as well as peaked P waves.
- Pneumothorax.
- Constrictive pericarditidis.
- Previous massive MI.
- End-stage dilated cardiomyopathy.
- Infiltrative myocardial diseases, i.e, restrictive cardiomyopathy due to amyloidosis, sarcoidosis, haemochromatosis.
- Scleroderma.
- Myxoedema, usually with bradycardia.
- Anasarca.

EKG Case 72

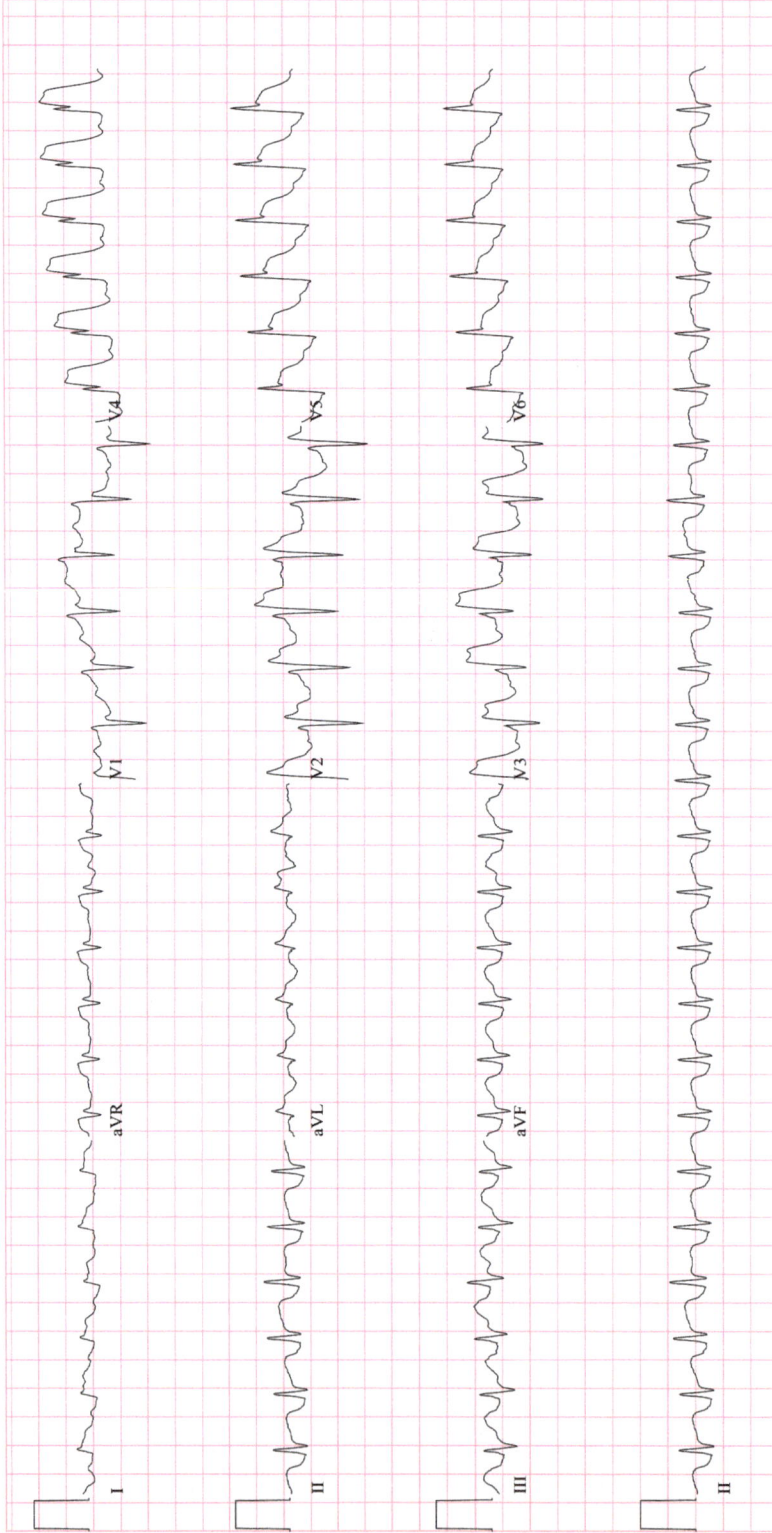

A 45-year-old male presents to the emergency room with the chief complaint of exertional dyspnea. He reports flu-like symptoms a week ago. Laboratory work reveals leukocytosis, elevated C-reactive protien, elevated creatinine kinase MB, and cardiac troponin I. An EKG is shown. What does it show?

DIAGNOSIS: Acute Myopericarditis

This EKG shows normal sinus rhythm at 150 bpm with ST segment elevation in V2- V6, I, II, III, aVF, and aVL - Q waves in V1-V3 consistent with diagnosis of acute myopericarditis.

- Myocardial inflammation in the absence of ischemia.

- Often associated with pericarditis, termed myopericarditis.

- Usually a self-limiting condition without serious long-term complications.

- In the acute setting can cause arrhythmias, cardiac failure, cardiogenic shock, and death.

- May result in delayed dilated cardiomyopathy.

Causes of Myocarditis include: *Viral* – including coxsackie B virus, HIV, influenza A, HSV, adenovirus. *Bacteria* – including mycoplasma, rickettsia, leptospira. *Immune mediated* – including sarcoidosis, scleroderma, SLE, Kawasaki's disease. *Drugs / toxins* – including clozapine, amphetamines etc.

EKG changes can be variable and include [1]

The EKG findings in patients with myocarditis vary from nonspecific T-wave and ST-segment changes to ST-segment elevation mimicking an acute myocardial infarction (as above). Also, atrial or ventricular conduction delays as well as supraventricular and ventricular arrhythmias can occur in patients with inflammatory heart disease. The presence of Q waves or a new left bundle branch block are associated with higher rates of cardiac death or need for heart transplantation. Recently, the prognostic role of EKG parameters was investigated in patients with suspected myocarditis[2]. The EKG recorded at the time of endomyocardial biopsy was predictive of cardiac outcome on long-term follow-up. Poor prognostic predictors include QTc prolongation > 440 ms, an abnormal QRS axis, and ventricular ectopic beats. A prolonged QRS duration of ≥ 120 ms was found to be an independent predictor for cardiac death or heart transplantation. Supportive care is the first line of treatment. A minority of patients who present with fulminant or acute myocarditis will require an intensive level of hemodynamic support and aggressive pharmacological intervention, including vasopressors and positive inotropic agents, similar to other patients with advanced heart failure due to profound left ventricular dysfunction.[3]

1   Kindermann, Ingrid, Christine Barth, Felix Mahfoud, Christian Ukena, Matthias Lenski, Ali Yilmaz, Karin Klingel et al. "Update on myocarditis." *Journal of the American College of Cardiology* 59, no. 9 (2012): 779-792

2   Ukena C., Mahfoud F., Kindermann I., Kandolf R., Kindermann M., Bohm M.; Prognostic electrocardiographic parameters in patients with suspected myocarditis. *Eur J Heart Fail.* 13 2011:398-405

3   Magnani, Jared W., and G. William Dec. "Myocarditis current trends in diagnosis and treatment." *Circulation* 113, no. 6 (2006): 876-890.

EKG Case 73

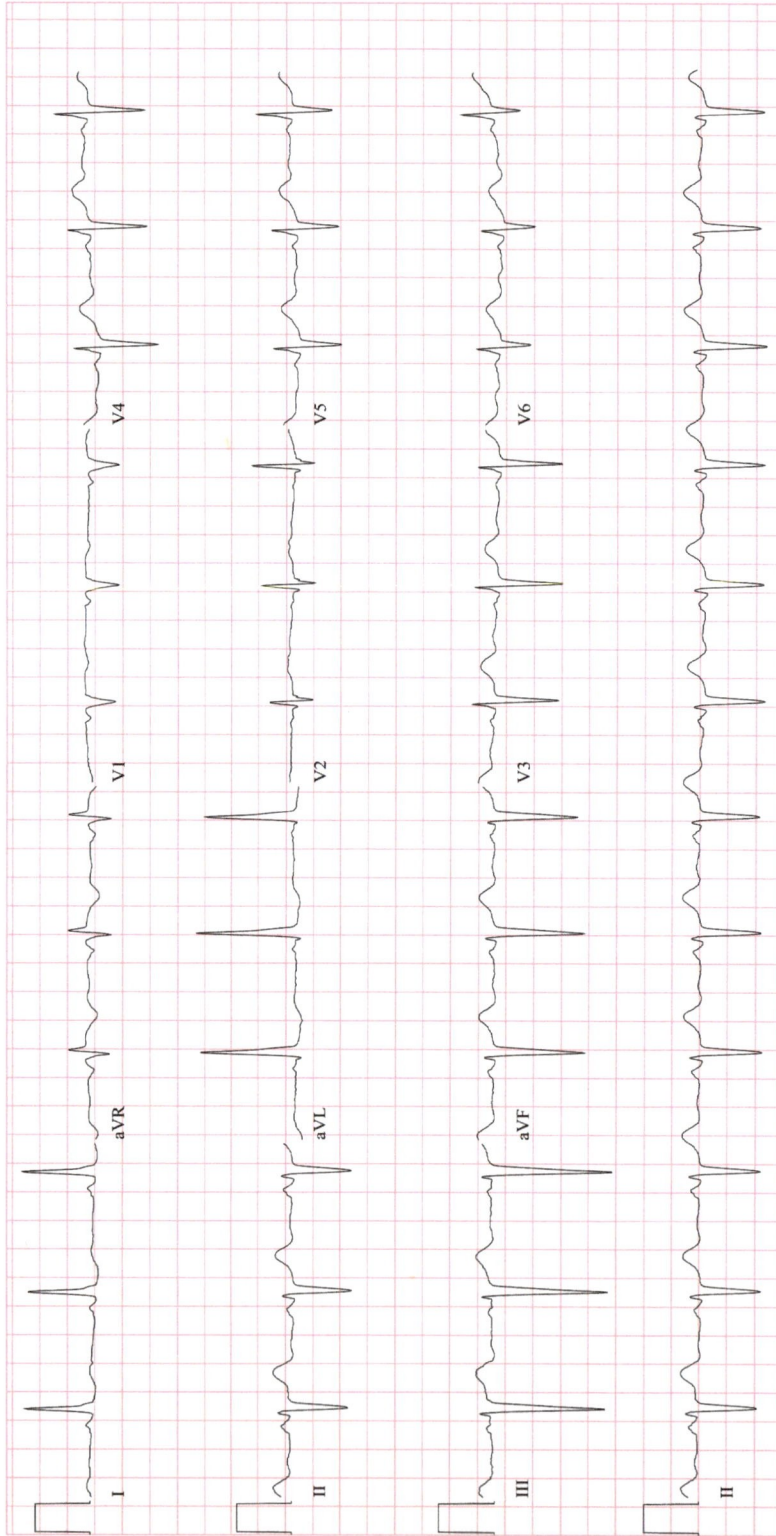

A 75-year-old male with history of end-stage renal disease is seen in the office for progressive shortness of breath. EKG is shown. What does it indicate?

DIAGNOSIS: Left Ventricular Hypertrophy (LVH) - Cornell Voltage Criteria.

The EKG demonstrates normal sinus rhythm with left anterior fascicular block, left axis deviation, and left ventricular hypertrophy by voltage criteria

The Cornell-criterion for LVH: (sensitivity = 22%, specificity = 95%) has different values in men and women:

- Amplitude of R in aVL, and S in V3 > 28 mm in men.
- Amplitude of R in aVL, and S in V3 > 20 mm in women.

Modified Cornell Criteria:

- Amplitude of R wave in lead I + S wave in lead III > 25 mm.
- Amplitude of R wave in aVL ≥ 11 mm *or*, if left axis deviation, R wave in aVL ≥ 13 mm *plus* S in III ≥ 15 mm.

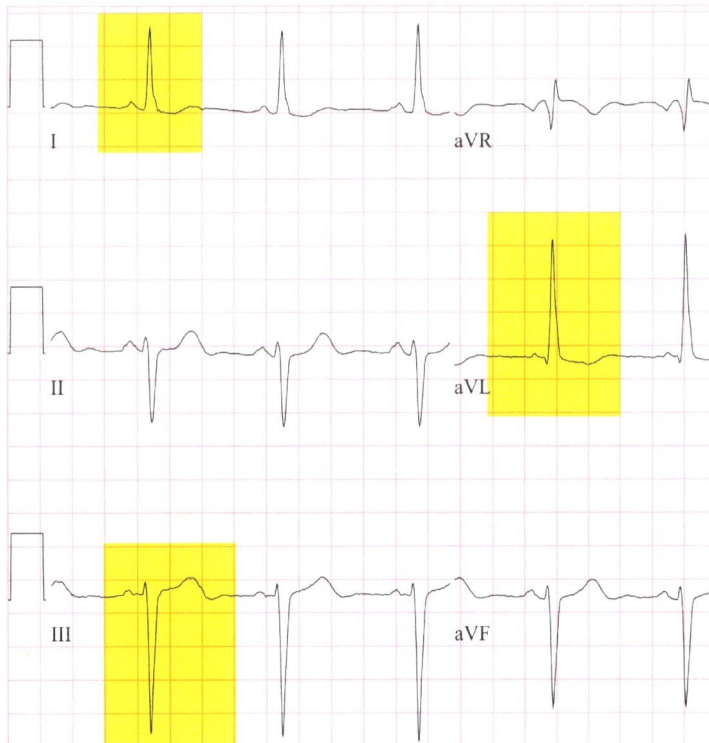

EKG Case 74

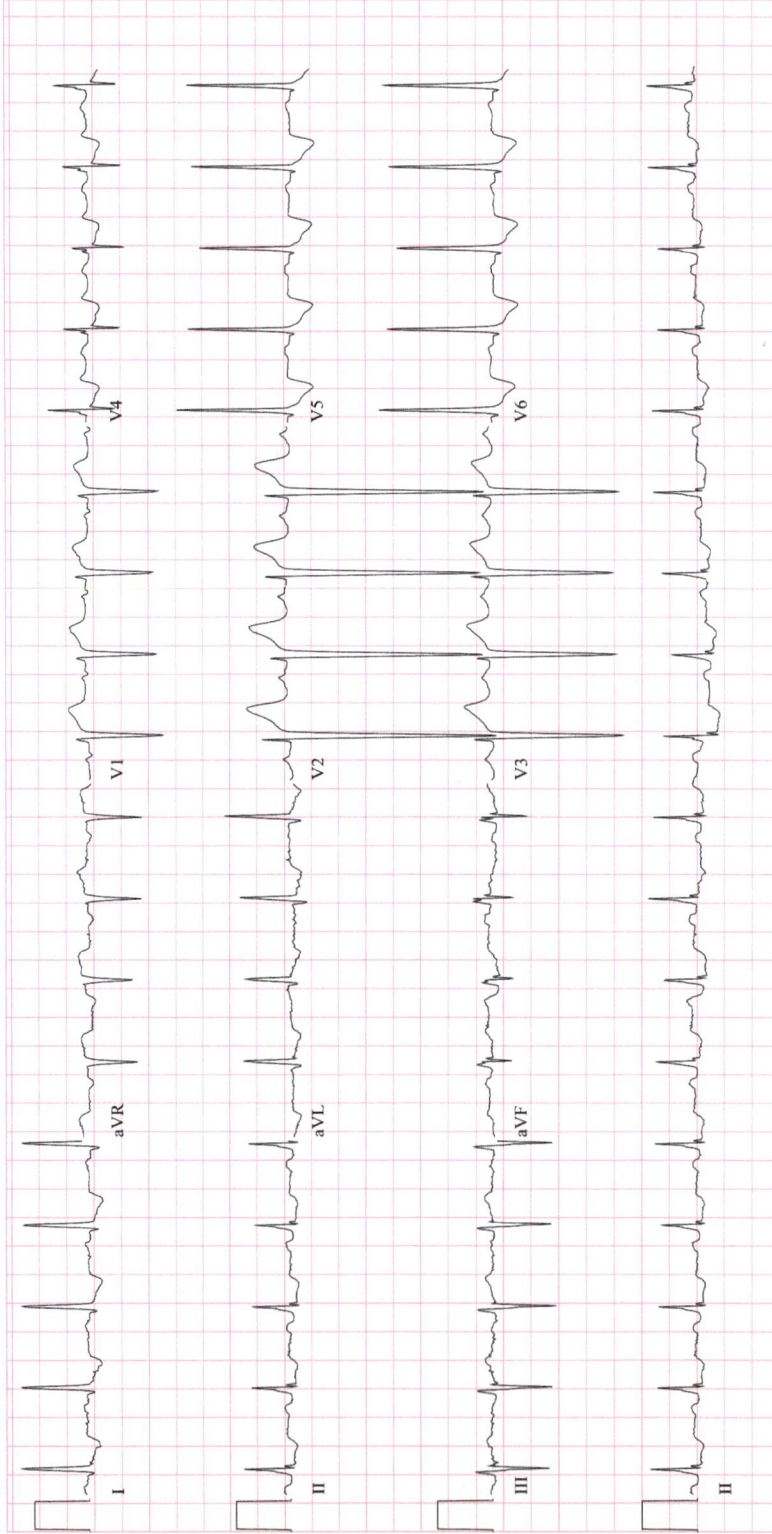

55-year-old male with a history of aortic stenosis presents to clinic with shortness of breath. He denies any chest pain. What does the EKG show?

DIAGNOSIS: Left Ventricular Hypertrophy (LVH) - Sokolov-Lyon Criteria

EKG shows sinus tachycardia with left ventricular hypertrophy and T wave inversions in lateral leads.

- Left ventricular hypertrophy can be diagnosed with EKG with good specificity. As the myocardium of left ventricle develops hypertrophy, there is a larger mass of myocardium for electrical activation, therefore the amplitude of QRS complex (ventricular depolarization) increases. This is especially true for leads V1- V6.

- Left ventricular strain pattern: These repolarization abnormalities can often mimic ischemic changes, including ST segment depression and T wave inversions in opposite direction to QRS complex — discordant change. This is known as strain pattern.

- There are numerous criteria for diagnosing LVH including Sokolow-Lyon criteria, Cornell voltage criteria, and Romhilt-Estes point score system. However, the most commonly used is the Sokolov-Lyon criteria, i.e, the amplitude of the S wave in lead V_1 or V_2 plus the amplitude of the R wave in V_5 or V_6 is > 35 mm.

- This EKG demonstrates left ventricular hypertrophy with strain pattern. S wave in V2 plus R wave in V6 > 35 mm, accompanied by T wave inversions in lateral leads.

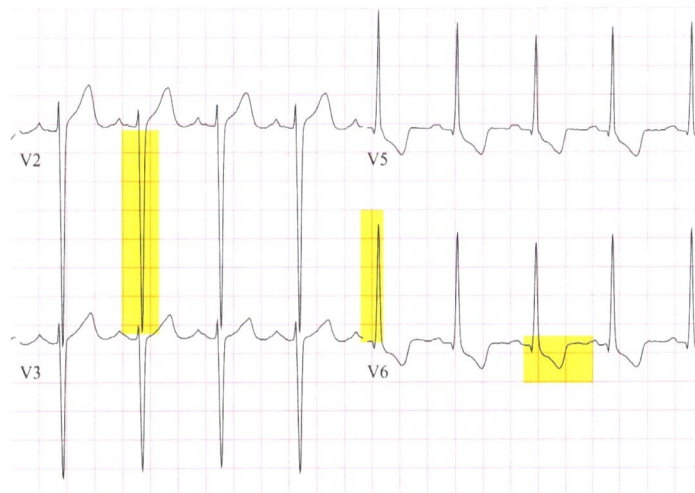

EKG Case 75

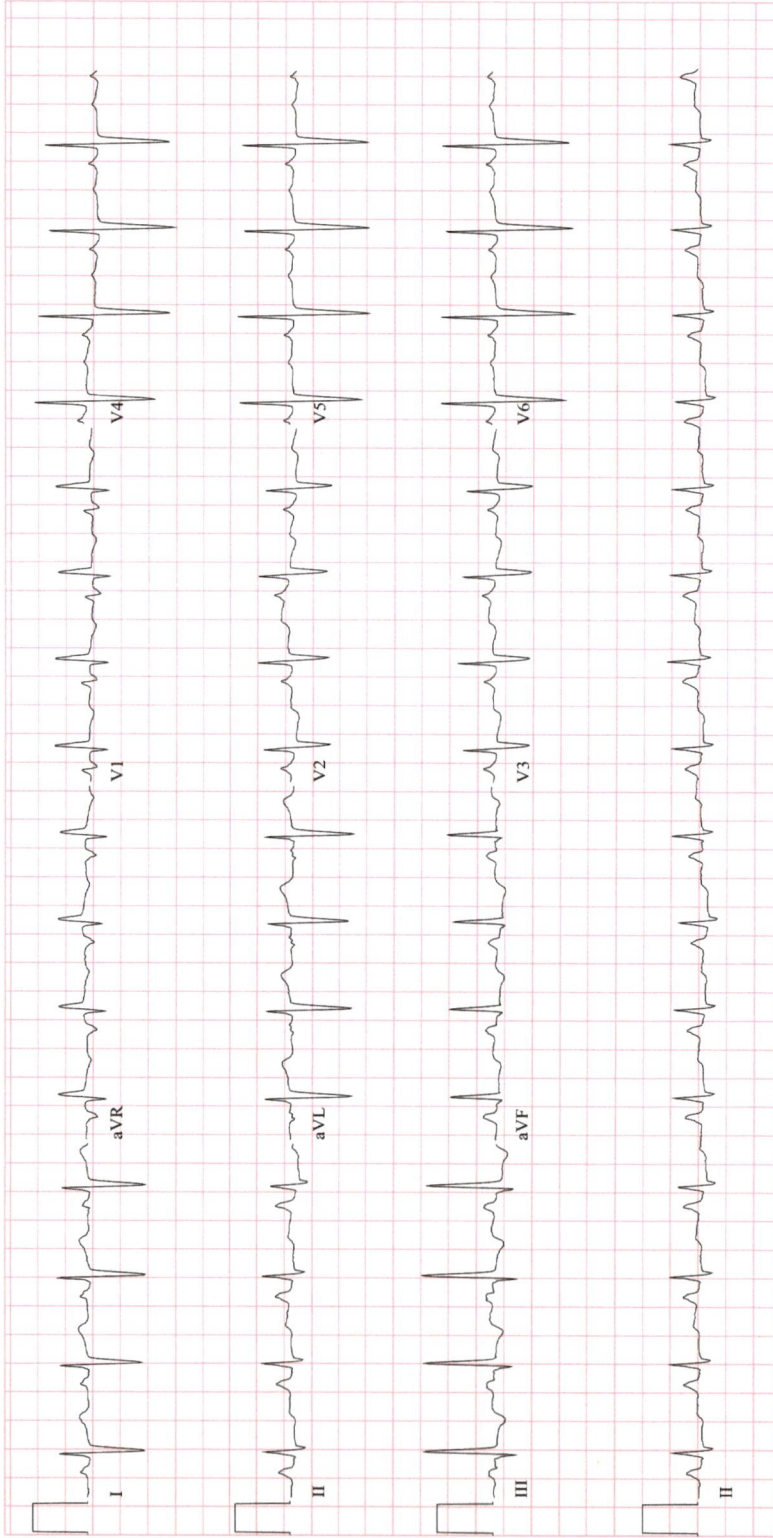

A 65-year-old female with a history of chronic deep vein thrombosis and recurrent pulmonary embolism presents with shortness of breath. An EKG is shown. What does it reveal?

DIAGNOSIS: Right Ventricular Hypertrophy (RVH) with RV Strain Pattern

EKG shows normal sinus rhythm, right axis deviation, RVH with strain pattern (see definition below), biatrial abnormality, and incomplete right bundle branch block.

Diagnostic criteria

- Right axis deviation.
- Dominant R wave in V1 (> 7 mm tall or R/S ratio > 1).
- Dominant S wave in V5 or V6 (> 7 mm deep or R/S ratio < 1).
- QRS duration < 120ms (i.e, changes not due to RBBB).

Supporting criteria

- Right atrial enlargement (P pulmonale) = > 2.5 mm in the inferior leads (II, III, and AVF) and > 1.5 mm in V1 and V2.
- Right ventricular strain pattern = ST depression / T wave inversion in the right precordial (V1-V4) and inferior (II, III, aVF) leads.
- S1,S2,S3 pattern = far right axis deviation with dominant S waves in leads I, II, and III.
- Deep S waves in the lateral leads (I, aVL, V5 - V6).

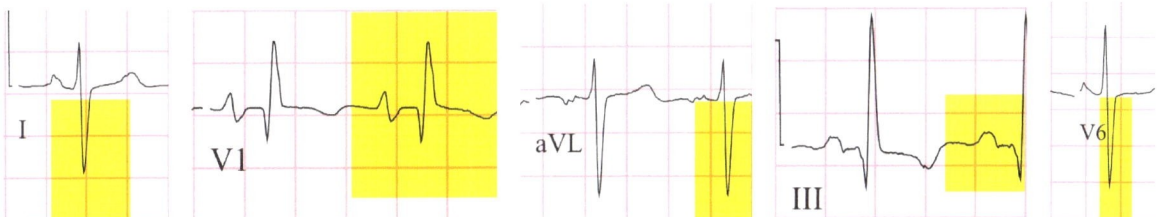

EKG Case 76

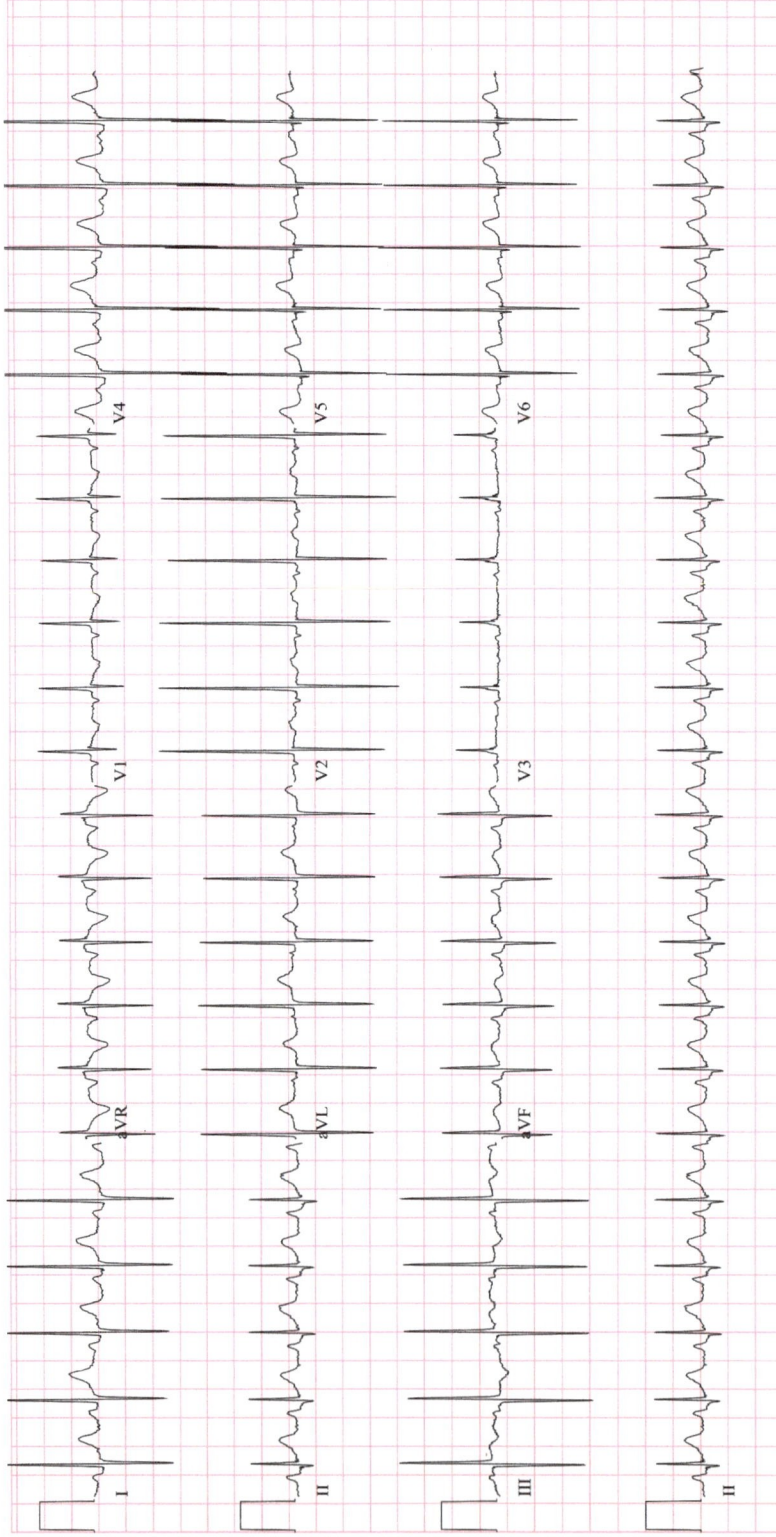

An 11 month old infant is evaluated for a heart murmur. His EKG is shown and an echocardiogram is ordered. What does the EKG show?

DIAGNOSIS: Biventricular Hypertrophy by Katz–Wachtel Sign / Phenomenon in Patient with Large Left to Right VSD Shunt.

- The EKG has a low sensitivity for the diagnosis of biventricular hypertrophy (BVH), as the opposing left and right ventricular forces tend to cancel each other out.

- There may be signs of both LVH and RVH on the same EKG, e.g, positive diagnostic criteria for LVH with some additional features suggestive of RVH.

- The *Katz Wachtel phenomenon* – large biphasic QRS complexes in V2- V5. This is the classic EKG pattern of BVH, most commonly seen in children with ventriculo-septal defect (VSD).

- This EKG shows sinus tachycardia with tall biphasic QRS complexes in multiple leads. (Tall R waves + deep S waves) in V2 - V5. It also demonstrates criteria for both LVH and RVH.

    ◊ LVH criteria: (S V2 + R V5 > 35 mm, R aVL > 11 mm).

    ◊ RVH criteria: Tall R waves in V1 with S waves in V5 - V6.

EKG Case 77

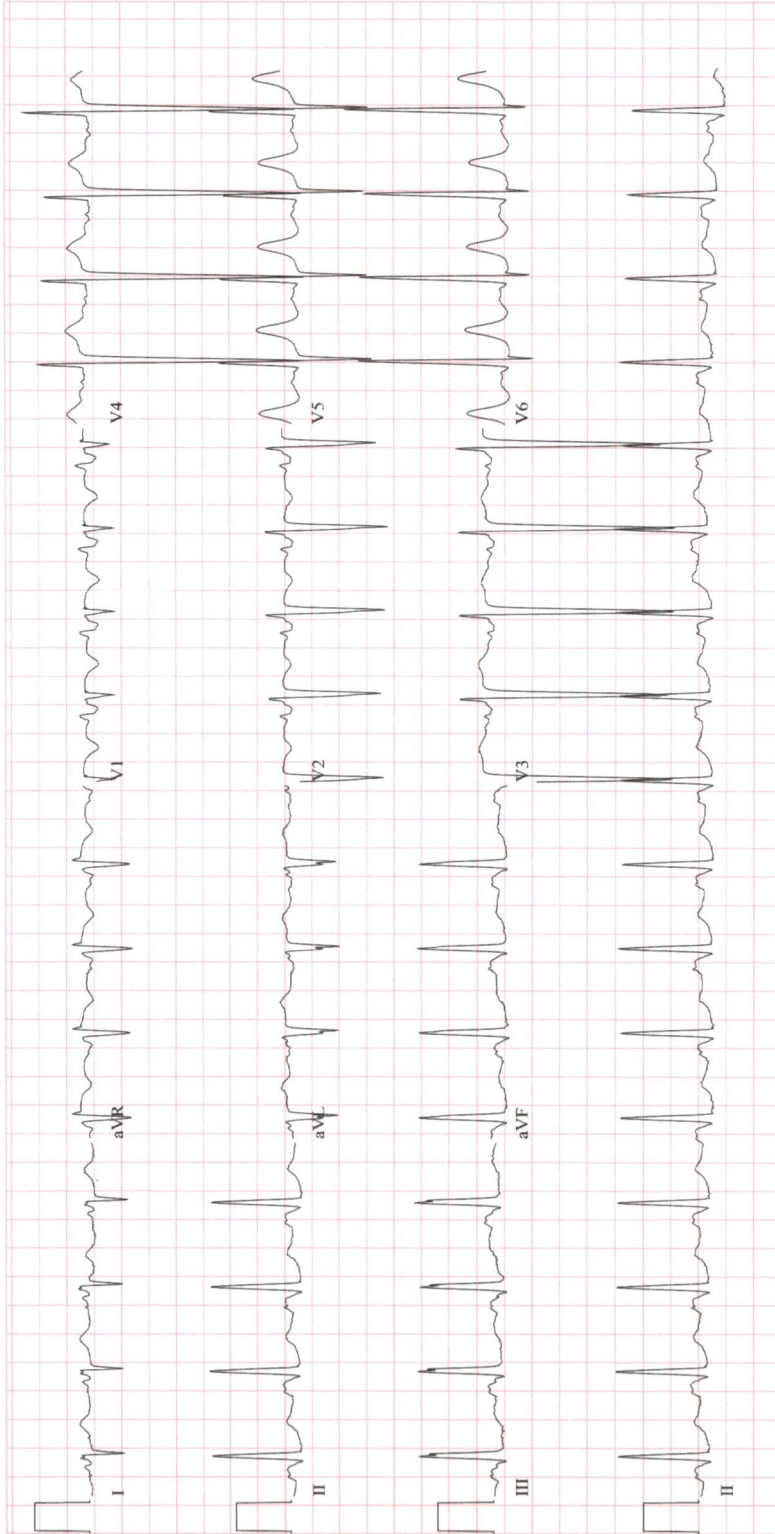

An 85-year-old female with a history of COPD, hypertension, sleep apnea, and pulmonary embolism is brought to the ER with progressive shortness of breath. An EKG is obtained. What does it show?

DIAGNOSIS: Cor Pulmonale - Biatrial and Biventricular Hypertrophy

- This EKG shows evidence of right ventricular (RV) overload with sinus tachycardia, right axis deviation, left posterior fascicular block, incomplete right bundle branch block with RSR' (or qR) in V1 and S waves in lateral chest leads. Absent R waves in the right precordial leads (SV1-SV2-SV3 pattern).

- Besides right ventricle hypertrophy, there is also evidence of left ventricle hypertrophy with deep S wave in V3 and tall R wave in V5.

- The EKG also shows biatrial hypertrophy. Right atrial enlargement produces a peaked P wave (*P pulmonale*) > 1.5 mm in V1 and V2.

- Left atrial enlargement, diagnostic criteria are as follows: in lead II, bifid P wave with > 40 ms between the two peaks. Total P wave duration > 110 ms. In V1, biphasic P wave with terminal negative portion > 40 ms duration and biphasic P wave with terminal negative portion > 1mm deep.

- This patient's history of underlying COPD, pulmonary hypertension, poorly controlled hypertension, sleep apnea, and thromboembolic disease is compatible with biatrial and biventricular enlargement.

EKG Case 78

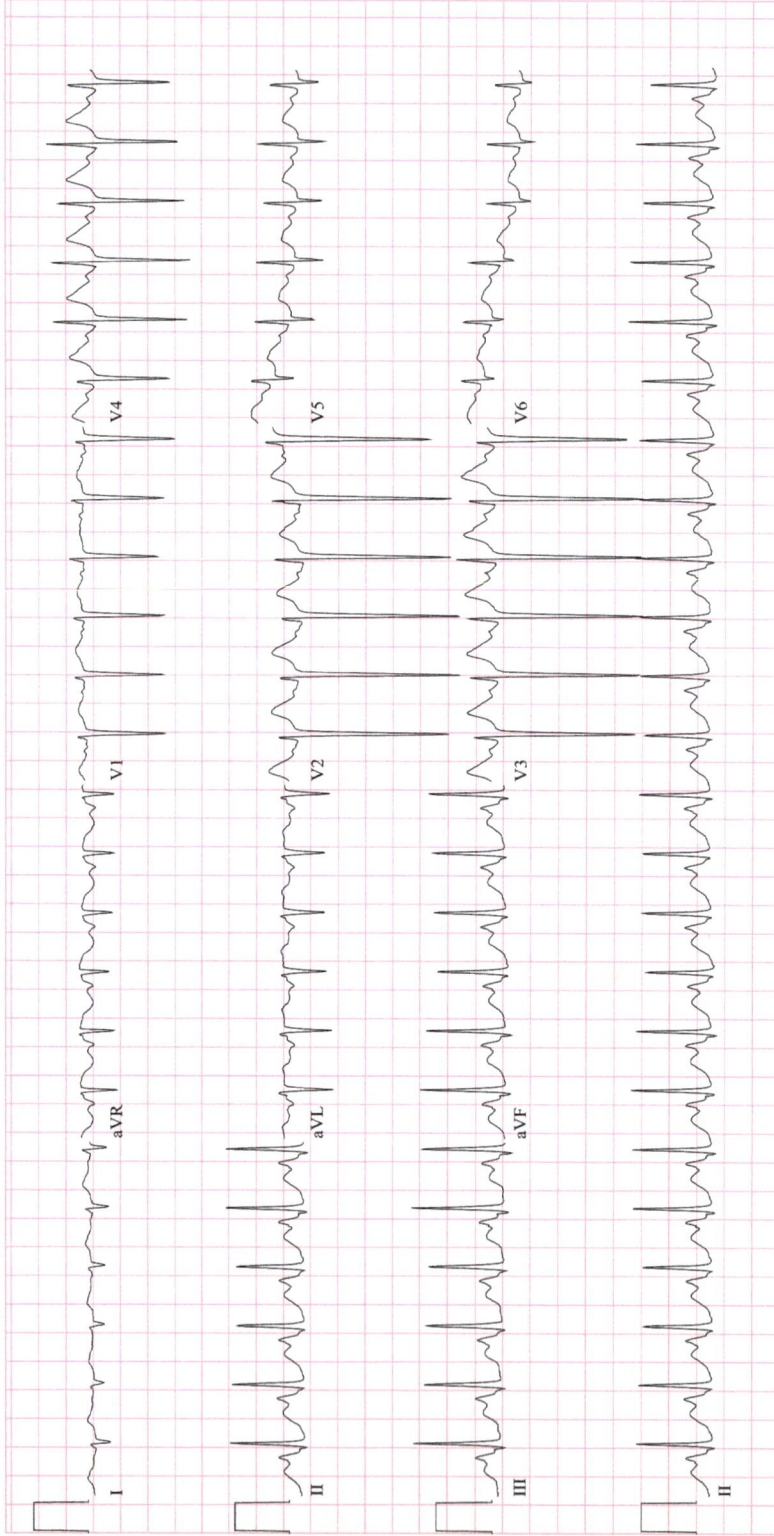

A 42-year-old female with a history of Hodgkin's disease status post radiation presents with severe shortness of breath. An EKG is obtained. What does it show?

DIAGNOSIS: Pulmonary Fibrosis with Cor Pulmonale

- The patient developed pulmonary fibrosis following radiotherapy for Hodgkin's disease, resulting in cor pulmonale.

- The EKG shows sinus tachycardia at 130 bpm with findings suggestive of right heart overload.

- Rightward QRS axis. Dominant R wave in leads III and aVF, and dominant S wave in leads I and aVL.

- Right atrial overload (*P Pulmonale*); P waves in leads II, III, and aVF are tall (> 2.5 mm), narrow ,and peaked.

- Cor pulmonale is defined as an alteration in the structure and function of the right ventricle caused by a primary disorder of the respiratory system. Pulmonary hypertension is the common link between lung dysfunction and the heart in cor pulmonale. In chronic cor pulmonale, RV hypertrophy (RVH) generally predominates (not seen in this EKG). In acute cor pulmonale, right ventricular dilatation mainly occurs. Chronic obstructive pulmonary disorder is the most common cause of cor pulmonale, but also some connective tissue disorders with pulmonary involvement may result in pulmonary hypertension and cor pulmonale. Other causes include: pulmonary hypertension, ARDS, increased blood viscosity secondary to blood disorders (e.g, polycythemia vera, sickle cell disease, macroglobulinemia), Idiopathic primary pulmonary hypertension, etc.

EKG Case 79

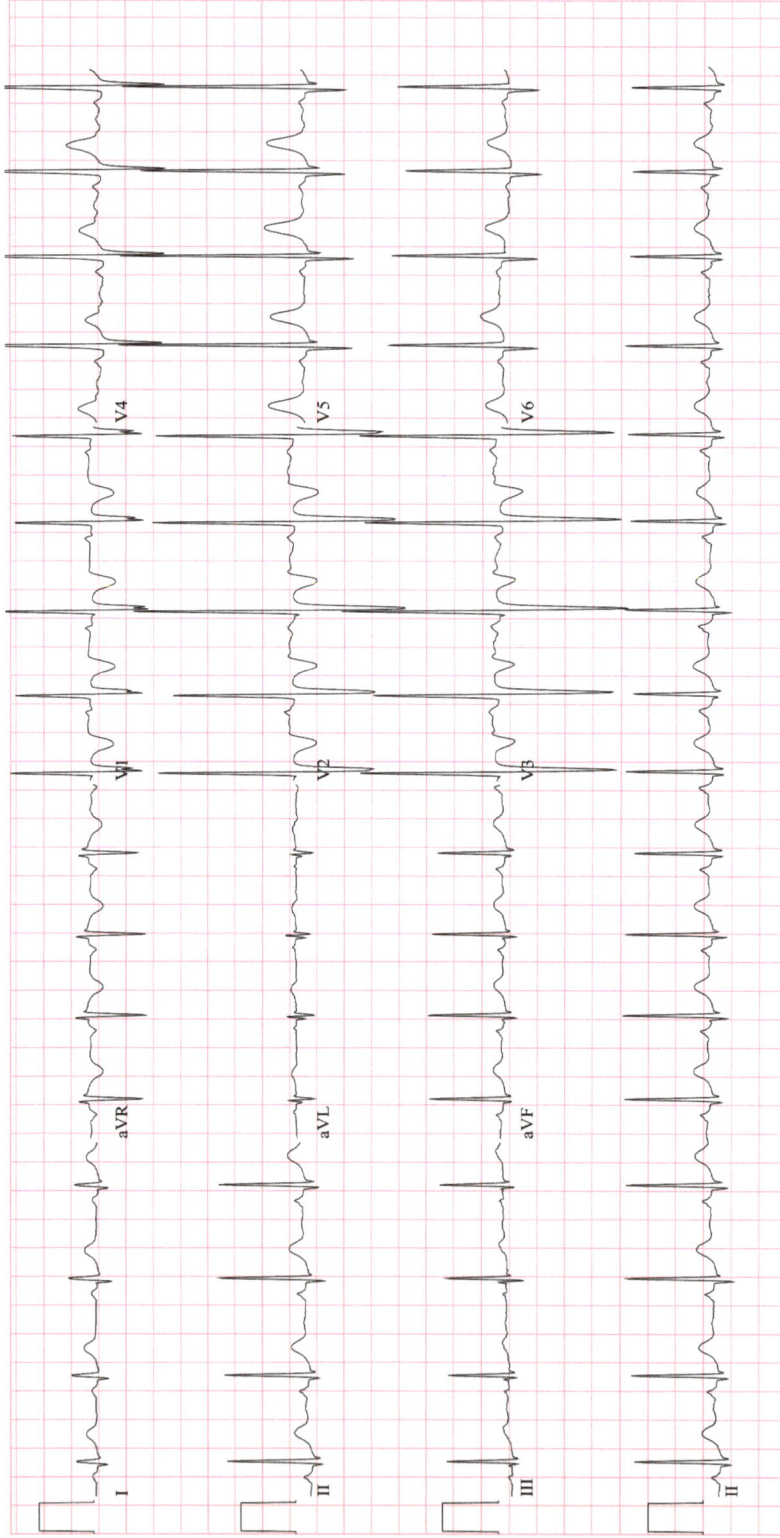

An 18-year-old male has a syncopal episode while playing football. He is brought to the emergency department and is asymptomatic upon arrival. Physical exam reveals systolic murmur at apex. An EKG is obtained. What does it show?

DIAGNOSIS: Hypertrophic Cardiomyopathy (HCM)

This EKG show sinus tachycardia and high left ventricular voltage with repolarizating T wave abnormalities. The hallmark of this EKG is presence of Q waves in lateral leads (V5, V6, I, and AVL)

- EKG findings in HCM are present in 85% of patients with HCM and include the following:

- Deep, narrow Q waves in inferior and lateral leads (described as dagger Q waves). These may mimic prior myocardial infarction, although the Q wave morphology is different since infarction Q waves are typically > 40 ms duration, while septal Q waves in HCM are < 40 ms. Lateral Q waves are more common than inferior Q waves in HCM.

- High left ventricular voltage and left atrial enlargement.

- Tall R waves in V1 (non-specific, mimics posterior MI).

- In general, the commonly used QRS voltage criteria for LVH apply to adults older than 35 years. Standards for patients aged 16-35 years are not as well-established, and the diagnosis of LVH based on voltage alone has a low specificity in this age group. The diagnosis of LVH in highly trained athletes is especially problematic.

- Comprehensive transthoracic echocardiography (TTE) with two-dimensional, color Doppler, spectral Doppler, and tissue Doppler imaging should be performed in all patients when considering a diagnosis of HCM.

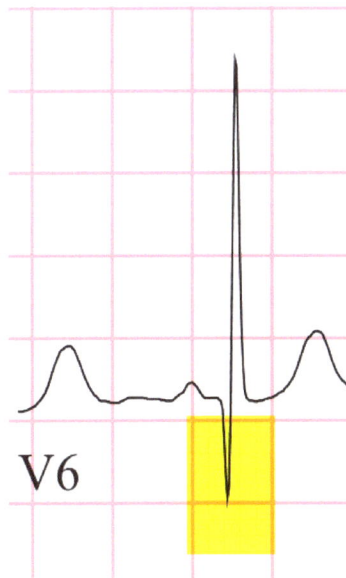

EKG Case 80

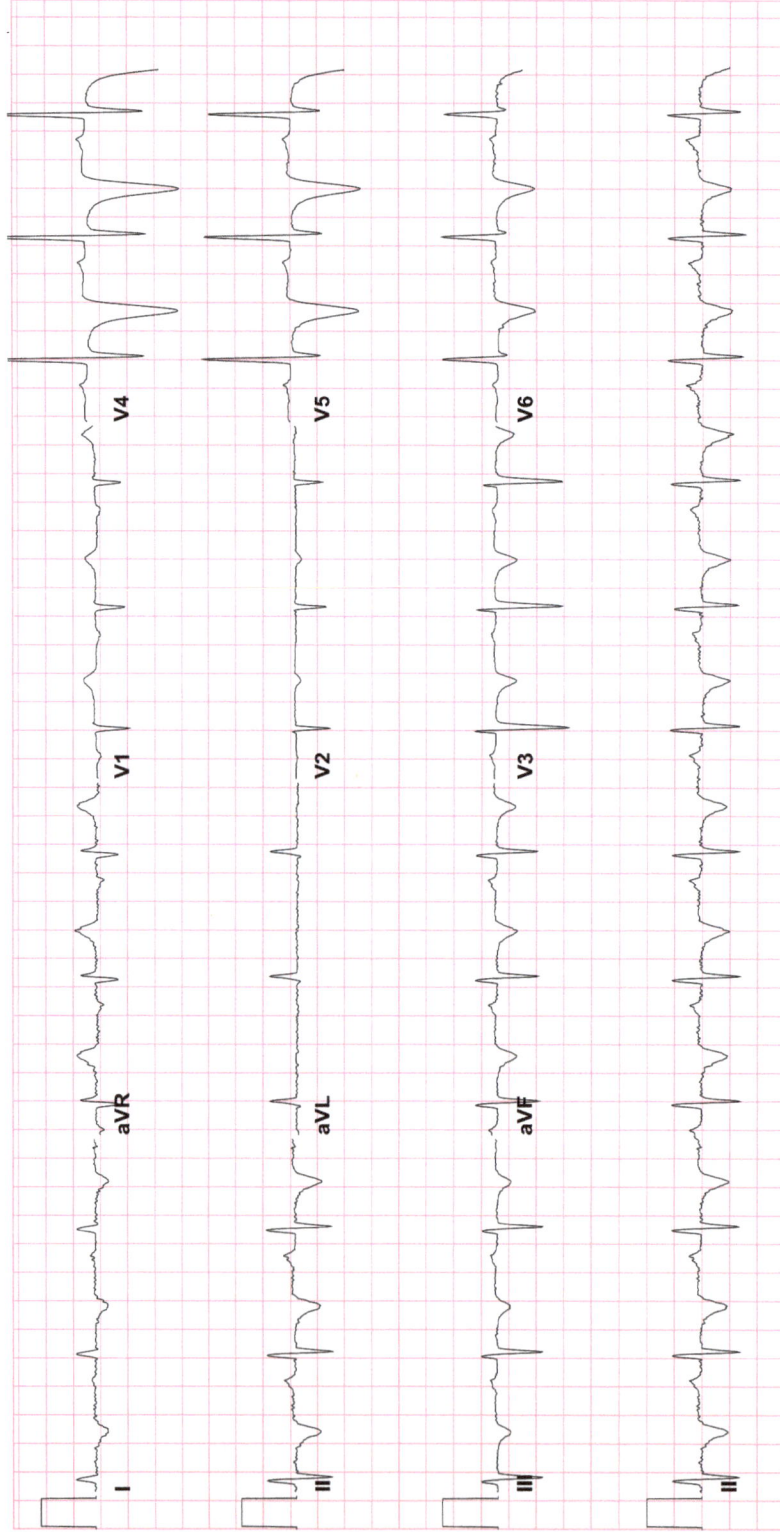

A 54-year-old male with a history of hypertension is admitted for hip fracture after sustaining a fall. An EKG obtained for a pre-op workup is shown above. Recent cardiac catheterization was negative for any occlusive disease. Previous EKGs from six months ago show similar pattern. Patient denies chest pain and cardiac troponin is negative. What does the EKG show?

DIAGNOSIS: Apical Hypertrophic Cardiomyopathy (AHCM)

EKG shows normal sinus rhythm, first degree AV block with diffusely inverted T waves in the V2, V3, V4, V5, V6, I, II, III, and aVF.

Apical hypertrophic cardiomyopathy (AHCM) is a rare form of hypertrophic cardiomyopathy (HCM) which usually involves the apex of the left ventricle and rarely involves the right ventricular apex or both.

About 54% of patients with AHCM are symptomatic and the most common presenting symptom is chest pain, followed by palpitations, dyspnea, and syncope. AHCM may also manifest as morbid events such as atrial fibrillation, myocardial infarction, embolic events, ventricular fibrillation, and congestive heart failure.[1]

The most frequent EKG findings are negative T waves in the precordial leads which are found in 93% of patients, followed by LV hypertrophy in 65% of patients. Negative T waves with a depth > 10 mm are found in 47% of patients with AHCM.

The diagnostic criteria for AHCM includes demonstration of asymmetric LV hypertrophy, confined predominantly to the LV apex, with an apical wall thickness ≥ 15 mm and a ratio of maximal apical to posterior wall thickness ≥ 1.5 mm, based on an echocardiogram or magnetic resonance imaging (MRI).

On imaging, AHCM may mimic other conditions, including apical cardiac tumors, LV apical thrombus, isolated ventricular non-compaction, and endomyocardial fibrosis (EMF). Chest pain in a patient with AHCM can be mistaken for ischemia from coronary artery disease. Frequently, these patients undergo a nuclear scan for abnormal EKG.

The prognosis of AHCM is usually benign.[2]

---

1   Eriksson MJ, Sonnenberg B, Woo A, Rakowski P, Parker TG, Wigle ED, Rakowski H. Long-term outcome in patients with apical hypertrophic cardiomyopathy. J Am Coll Cardiol. 2002;39:638–645.

2   Yusuf, Syed Wamique, Jaya D. Bathina, Jose Banchs, Elie N. Mouhayar, and Iyad N. Daher. "Apical hypertrophic cardiomyopathy." World journal of cardiology 3, no. 7 (2011): 256

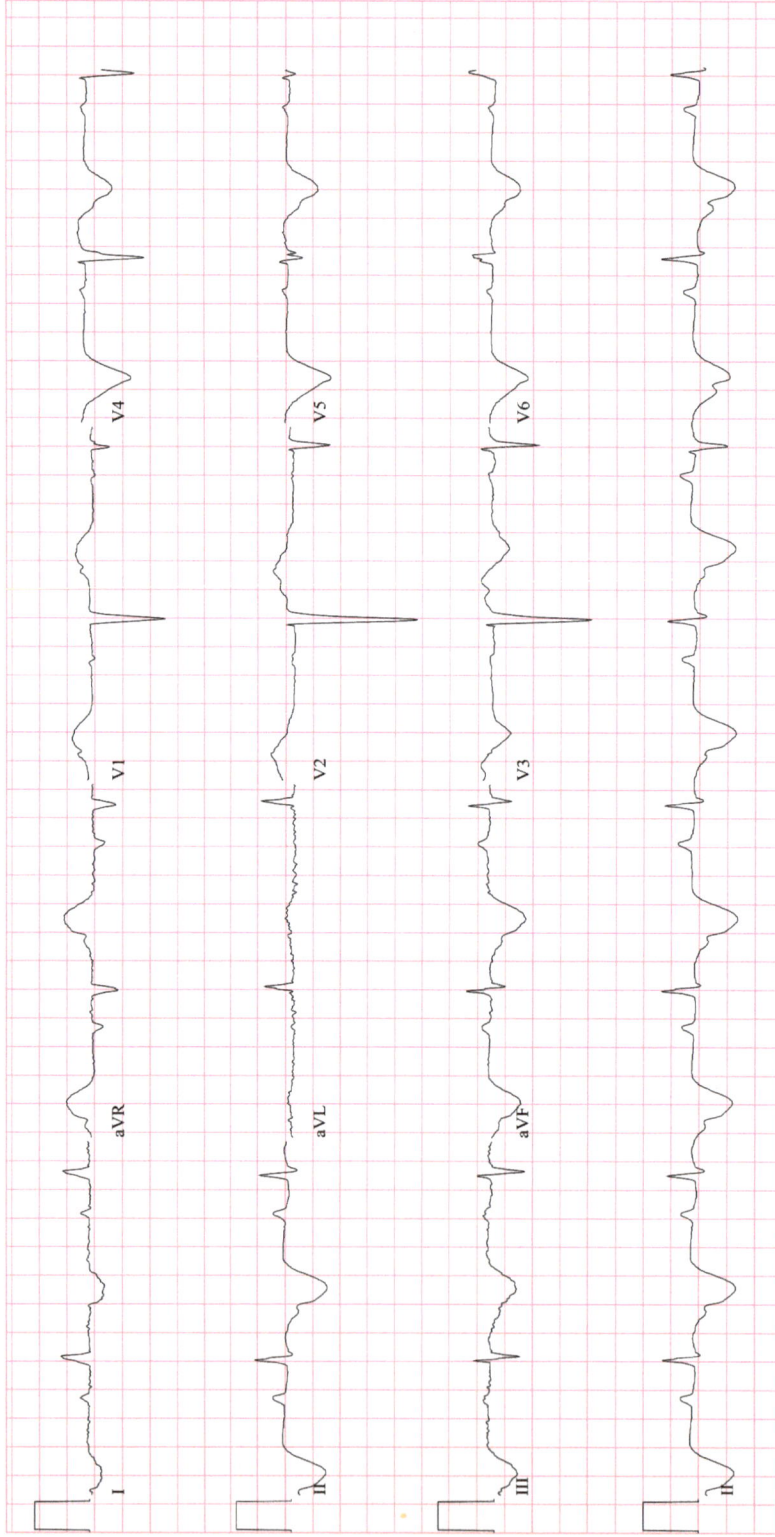

A 65-year-old female with a history of severe depression presents to the hospital after an out-of-hospital witnessed ventricular fibrillation and cardiac arrest. Patient was successfully resuscitated and brought to the hospital. On arrival, troponins were 0.61 ng/mL. Bedside echocardiogram showed severe hypokinesis of the entire apical segment, with a hyperkinetic base. Coronary angiogram was performed which did not show significant coronary artery disease. What does this EKG show?

DIAGNOSIS: Takotsubo Cardiomyopathy

- This EKG shows normal sinus rhythm at 50 bpm with 2:1 second degree AV block with non-conducted P waves (presumably due to the refractoriness of the ventricles) superimposed at the end of the T waves. Global deep T wave inversion is seen. QTc is prolonged and is measured at 620 ms.

- Takotsubo cardiomyopathy (TCM) is a disorder characterized by temporary left ventricular apical ballooning in the absence of significant left main or left anterior descending coronary artery disease.

- In the setting of TCM, the risk of TdP increases as the QTc prolongs.

- The initial EKG in Takotsubo cardiomyopathy can mimic an acute, anterior ST-segment elevation myocardial infarction, but can also present with deep T wave changes as in the present EKG.

- Given the consequences of missing the diagnosis of an acute anterior STEMI, the accuracy of a diagnosis based solely on EKG is insufficient as it cannot reliably distinguish between patients with TCM and those with acute anterior STEMI. Coronary angiography, which remains the gold standard, is therefore needed.[1]

---

1   Vervaat, Fabienne E., Thomas E. Christensen, Loes Smeijers, Lene Holmvang, Philip Hasbak, Balázs M. Szabó, Jos WMG Widdershoven, Galen S. Wagner, Lia E. Bang, and Anton PM Gorgels. "Is it possible to differentiate between Takotsubo cardiomyopathy and acute anterior ST-elevation myocardial infarction?." *Journal of electrocardiology* (2015).

EKG Case 82

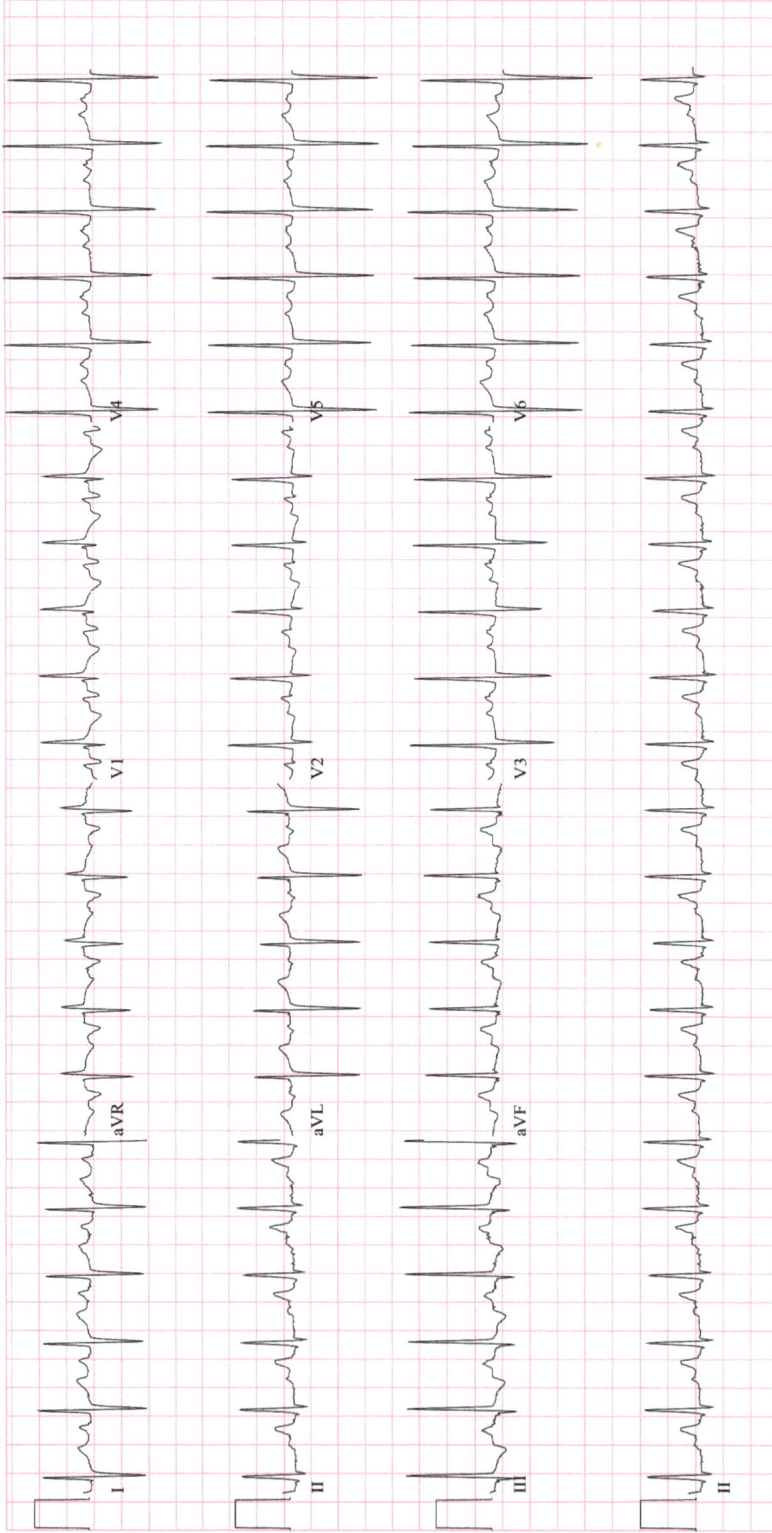

A 35-year-old female with a history of antiphospholipid syndrome presents to the ER with chief complaint of recurrent chest pains, shortness of breath, and palpitations. She is found to be hypoxic on room air. An EKG is obtained. What does it show?

DIAGNOSIS: Acute Pulmonary Embolism

The EKG shows sinus tachycardia. Right axis deviation, right ventricular strain pattern, right atrial enlargement (*P pulmonale*), and S1Q3T3 pattern suggestive of acute pulmonary embolism

EKG features include:

- Sinus tachycardia: the most common abnormality; seen in 44% of patients.
- Complete or incomplete RBBB: associated with increased mortality; seen in 18% of patients.
- Right ventricular strain pattern: T wave inversions in the right precordial leads (V1-4) ± the inferior leads (II, III, aVF). This pattern is seen in up to 34% of patients and is associated with high pulmonary artery pressures.
- Right axis deviation: seen in 16% of patients. Extreme right axis deviation may occur, with axis between zero and -90 degrees, giving the appearance of left axis deviation ("pseudo left axis").
- Dominant R wave in V1: a manifestation of acute right ventricular dilatation.
- Right atrial enlargement (*P pulmonale*): peaked P wave in lead II > 2.5 mm in height. Seen in 9% of patients.
- S1Q3T3 pattern: deep S wave in lead I, Q wave in III, inverted T wave in III. This "classic" finding is neither sensitive nor specific for pulmonary embolism; found in only 20% of patients with PE – (highlighted below).
- Clockwise rotation: shift of the R/S transition point towards V6 with a persistent S wave in V6 ("pulmonary disease pattern"), implying rotation of the heart due to right ventricular dilatation.
- Atrial tachyarrhythmias: AF, flutter, atrial tachycardia. Seen in 8% of patients.
- Nonspecific ST segment and T wave changes, including ST elevation and depression. Reported in up to 50% of patients with PE.
- The EKG is neither sensitive nor specific enough to diagnose or exclude PE.
- Around 18% of patients with PE will have a completely normal EKG.
- However, with a compatible clinical picture (sudden onset pleuritic chest pain, hypoxia), an EKG showing new RAD, RBBB, or T wave inversions should raise the suspicion of PE and prompt further diagnostic testing and therapy.

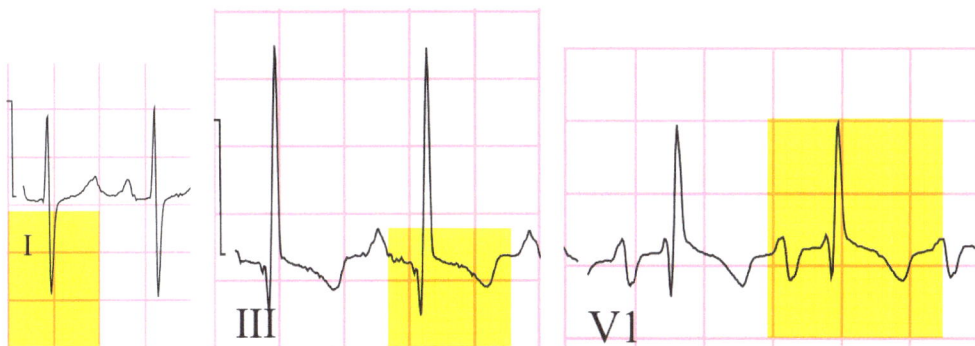

EKG Case 83

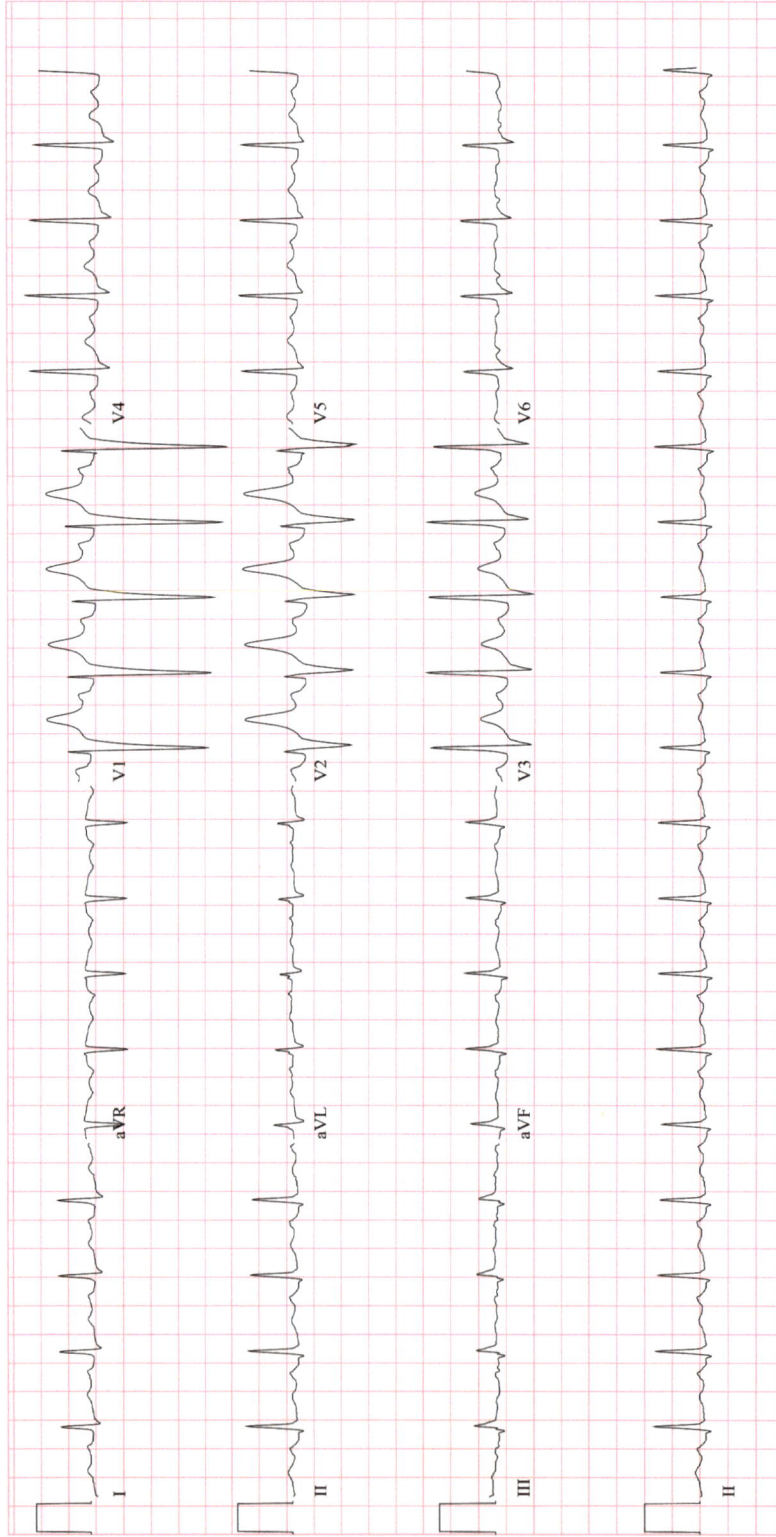

I, II, III, aVR, aVL, aVF, V1, V2, V3, V4, V5, V6, II

A 49-year-old female with a history of Hodgkin's lymphoma presents with a change in mental status and lethargy. She has a one week history of vomiting and loss of appetite. An EKG is obtained. What is the diagnosis and how should it be treated?

DIAGNOSIS: Hyperkalemia

This EKG shows sinus tachycardia with tall and tented T waves in the precordial leads.

- Potassium is important for the normal electric activity of heart. Hyperkalemia leads to progressive of EKG changes with increasing potassium levels.

- Serum potassium > 5.5 mEq/L is associated with repolarization abnormalities. Increased amplitude and peaking of the T wave; tall "tented" T waves.

- Higher level of potassium can lead to PR prolongation, loss of P waves, QRS widening and merger with T waves (sine waves), ventricular fibrillation, and eventually cardiac arrest.

- The patient was dehydrated with acute renal failure. Her potassium level was 5.9 mEq/L. She received IV fluids with bicarbonate, calcium gluconate, and sodium polystyrene sulfonate (Kayexalate). Follow up labs and EKG showed resolution of hyperkalemia and normal EKG.

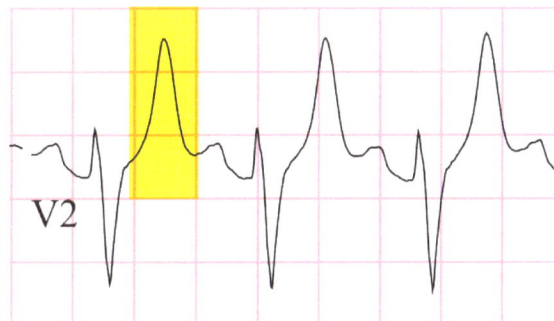

EKG Case 84

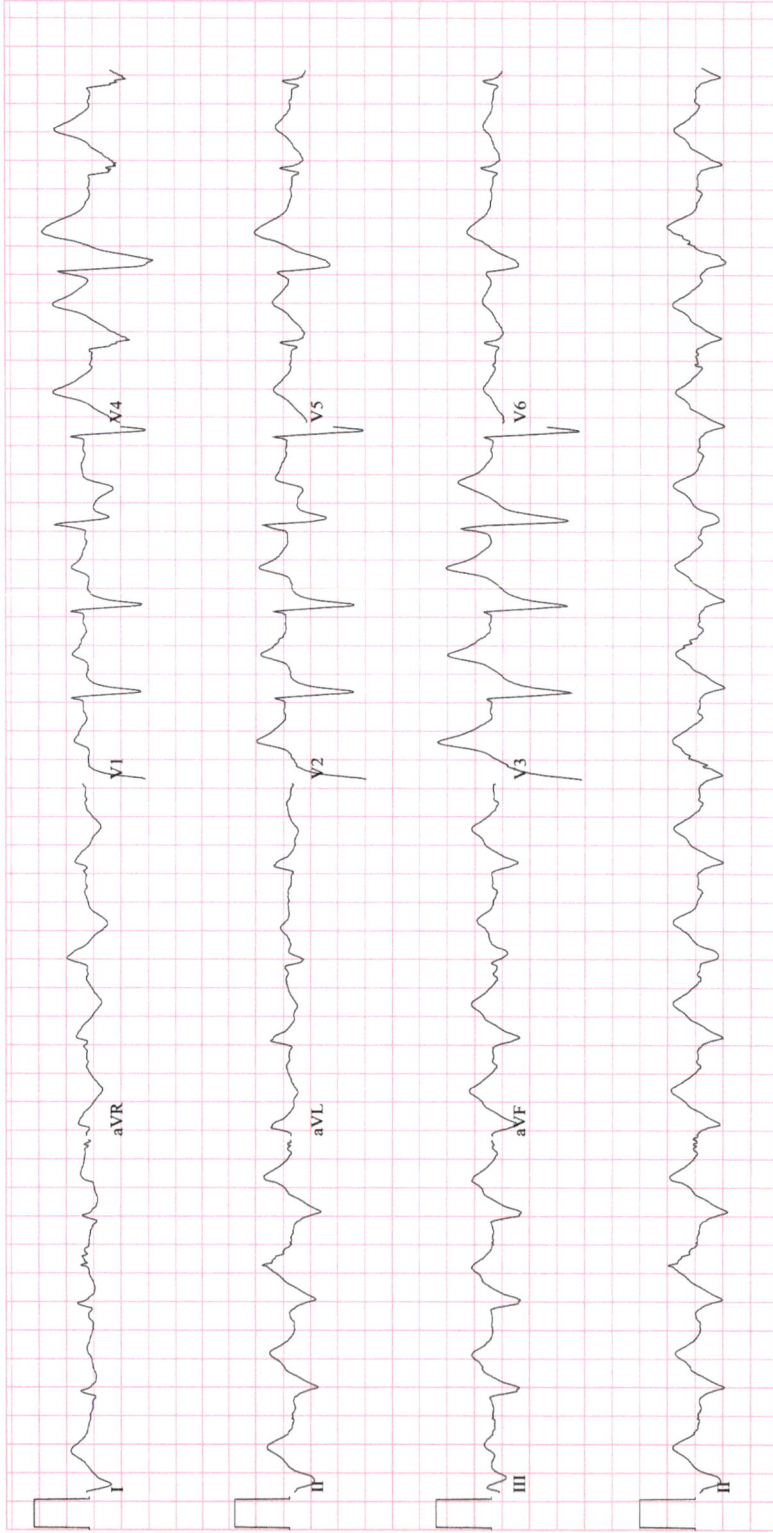

A 78-year-old patient with end-stage renal disease on hemodialysis is found on the floor at her residence by the EMS. When found, she had been on the ground for five days. What does the EKG show?

DIAGNOSIS: Hyperkalemia and Sine Waves

This EKG shows peaked T waves, QRS prolongation, and an absence of P waves in the setting of hyperkalemia due to rhabdomylosis and kidney failure.

- Potassium is important for the normal electric activity of heart; hyperkalemia leads to sequence of EKG changes for different potassium levels.

- Serum potassium > 5.5 mEq/L is associated with repolarization abnormalities: increased amplitude and peaking of the T wave; tall, "tented" T waves - as discussed in previous case.

- Serum potassium > 6.5 mEq/L is associated with progressive paralysis of the atria resulting in widening of P wave, followed by PR interval prolongation, and eventually loss of P waves.

- Serum potassium > 7.0 mEq/L is associated with conduction abnormalities and bradycardia: prolonged QRS interval with bizarre QRS morphology, high-grade AV block with slow junctional and ventricular escape rhythms, any kind of conduction block (bundle branch blocks, fascicular blocks), The QRS complex widens until it merges with T waves, forming the sine wave pattern.

- Serum potassium level of > 9.0 mEq/L can cause cardiac arrest due to: asystole, ventricular fibrillation, and PEA.

- When the diagnosis of hyperkalemia is confirmed by serum levels, the underlying cause needs to be addressed, e.g acute on chronic renal failure — our patient required emergent hemodialysis.

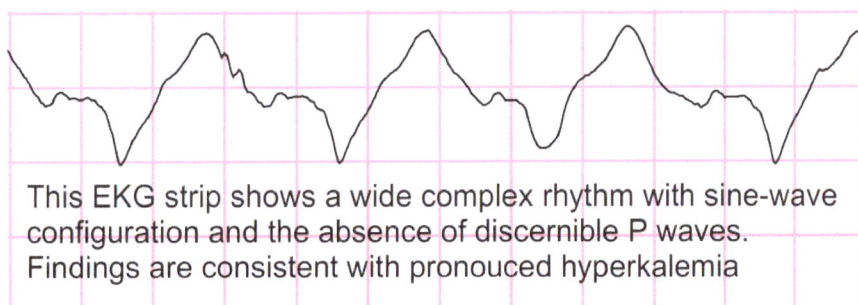

This EKG strip shows a wide complex rhythm with sine-wave configuration and the absence of discernible P waves.
Findings are consistent with pronouced hyperkalemia

EKG Case 85

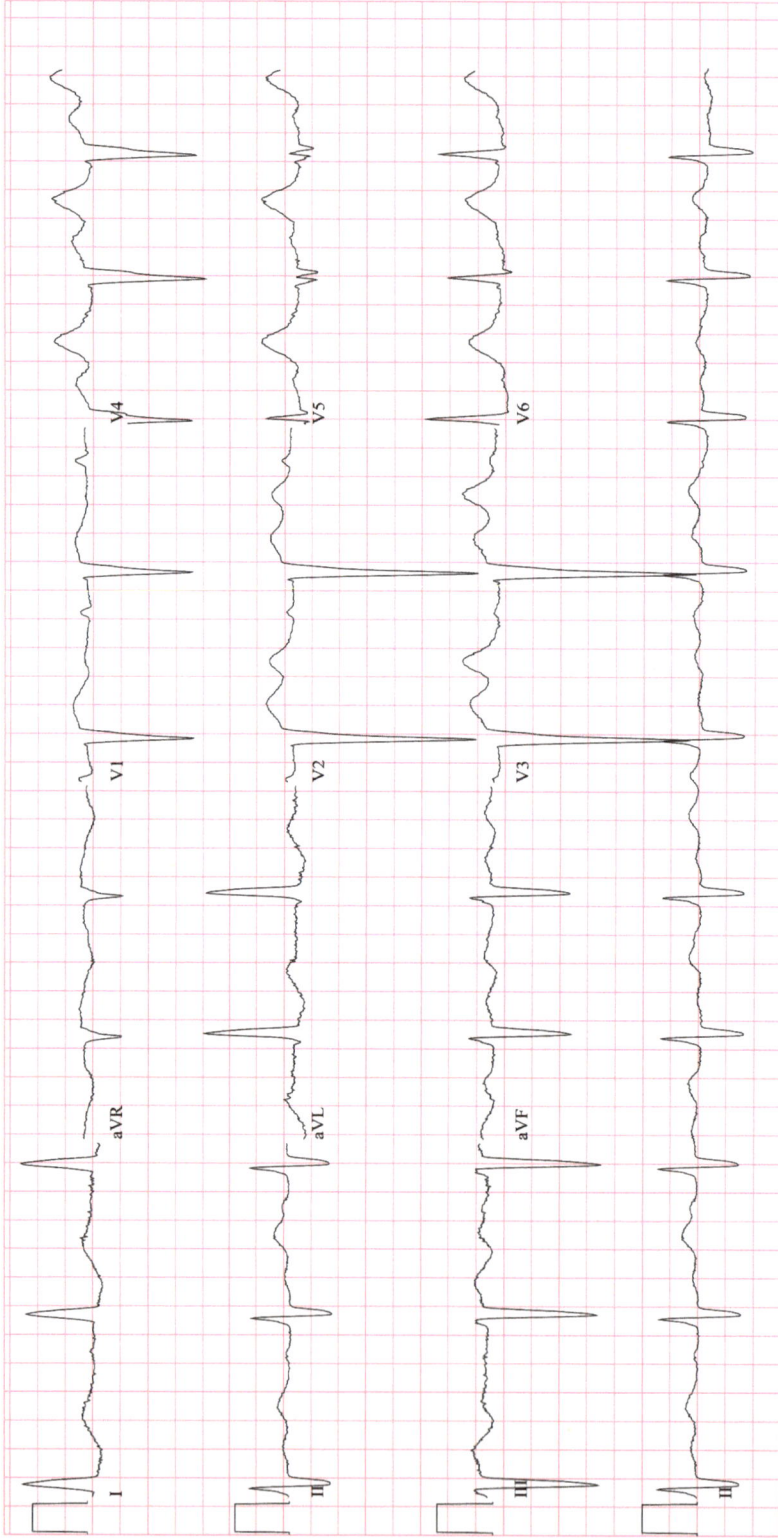

A 70-year-old female with a history of coronary artery disease, hypertension, and congestive heart disease is admitted to the hospital for volume overload. An EKG is obtained on the third day of admission. What prominent feature of electrolyte imbalance could be identified?

DIAGNOSIS: Prominent "U" Waves in Hypokalemia

The EKG shows, normal sinus rhythm with first degree AV block, left axis deviation, left anterior fasicular block, presence of prominent U waves (best seen in lead V2), left ventricular hypertrophy and deep Q waves in anterior leads likely secondary to prior anterior wall MI.

Normally, the U wave is a small (0.5 mm) deflection immediately following the T wave, usually in the same direction as the T wave. It is best seen in leads V2 and V3. U waves generally become visible when the heart rate falls below 65 bpm. The voltage of the U wave is normally < 25% that of the T wave voltage. Disproportionately large U waves are abnormal. Maximum normal amplitude should not exceed 1- 2 mm.

Abnormalities of the U wave can be broadly classified as Prominent U waves and Inverted U waves.

Prominent U Waves

* U waves are prominent if > 1- 2mm or 25% of the height of the T wave. The most common cause of prominent U waves is bradycardia. Abnormally prominent U waves are characteristically seen in severe hypokalemia, as in this case with the potassium of 1.9 mE/L. Other causes of prominent U waves include hypocalcaemia, hypomagnesaemia, hypothermia, raised intracranial pressure, left ventricular hypertrophy, and hypertrophic cardiomyopathy.

Inverted U Waves

U wave inversion is abnormal (in leads with upright T waves). A negative U wave is highly specific for the presence of underlying heart disease, such as coronary artery disease, hypertension, valvular heart disease, congenital heart disease, or cardiomyopathy.

Other EKG features include:

* ST depression, which usually is more pronounced in the lateral leads.
* QTc prolongation, but accurate QT interval measurement is challenging when the T and U waves are fused.
* Prolongation of the PR interval (above 250 ms), premature supraventricular ectopic beats, and sustained atrial fibrillation or flutter.
* Hypokalemia when unchecked can lead to life-threatening ventricular arrhythmias, e.g, VT, VF, and Torsades de Pointes.
* Hypokalaemia is often associated with hypomagnesaemia, which increases the risk of malignant ventricular arrhythmias
* Treatment involves aggressive potassium replacement and addressing the underlying cause.

EKG Case 86

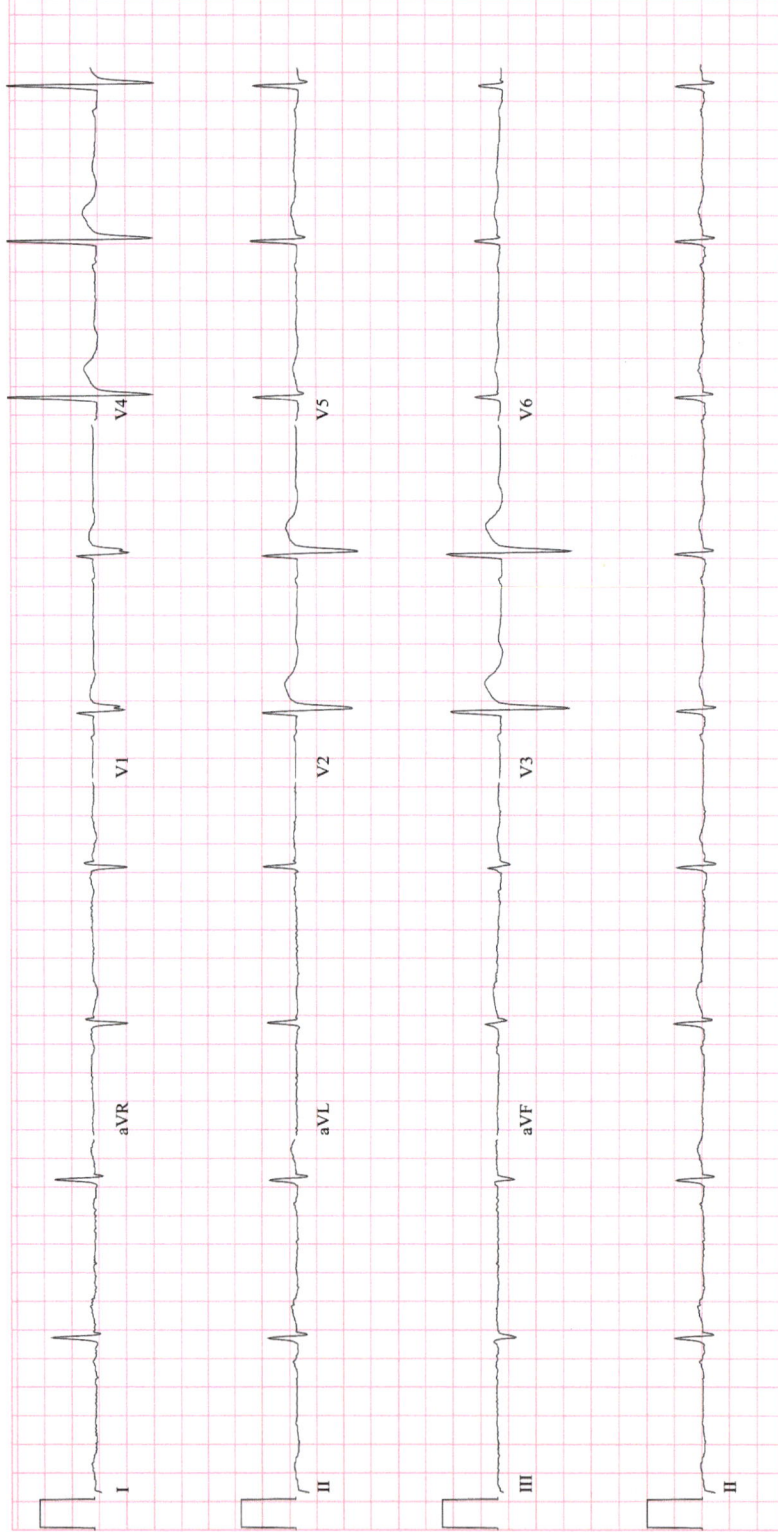

A 79-year-old male with a history of primary hyperparathyroidism is brought to the hospital with a change in mental status. Lab work reveals serum creatinine of 1.49 mg/dl, serum calcium of 15.8 mg/dl, and PTH of 453 pg/ml. An EKG is obtained. What EKG findings of hypercalcemia could be identified?

DIAGNOSIS: Hypercalcemia

The above EKG shows many changes typical of hypercalcemia, including sinus bradycardia at 55 bpm and short QT and QTc intervals of 374 ms and 357 ms, respectively.

High and low levels of ionized serum calcium concentration can produce characteristic changes on the electrocardiogram. These changes are almost entirely limited to the duration of the ST segment, with no change in the QRS complexes or T waves. High ionized serum calcium shortens the ST segment, and low ionized serum calcium prolongs the ST segment.

EKG changes in hypercalcemia:

- The main EKG abnormality seen with hypercalcemia is shortening of the QT interval.
- In severe hypercalcemia, Osborn waves (J waves) may be seen.
- Ventricular irritability and VF arrest have been reported with extreme hypercalcemia.

Some of the causes of hypercalcemia include:

- Hyperparathyroidism
- Multiple Myeloma
- Bone metastases
- Paraneoplastic syndromes
- Milk-alkali syndrome
- Sarcoidosis
- Excess vitamin D (e.g, iatrogenic)

QTc measurement is discussed further in case 89.

EKG Case 87

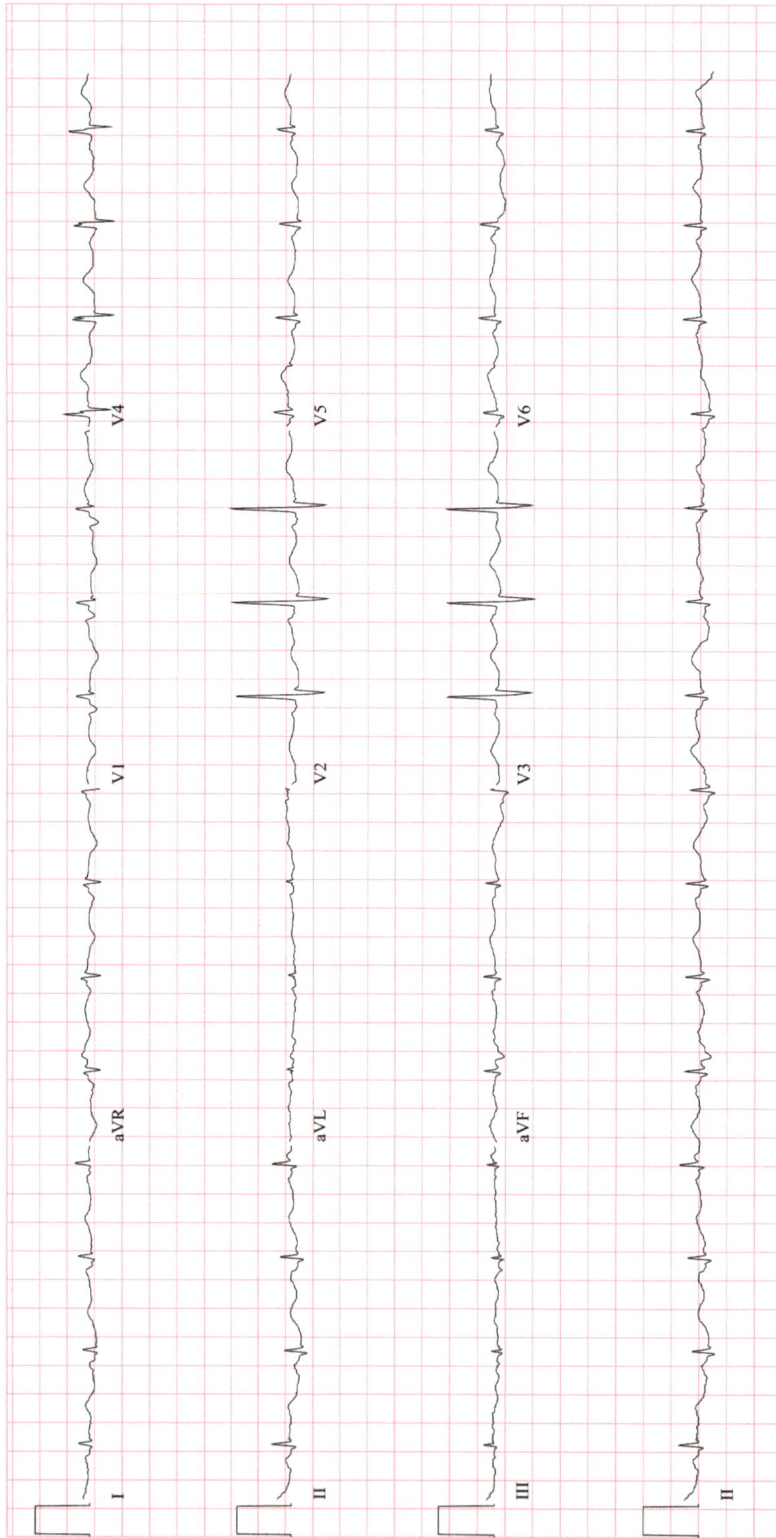

A 35-year-old female is admitted to the hospital for acute pancreatitis. Patient is complaining of abdominal pain. Based on the above EKG can you spot an electrolyte imbalance?

I   aVR   V1   V4
II   aVL   V2   V5
III aVF   V3   V6
II

DIAGNOSIS: Hypocalcemia and Prolonged QTc

This EKG shows normal sinus rhythm with prolonged QTc of 516 ms seen in the context of hypocalcemia. In above patient, the ionized calcium was 0.9 mMol/L.

EKG features include:

- QTc prolongation primarily due to prolonging the ST segment.
- T wave is typically unchanged.
- Torsades de pointes may occur, but is much less common than with hypokalemia or hypomagnesaemia.

Causes of hypocalcemia include:

- Hypoparathyroidism
- Vitamin D deficiency
- Acute pancreatitis
- Hyperphosphataemia
- Hypomagnesaemia
- Diuretics use (e.g, furosemide)
- Pseudohypoparathyroidism
- Congenital disorders (e.g, DiGeorge syndrome)
- Critical illness (e.g, sepsis)
- Factitious (e.g, EDTA blood tube contamination)

EKG Case 88

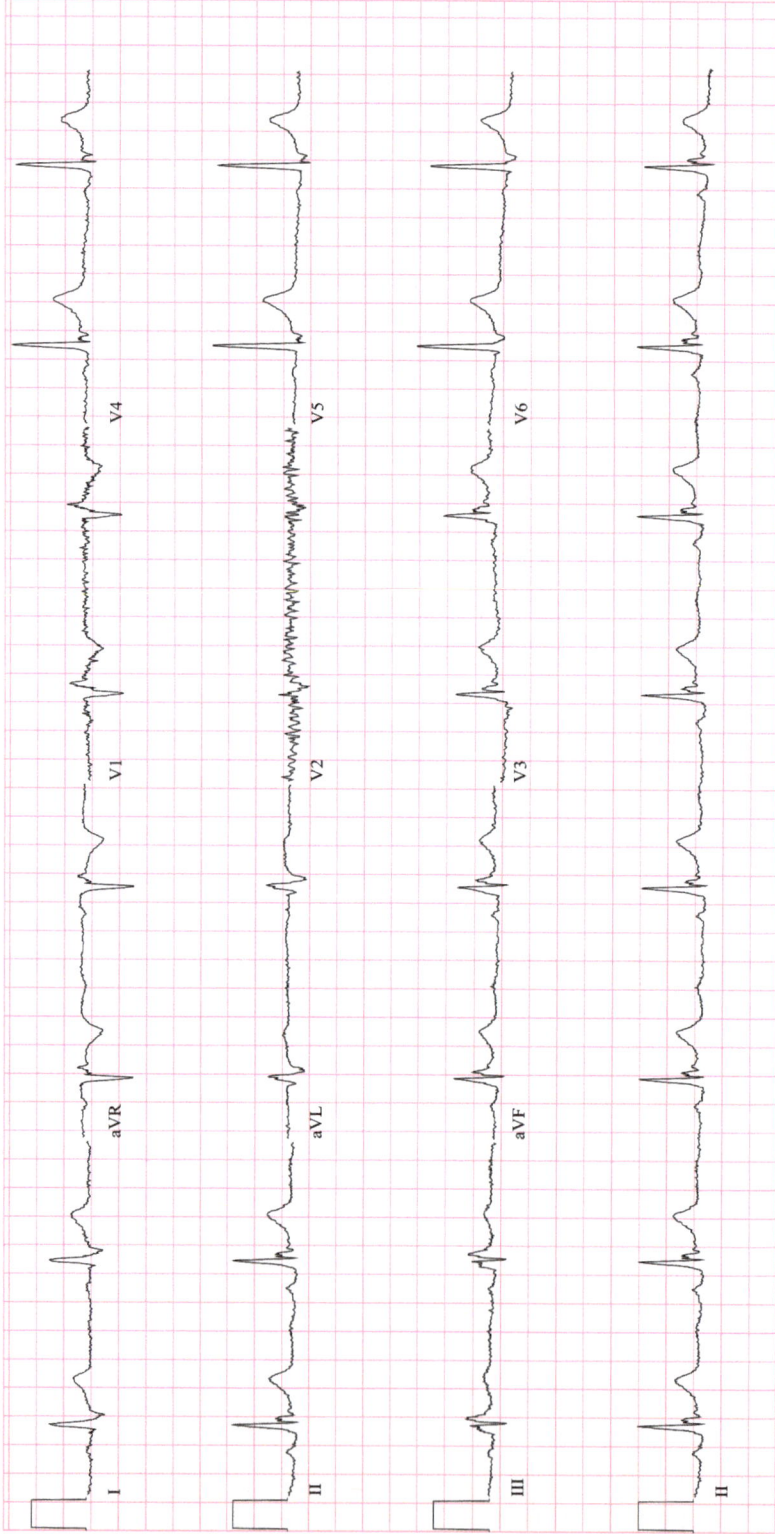

A 65-year-old homeless male with a history of alcoholism is found unconscious by EMS. On arrival to the ER, his core body temperature is 33.7 °C (92.7 °F). What characteristic signs of hypothermia could be identified on this EKG?

DIAGNOSIS: Hypothermia and Osborn Waves

This EKG shows normal sinus rhythm with J point elevation in leads II, III, aVF, V2, V3, V4, and V5.

- Hypothermia, a potentially fatal condition is defined by core body temperature dropping below 35°C (95°F).

- Osborne waves[1] also known as camel-hump waves or hypothermic waves, refer to distinctive J point elevation seen in hypothermia. They are best seen in the inferior leads and in the lateral precordial leads.

- They are formed by an abrupt J point elevation followed by sudden "plunge" back to baseline.

- The height of the J wave is roughly proportional to the degree of hypothermia.

- Shivering waves and muscle tremor artifact can also be seen (lead V2).

- In the initial stages of hypothermia, sinus tachycardia develops as part of the general stress reaction.

- At temperature ~ 32°C, all intervals of the EKG including RR, PR, QRS, and QT lengthen.

- At temperature ~ 30°C, atrial ectopic activity is noted which can progress to atrial fibrillation and widening of QRS complex. This could lead to ventricular fibrillation and eventually to asystole.

- J waves can be seen in a number of other conditions, e.g., normal variant, early repolarization, hypercalcemia, intracranial hypertension, Le syndrome d'Haïssaguerre (idiopathic VF).

- After rewarming our patient, normal sinus rhythm was reestablished with resolution of Osborn waves.

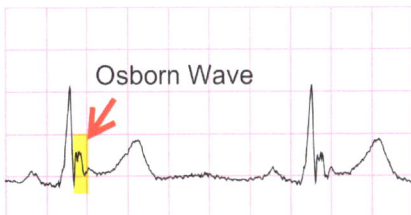

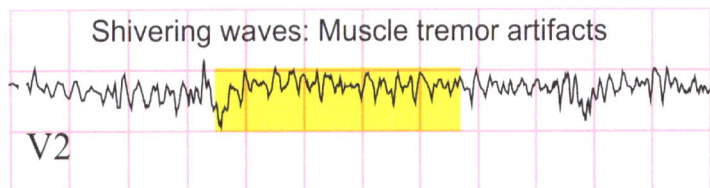

Osborn Wave

Shivering waves: Muscle tremor artifacts

V2

1   Alhaddad, Imad A., Mohammed Khalil, and Edward J. Brown. "Osborn waves of hypothermia." *Circulation* 101, no. 25 (2000): e233-e244

EKG Case 89

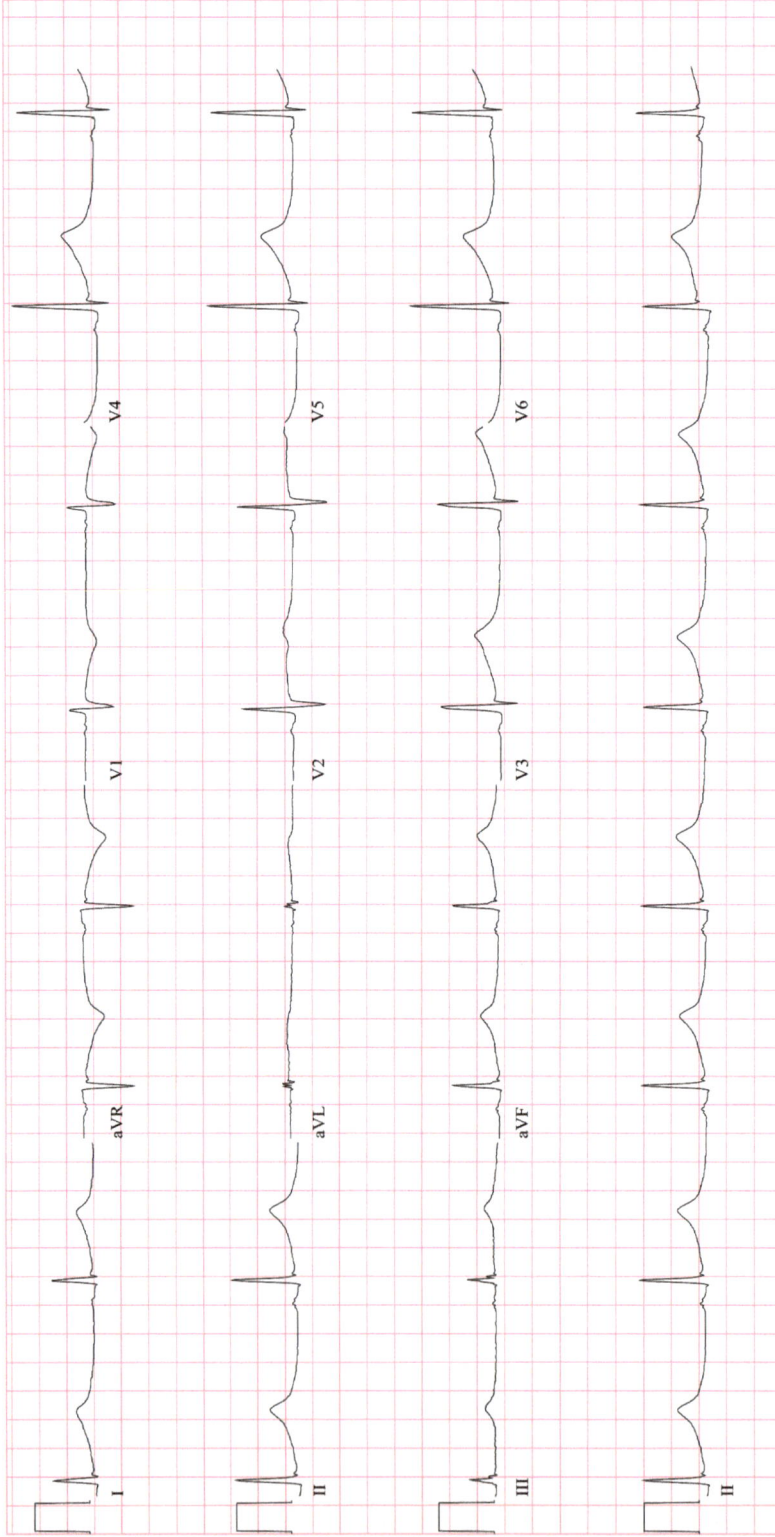

An 18-year-old female with a history of depression, seizures, and recurrent falls is being evaluated at your office for dizziness. An EKG is obtained. What does it show?

DIAGNOSIS: Congenital Long QT Syndrome

This EKG demonstrates sinus bradycardia with very prolonged QT interval of 640 ms (QTc of 540 ms).

- The long QT syndrome (LQTS) is a disorder of ventricular myocardial repolarization characterized by a prolonged QT interval on the electrocardiogram that can lead to symptomatic ventricular arrhythmias and an increased risk of sudden cardiac death. This syndrome is associated with an increased risk of a characteristic life-threatening cardiac arrhythmia, known as torsades de pointes or "twisting of the points". The main symptoms of LQTS patients include palpitations, syncope, seizures, and cardiac arrest.[1]

- The long QT syndrome may be congenital or acquired.

- Acquired LQTS usually results from drug therapy or electrolyte disturbances.

- Multiple medications such as sotalol, erythromycin, metoclopramide, quinidine, haloperidol, droperidol, methadone, ondansetron, fluoxetine, amitriptyline, etc., can cause acquired LQTS also increasing the risk of torsade de pointes and sudden death.[2]

- Prolongation of the QT interval is an essential component of the diagnosis of LQTS. Other EKG features, such as T wave morphology, bradycardia, and QT dispersion may be useful in the evaluation of the patient with suspected LQTS, but the corrected QT interval appears to be the most useful diagnostic and prognostic parameter.[3]

- QTc is prolonged if > 440 ms in men or > 460 ms in women. QTc > 500 is associated with increased risk of torsades de pointes. QTc is abnormally short if < 350 ms, such as in short QT syndrome which is also associated with increased risk of sudden death. The correction of the QT interval for heart rate poses a number of challenges and controversies. There are multiple formulas used to estimate QTc including:
    - Bazett's formula: $QTC = QT / \sqrt{RR}$
    - Fredericia's formula: $QTC = QT / RR\ 1/3$
    - Framingham formula: $QTC = QT + 0.154\ (1 - RR)$
    - Hodges formula: $QTC = QT + 1.75\ (\text{heart rate} - 60)$

Bazett's formula is the most commonly used. It overcorrects at heart rates > 100 bpm and under-corrects at heart rates < 60 bpm, but provides an adequate correction for heart rates in the range of 60 — 100 bpm. Outside that range, the Fredericia or Framingham corrections are more accurate and should be used instead. Several Online and mobile apps for QTc calculations are now available.[4]

- Patients at high risk of recurrent syncope or sudden death are usually considered for implantable cardioverter defibrillator therapy along with beta blockade.

---

1 Moss, Arthur J. "Long QT syndrome." *JAMA* 289, no. 16 (2003): 2041-2044.

2 Yap, Yee Guan, and A. John Camm. "Drug induced QT prolongation and torsades de pointes." *Heart* 89, no. 11 (2003): 1363-1372.

3 Mönnig, Gerold, Lars Eckardt, Horst Wedekind, Wilhelm Haverkamp, Joachim Gerss, Peter Milberg, Kristina Wasmer et al. "Electrocardiographic risk stratification in families with congenital long QT syndrome." *European heart journal* 27, no. 17 (2006): 2074-2080.

4 http://www.mdcalc.com/corrected-qt-interval-qtc/

EKG Case 90

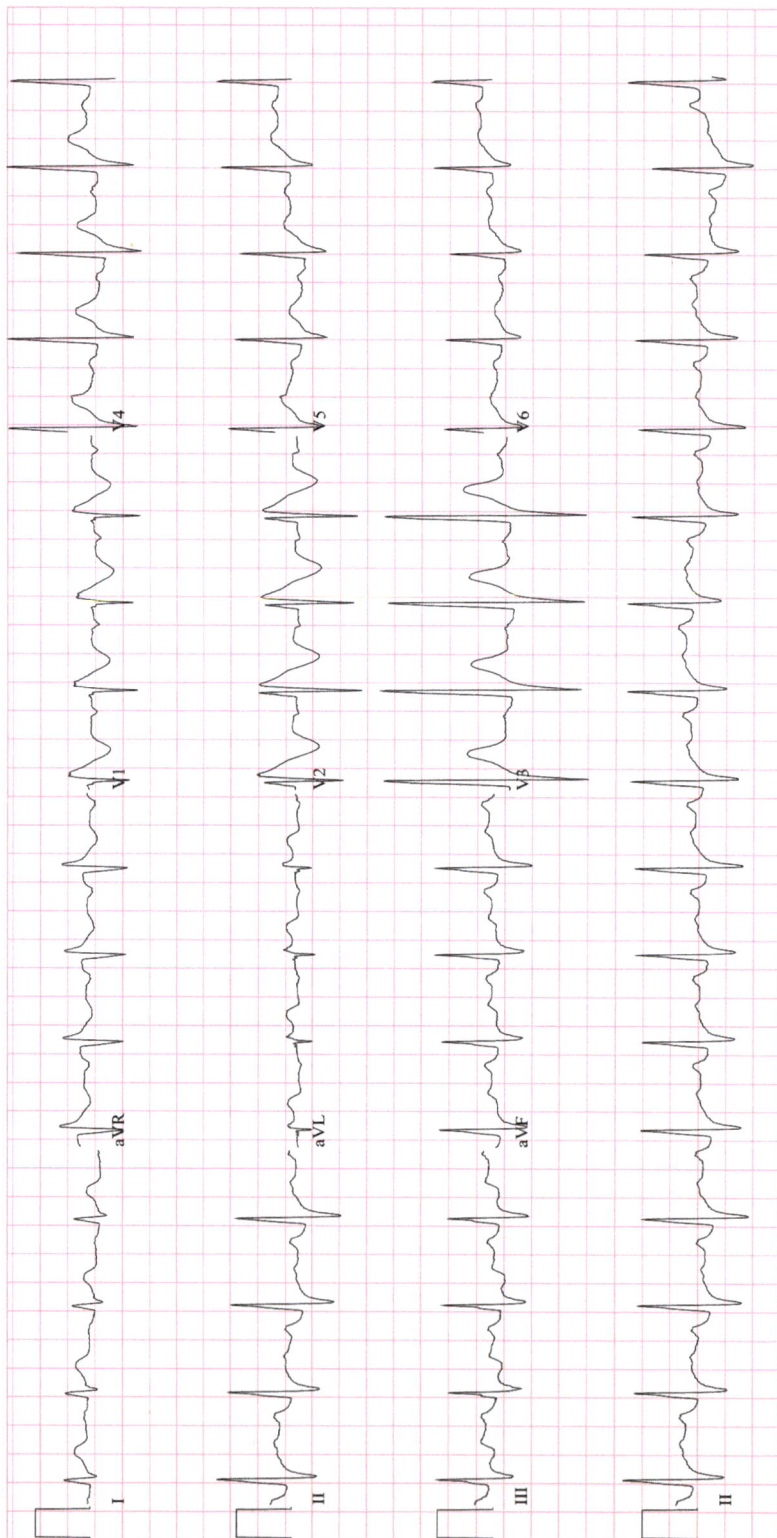

A 35-year-old Asian man with a history of frequent presyncopal spells is brought to the emergency department after an episode of syncope. An EKG is obtained in the ER. What does it show?

DIAGNOSIS: Brugada Syndrome Type I

The EKG shows sinus tachycardia with prominent coved ST elevation in V1- V2, followed by a negative (inverted) T wave.

The Brugada syndrome, first described in 1953, was recognized as a clinical syndrome in 1992 by Brugada et al.[1] when it was associated with sudden cardiac death. Brugada syndrome is an inherited sodium channelopathy, associated with sudden death and syncope due to polymorphic VT or VF. It is predominantly seen in the male Asian population with mean age of 41. Three different types have been described as types 1, 2, and 3 based on the EKG appearance. Importantly, the pattern is dynamic and all three types could be seen in a single patient at different times.

- **Type 1:** It is characterized by a prominent coved ST segment elevation displaying J point amplitude or ST segment elevation ≥2 mm in V1- V3, followed by a negative (inverted) T wave. Type 1 is most associated with ventricular arrhythmias.

- **Type 2:** It has ≥2 mm J point elevation, ≥1 mm ST segment elevation and a saddleback appearance, followed by a positive (upright) or biphasic T wave.

- **Type 3:** It has either a saddleback or coved appearance, but with an ST segment elevation <1 mm.

In conjunction with these EKG features, at least one of the following features are needed to make a diagnosis of Brugada syndrome:

- Documented VF or polymorphic VT , family history of sudden cardiac death at age < 45 years, coved ST elevation EKG in family members, inducibility of VT with programmed electrical stimulation, history of syncope, nocturnal agonal respiration.

- The only available therapy is an implantable cardioverter - defibrillator (ICD) for protection against sudden cardiac death. Quinidine has been proposed as an alternative in settings where ICD's are unavailable or where they would be inappropriate (e.g., neonates). Quinidine can also be used as adjunctive therapy to ICD in case of multiple shocks for ventricular arrhythmias.

- Some drugs may induce VF/VT and a comprehensive list can be found at:
  http://www.brugadadrugs.org

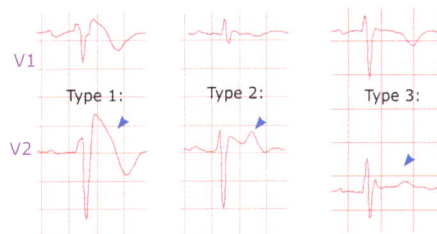

V1 · V2 · Type 1: · Type 2: · Type 3:

---

1   Brugada P., Brugada J.; Right bundle branch block, persistent ST- segment elevation and sudden cardiac death. a multicenter report. J Am Coll Cardiol. 20 1992:1391-1396.

EKG Case 91

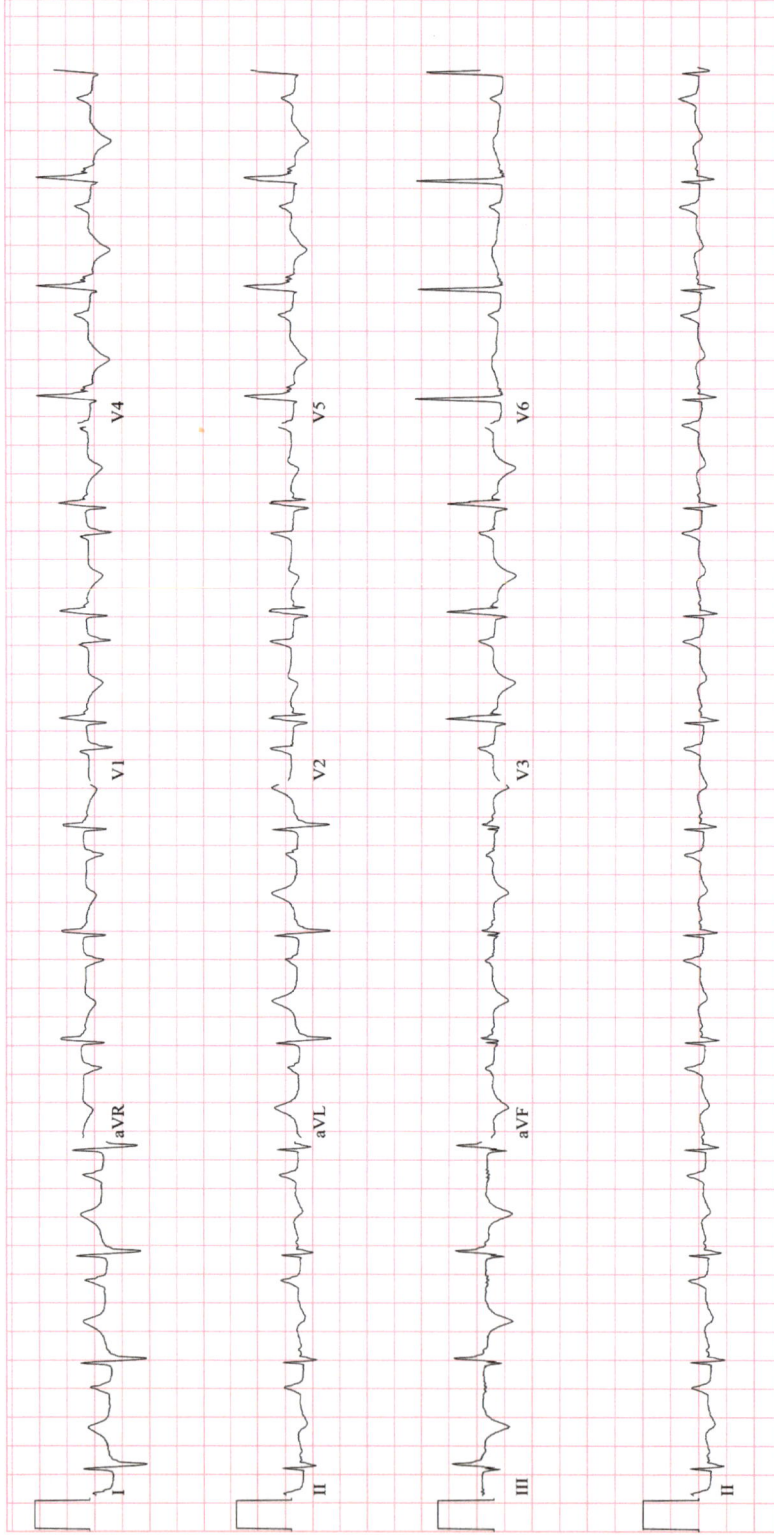

A 10-year-old girl is brought to the ER with complaints of shortness of breath. Heart auscultation reveals wide and fixed split S2 with loud P2. An EKG is obtained. What does it show?

DIAGNOSIS: Ostium Secundum – Atrial Septal Defect (ASD)

This EKG shows normal sinus rhythm with first degree AV block (PR interval of 200 ms). It also shows right axis deviation, right bundle branch block (rsR' pattern in lead V1), and biatrial enlargement.

The EKG findings and clinical scenario is consistent with atrial septal defect - ostium secundum type.

- There are three major types of ASDs or interatrial communications: ostium secundum, ostium primum, and sinus venosus defects.[1]

- The **ostium secundum** is a true defect of the atrial septum and involves the region of the fossa ovalis.

- The ostium primum defect falls within the spectrum of the atrioventricular (AV) septal defects, also known as endocardial cushion defects, which include ventricular septal defects and common AV valves.

- The sinus venosus defect is usually located at the junction of the right atrium and superior vena cava and is almost always associated with partial anomalous pulmonary venous return.

Many patients with ASDs are free of overt symptoms, although most will become symptomatic at some point in their lives. The age at which symptoms appear is highly variable and correlates — although not exclusively — with the size of the shunt. A pansystolic murmur of "mitral" regurgitation is characteristic of the patient with a primum ASD.

The EKG may be an important clue to diagnosis. The rhythm may be sinus, atrial fibrillation, or atrial flutter. Inverted P waves in the inferior leads suggest an absent or deficient sinus node, as may be seen in a sinus venosus defect[2]. Right atrial overload is often present. First-degree heart block suggests a primum ASD[3] but may be seen in older patients with a secundum ASD. The QRS axis is typically rightward in secundum ASD, markedly so if pulmonary hypertension is present.

The QRS axis is leftward or extremely to the right in ostium primum ASDs (due to absence of a left anterior fascicle). Voltage evidence of right ventricular hypertrophy may be seen in all ASDs, often in the form of "incomplete" right bundle branch block, with the more extreme forms usually found in patients with pulmonary hypertension. Patients with mitral valve insufficiency may have left ventricular hypertrophy or left atrial overload.

Transthoracic echocardiogram and cardiac MRI are required to establish the diagnosis and to assess its severity.

---

1   Webb, Gary, and Michael A. Gatzoulis. "Atrial septal defects in the adult recent progress and overview." *Circulation* 114, no. 15 (2006): 1645-1653.

2   Davia, James E., Melvin D. Cheitlin, and Julius L. Bedynek. "Sinus venosus atrial septal defect: analysis of fifty cases." *American heart journal* 85, no. 2 (1973): 177-185.

3   Fournier A, Young ML, Garcia OL, Tamer DF, Wolff GS. Electrophysiologic cardiac function before and after surgery in children with atrioventricular canal. Am J Cardiol. 1986; 57: 1137–1141

EKG Case 92

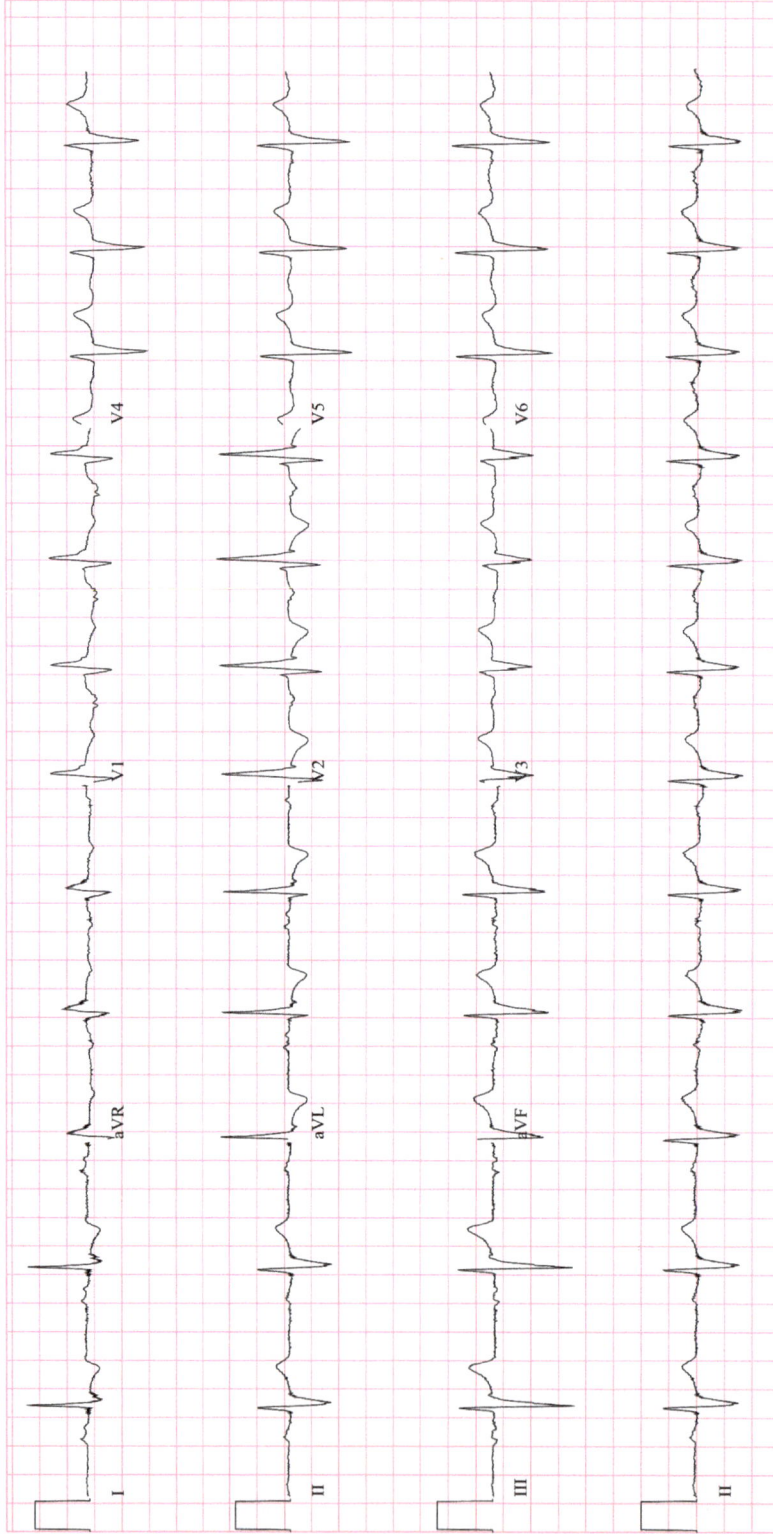

A 30-year-old male recently emigrated from Africa with history of atrial fibrillation, hypertension, and "cardiac murmur" presents to the office to establish care. Chest auscultation reveals pansystolic murmur. An EKG is obtained. What does it show?

DIAGNOSIS: Ostium Primum - Atrial Septal Defect (ASD)

This EKG shows normal sinus rhythm with sinus arrhythmia and first degree AV block (PR interval of 220 ms). It also shows left axis deviation, right bundle branch block (rsR' pattern in lead V1), and left atrial enlargement (P wave duration ≥ 0.12 s in lead II).

The EKG findings (as discussed in previous case) and clinical scenario are consistent with atrial septal defect - ostium primum type.

Ostium primum ASDs may also be associated with DiGeorge syndrome and Ellis-Van Creveld syndrome. Most primum ASDs are relatively large and lead to right heart dilation.

EKG features of ostium primum ASD include:

- rsR' pattern in lead V1.
- Left axis deviation (due to absence of the left anterior fascicle).
- Left axis deviation persists even after closure of the defect.
- Determination of QRS axis is very important in the differential diagnosis of ostium secundum and ostium primum ASD. Right axis deviation is not observed in ostium primum ASD.
- Left atrial abnormality.
- Complete or incomplete RBBB.
- Prolongation of the PR interval (first degree atrioventricular block).

EKG Case 93

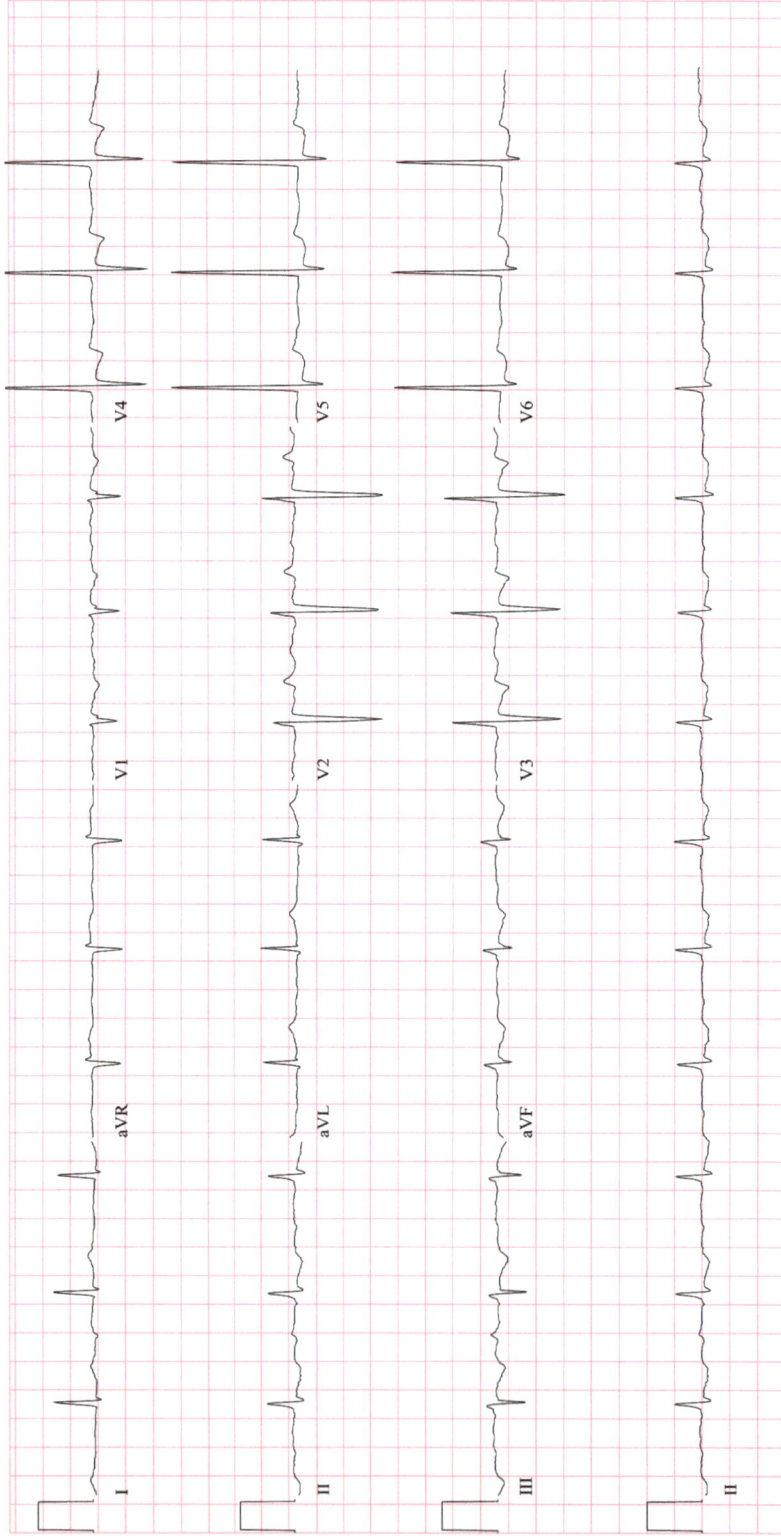

A 75-year-old white female with a history of CHF and atrial fibrillation presents to the ER with the chief complaint of nausea, vomiting, and blurry vision. She was seen in the ER five days ago and was started on antibiotics for urinary tract infection. Her resting EKG is shown. What does the EKG reveal and what tests should be ordered for further evaluation?

DIAGNOSIS: Digoxin Toxicity

This EKG shows atrial fibrillation with accelerated junctional rhythm. Digoxin effect is seen with sagging ST and T waves ("scooping"). This is most notable in EKG leads with tall R waves.

- T waves are inverted with short QT intervals. This classical presentation is known as "reverse tick", "hockey stick", or "Salvador Dali's moustache".

- Digoxin toxicity can cause many arrhythmias, due to increased automaticity (increased intracellular calcium) and decreased AV conduction (increased vagal effects at the AV node). This could therefore lead to "atrial tachycardia with AV block".

- Other arrhythmias associated with digoxin toxicity include ventricular bigeminy and trigeminy and sinus bradycardia with prominent of U waves.

- Differential diagnosis of ST segment depression includes drugs (e.g, digoxin, quinidine), myocardial ischemia, and left ventricular hypertrophy with "strain".

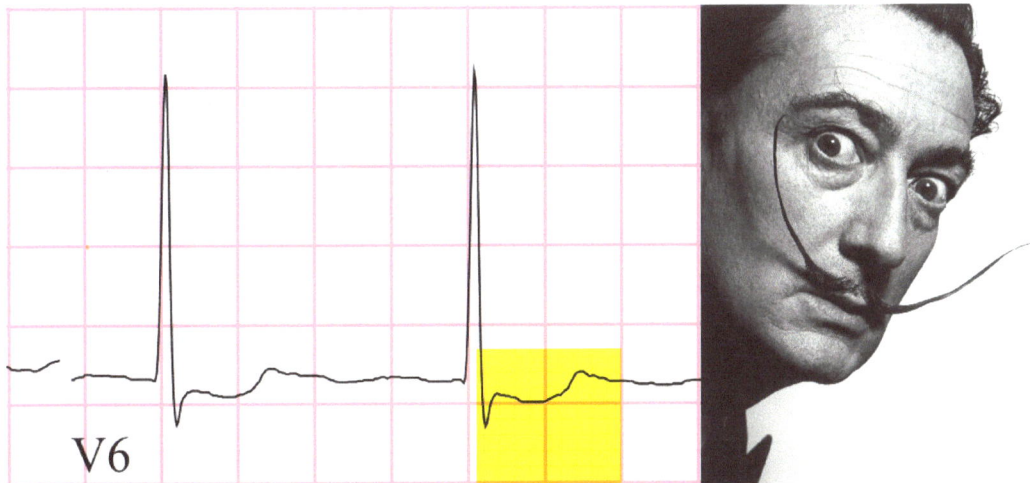

V6

[1]

---

1   Salvador Domingo Felipe Jacinto Dalí i Domènech, Marqués de Dalí de Pubol, known as Salvador Dalí,
     was a prominent Spanish surrealist painter born in Figueres, Catalonia, Spain

EKG Case 94

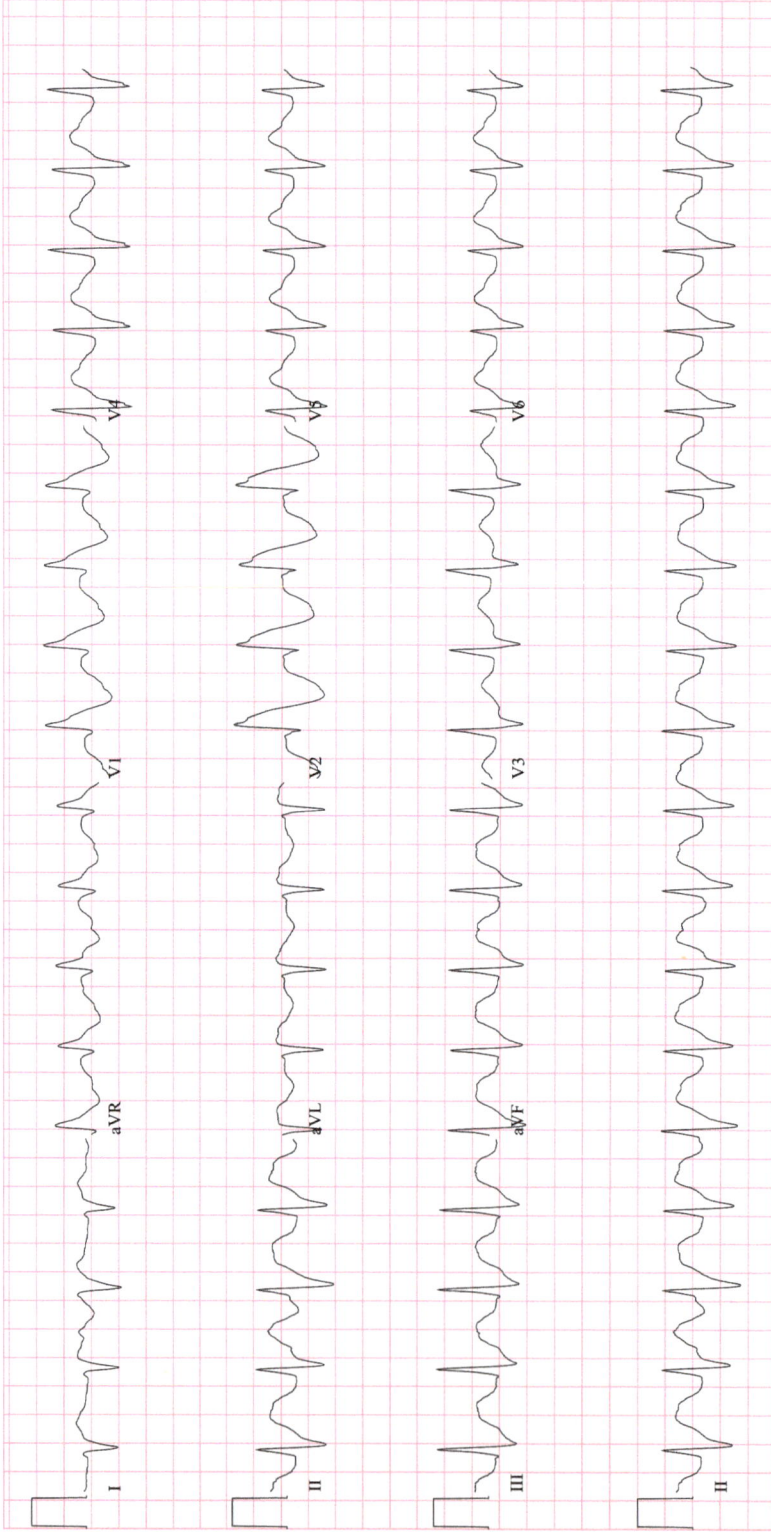

32-year-old female with a history of depression is brought to the ER by EMS after an attempt to commit suicide by ingesting an unknown drug. An EKG is obtained. What does it show and how should it be treated?

DIAGNOSIS: Sodium-Channel Blocker Toxicity

- This EKG shows sinus tachycardia, wide QRS complexes, and positive R' wave in aVR.

- Tricyclic antidepressants (TCA) exhibit their cardiotoxic effects via blockade of myocardial fast sodium channels (QRS prolongation, tall R wave in aVR), inhibition of potassium channels (QTc prolongation) and direct myocardial depression. Other toxic effects are produced by blockade of muscarinic (M1), histamine (H1), and beta 1-adenergic receptors.

EKG features include:

1. Broad complex dysrhythmias. The degree of QRS broadening on the EKG is correlated with adverse events: QRS > 100 ms is predictive of seizures and QRS > 160 ms is predictive of ventricular arrhythmias.

2. Right axis deviation of the terminal QRS: TCA toxicity is also supported by the presence of deep S waves in lead I and prominent (> 3 mm) terminal R waves in lead aVR. R/S ratio > 0.7 in aVR.

- Management includes correcting acidemia with IV sodium bicarbonate and electrolyte imbalances, protecting airway, and IV benzodiazepine for seizures. Avoid class Ia (e.g., procainamide) and class Ic (e.g., Flecainide) agents, beta blockers, and amiodarone as they may worsen hypotension and conduction abnormalities.

- Other sodium channel blocking medications which could produce similar EKG findings in overdose include: type Ia antiarrhythmic drug (e.g, quinidine, procainamide, disopyramide), Type Ic antiarrhythmics drugs (e.g., flecainide and propafenone), local anaesthetics (e.g., bupivacaine), Antimalarial drug (e.g., chloroquine, hydroxychloroquine), dextropropoxyphene, propranolol, carbamazepine and quinine.

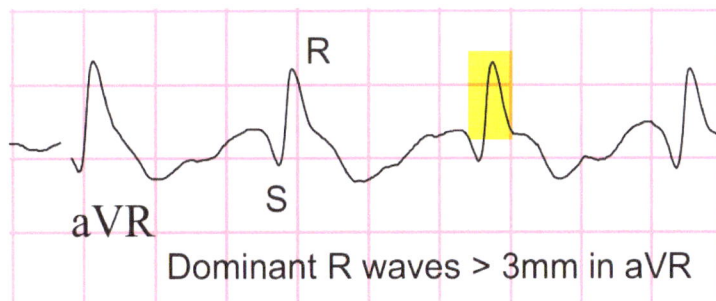

Dominant R waves > 3mm in aVR

EKG Case 95

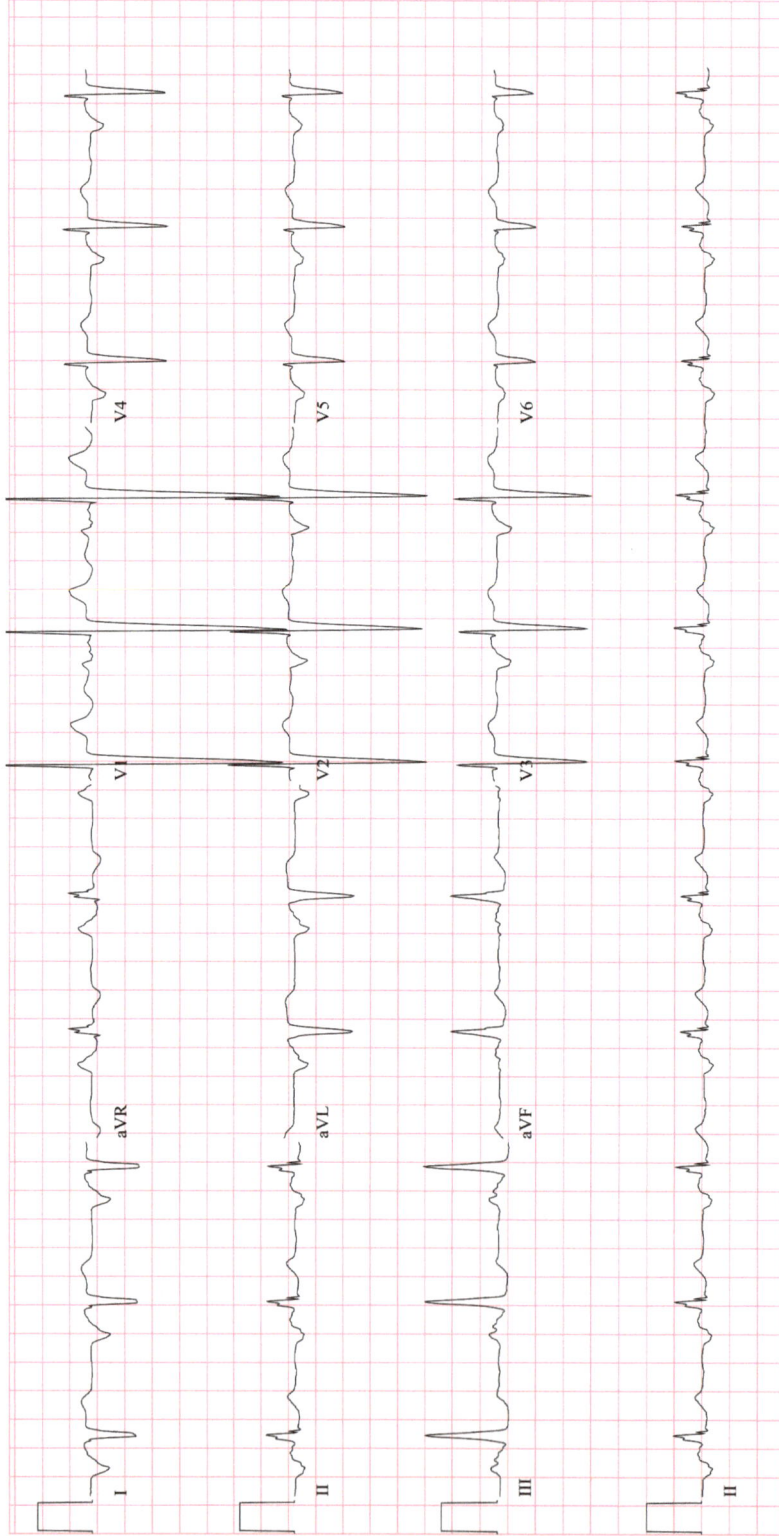

A 26-year-old female with a history of complex, cyanotic, congenital heart disease including right atrial isomerism and dextrocardia presents to the clinic for the first time. An EKG is obtained. What does it show?

DIAGNOSIS: Dextrocardia

In dextrocardia, the electrical axis of the heart is directed inferiorly and to the right. The EKG has the appearance of a tracing in which the left and right arm electrodes are reversed. It has the following features:

- In lead I, all electric waves are inverted i.e, negative P wave, QRS complex, and T wave.
- Positive QRS complex with upright P and T waves in aVR.
- Right axis deviation.
- Due to position of heart, the normal R-wave progression in the chest leads is missing, leading to dominant S waves in all precordial leads.

These changes can be corrected by reversing the left and right arm electrodes and by recording the precordial leads in a mirror image position on the right side of the chest, i.e, progressing from V1R (which is in fact lead V2) to V6R.

Differential Diagnosis:

Accidental reversal of the left and right arm electrodes may produce a similar picture to dextrocardia in the limb leads (but with normal appearances in the precordial leads).

EKG Case 96

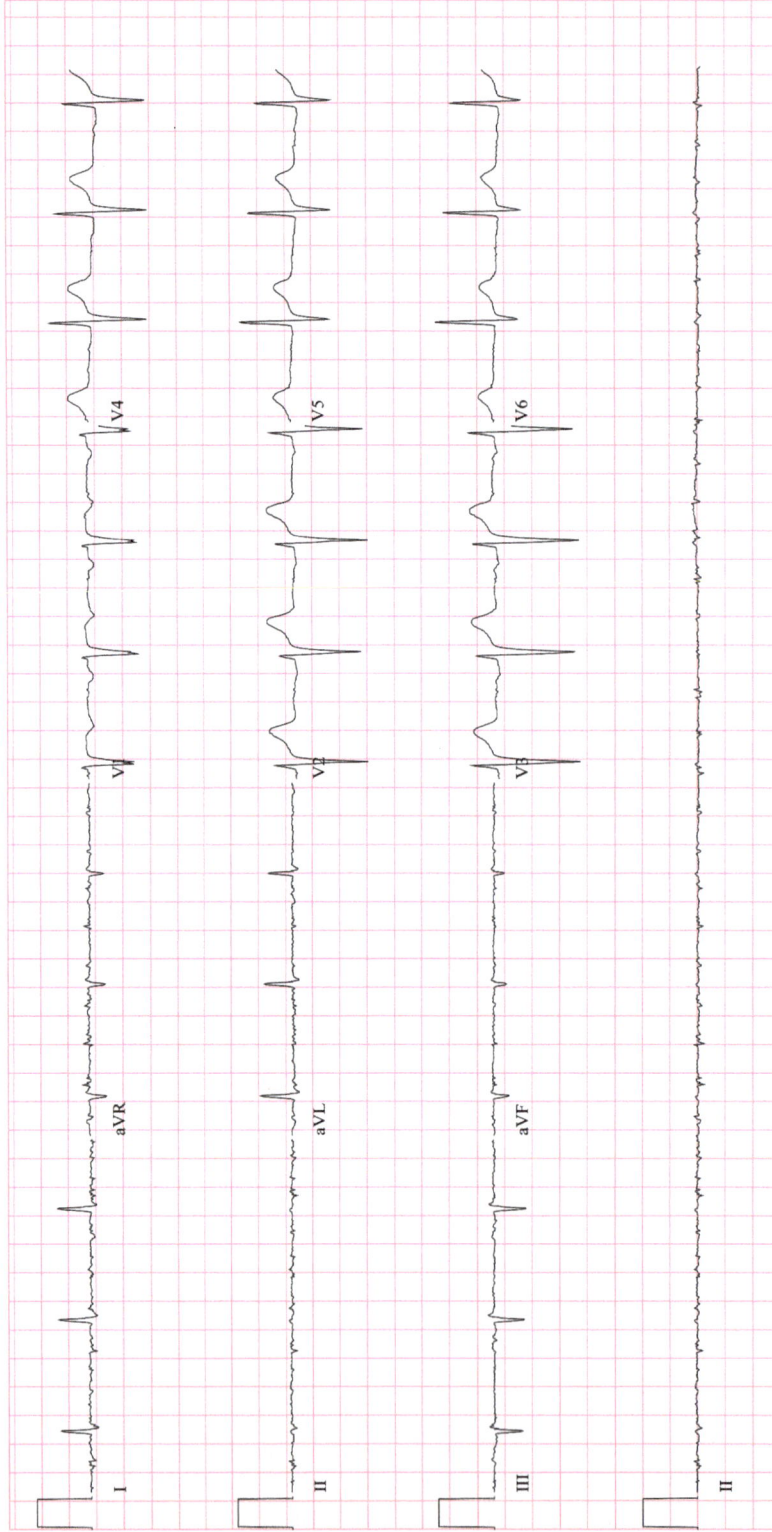

This routine EKG was recorded from a 60-year-old man who had no symptoms but who was found to have high blood pressure on routine examination. What does it show?

DIAGNOSIS: Lead Misplacement (Right Arm and Right Leg)

- The EKG shows right arm and right leg reversal and cannot be reliably interpreted.

Left arm or right arm and right leg reversal.[1]

- When one of the arms is connected to the leg electrodes, this gives a zero signal in that specific arm vector (left arm lead III and right arm lead II).

- This results in a "flat-line" or pseudoasystole of an isolated lead.

- Reversal of the left arm and right leg will result in pseudo-asystole in lead III.

- Similarly, reversal of the right arm and right leg results in pseudoasystole in lead II (as shown above).

- Leg-arm lead reversal could mimic low voltage conditions such as a pericardial effusion or amyloidosis. With lead reversal, this finding is however isolated to one lead.

In the case presented here, the low voltage is only seen in lead II. Furthermore, the precordial leads are all normal, making a lead reversal the most likely diagnosis.

---

1   Baranchuk, Adrian, Catherine Shaw, Haitham Alanazi, Debra Campbell, Kathy Bally, Damian P. Redfearn, Christopher S. Simpson, and Hoshiar Abdollah. "Electrocardiography pitfalls and artifacts: the 10 commandments." *Critical care nurse* 29, no. 1 (2009): 67-73.

EKG Case 97

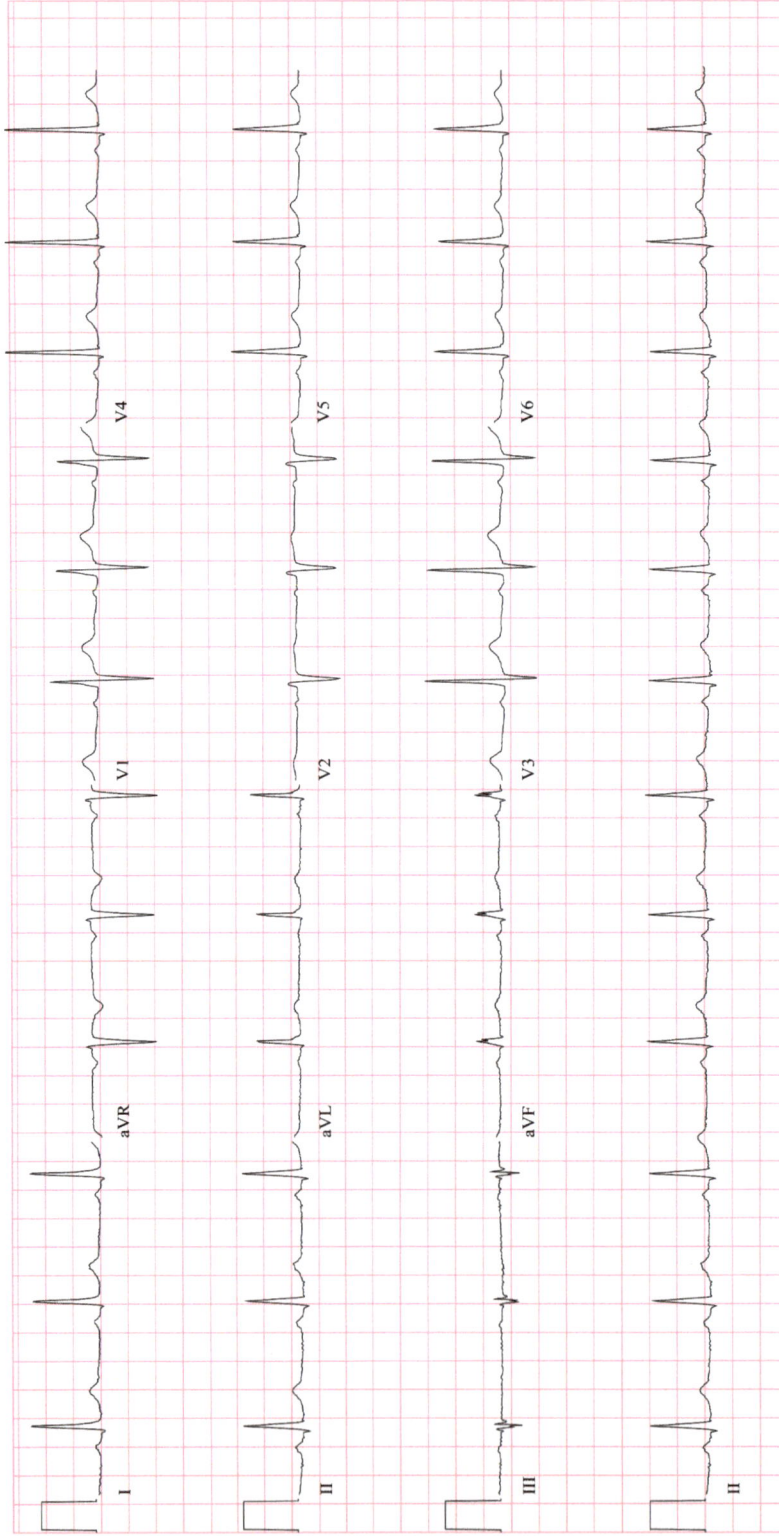

An EKG is recorded on a 25-year-old woman admitted to the ER. Can you spot anything abnormal in this EKG tracing?

DIAGNOSIS: Precordial Leads (V1 - V2) Misplacement - Pseudoinfarction Due to Misplacement of the Precordial Electrodes

This EKG shows normal sinus rhythm at 80 bpm. Close inspection of EKG reveals regressing R/S wave amplitude between V1 and V2. The EKG is otherwise within normal limits.

- It is difficult to ascertain the diagnosis of precordial lead misplacement or misconnection by analyzing a single tracing.

- Precordial lead misplacements are common. They are more likely to happen in obese patients and in women.

- Normally, there should be a gradual transition of R wave increase and S wave decrease in amplitude moving from V1 to V6. Disruption of this gradual transition will result if two precordial electrodes are reversed.

- Improper positioning of the precordial electrodes may result in a pseudo-infarction pattern.

- Cardiac ischemia virtually never occurs in one lead, so such an aberration is suggestive of precordial electrode reversal.

- After the EKG was repeated with careful attention to precordial electrode connections, this finding disappeared.

EKG Case 98

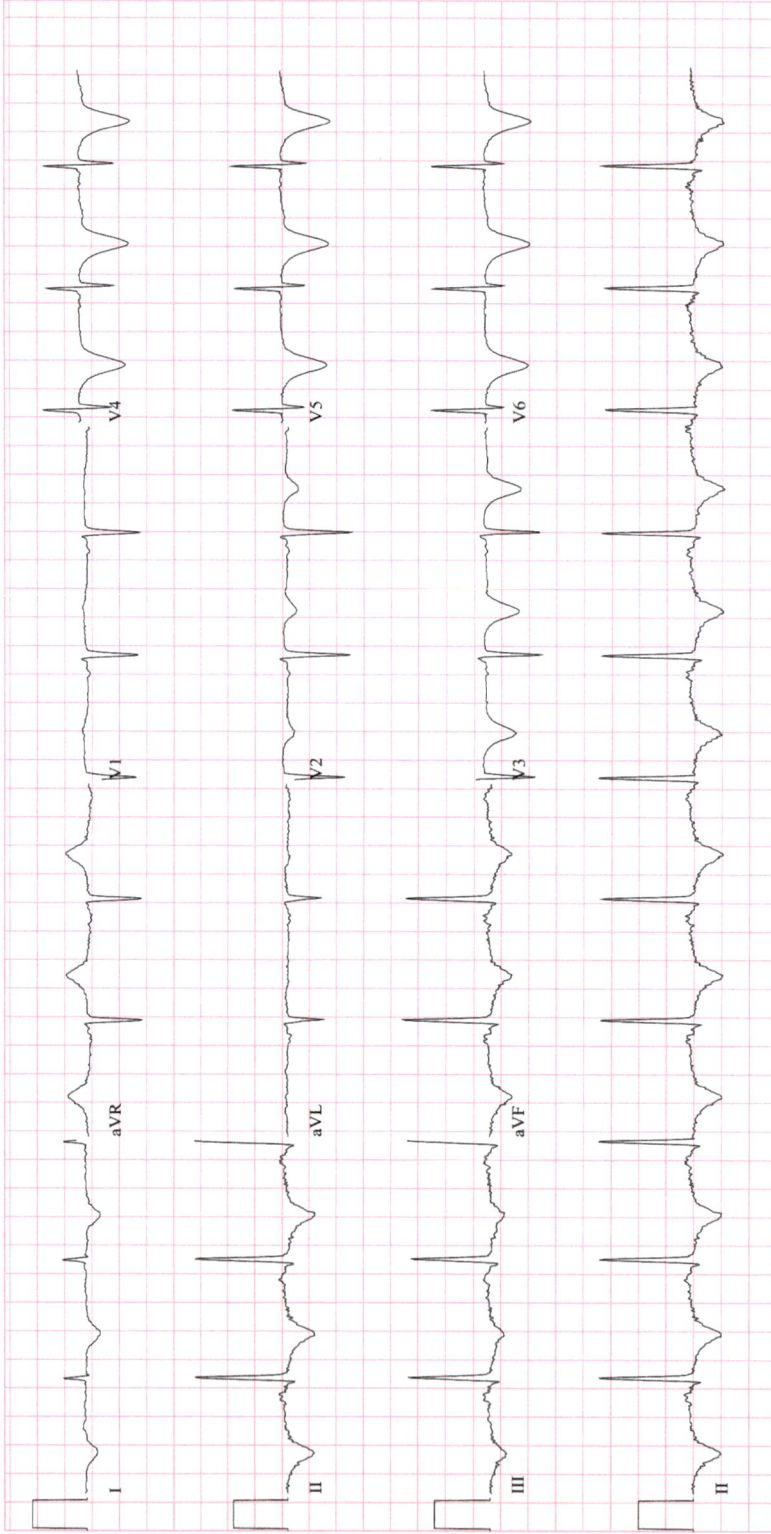

A 52 year-old female presents to the emergency room with chief complaint of severe headache over the last six hours. CT scan of the head is ordered and is pending. Meanwhile, an EKG is obtained and is shown above. What does the EKG show?

DIAGNOSIS: Cerebral T Waves - Changes associated with Acute Subarachnoid Hemorrhage

The EKG shows normal sinus rhythm with diffuse deep T wave inversions and prolonged QTc of 518 ms. This EKG pattern could easily be mistaken for myocardial ischemia, however her CT scan showed massive subarachnoid hemorrhage with normal troponins in the absence of chest pain.

EKG changes due to increased intracranial pressure are most commonly seen with intracranial hemorrhages like subarachnoid hemorrhages or hemorrhagic strokes. The most common EKG findings are:

- Widespread deep T wave inversions known as "cerebral T waves".

- Prolongation of QTc interval.

- Sinus bradycardia (the Cushing reflex - indicates imminent brainstem herniation).

- Other findings include, ST segment depression and increased U wave amplitude.

EKG Case 99

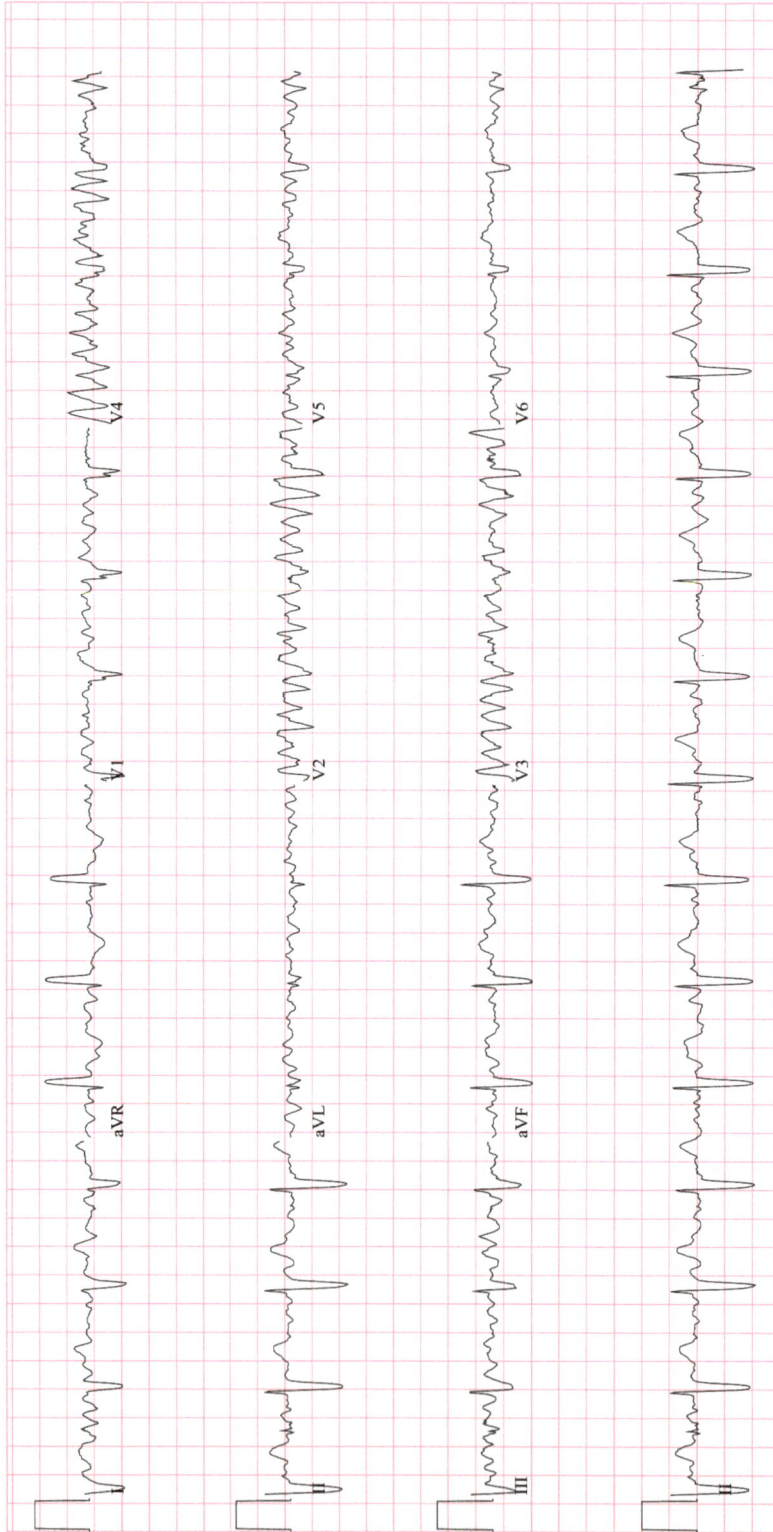

A 65-year-old male with a history of recent heart transplant presents to the office for follow up. He complains of occasional fatigue but otherwise feels good. An EKG is obtained. What does it show?

DIAGNOSIS: Heterotopic Heart Transplant

This EKG shows an example of heterotopic heart transplant. The native (recipient's) rhythm is ventricular fibrillation whereas donor's rhythm is normal sinus rhythm.

Key considerations in orthotropic heart transplant patients:

- The recipient retains the posterior walls of their own atria.

- The transplanted heart is denervated and lacks autonomic neural control.

- The EKG changes in these patients are mainly due to the remnant activity of the recipient's atria, injury to the donor heart during the transplant procedure, and increased PVR (pulmonary vascular resistance) in the recipient.

- Atrial arrhythmias and ventricular conduction defects are common.

- Role of the EKG in acute rejection is controversial.

EKG Features Include:

- The recipient's native P waves are usually of a small amplitude.

- Donor P waves have normal amplitude and configuration.

- The suture line between the donor and the recipient atria blocks any interchange of the electrical impulses from the two sources. Atrial dissociation is present. The donor P wave is conducted and stimulates the ventricles. The recipient's atrial impulses are not conducted.

- P waves of the recipient atrial remnants may not be seen because of their small amplitude or the presence of sinus node dysfunction or atrial fibrillation prior to the transplantation. May also lose the sinus node artery during surgery.

- Atrial fibrillation or flutter may be present in one set of atria while NSR is present in the other pair, making interpretation difficult.

- The other most prevalent EKG abnormalities are: incomplete or complete right bundle branch block, shift of QRS axis to the left, shorter QT interval, decreased precordial voltage.

Orthotopic Approach. The more common of the two procedures, the orthotopic approach, requires replacing the recipient heart with the donor heart. **Heterotopic Approach**. Heterotopic transplantation, also called "piggyback" transplantation, is accomplished by leaving the recipient's heart in place and connecting the donor heart to the right side of the chest (as in the present case).

EKG Case 100

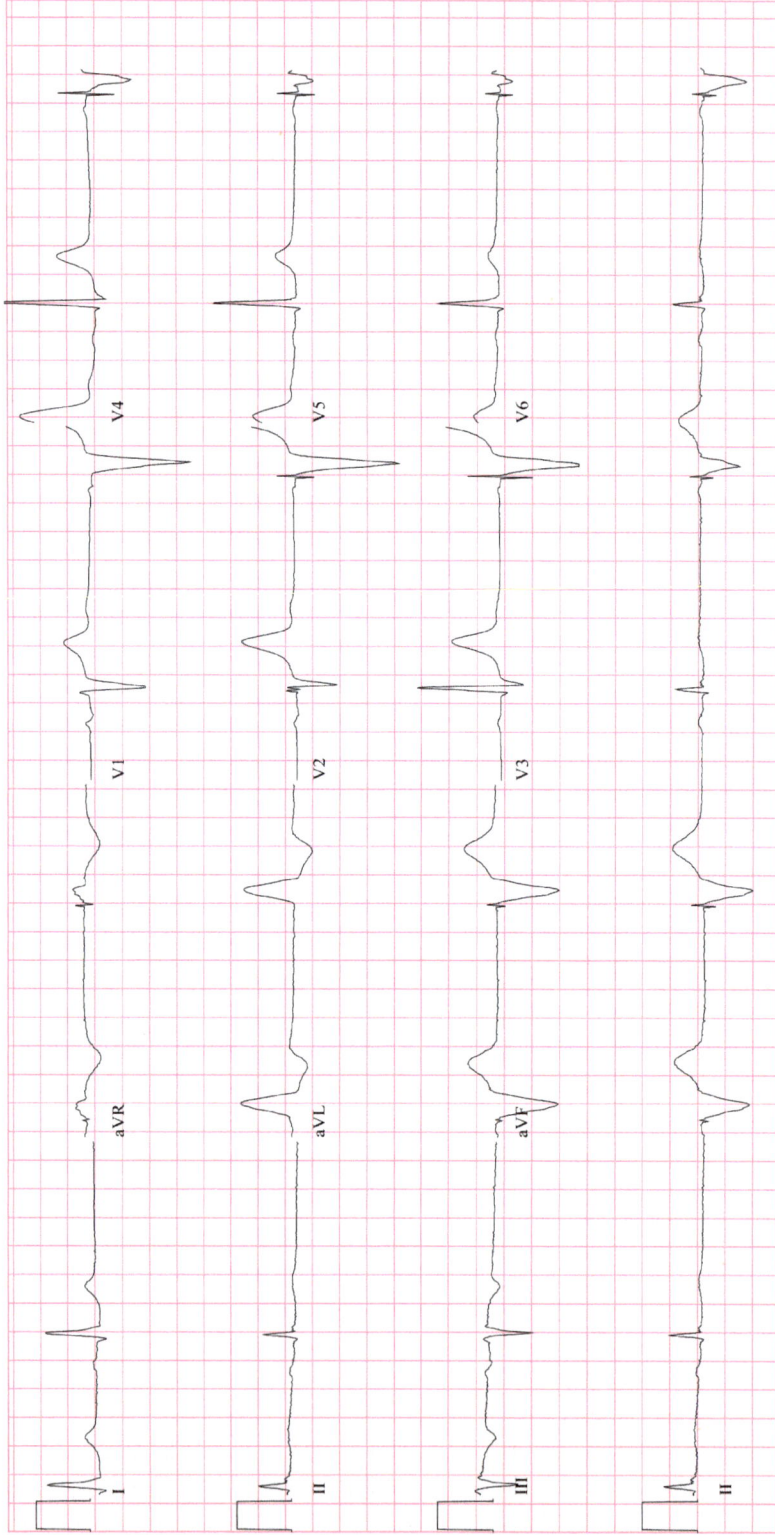

A 70-year-old female with a history of non-ischemic cardiomyopathy presents to the office for a routine checkup. An EKG is obtained. What does it show?

DIAGNOSIS: Right Ventricular Pacing in VVI (Demand) Mode and Fusion Beats. Underlying Rhythm Sinus Bradycardia with First Degree AV Block

- In ventricular pacing, spike precedes the QRS complex.

- Right ventricle pacing lead placement at the apex results in a QRS morphology similar to LBBB with superior axis. Left ventricular pacing lead placement results in a QRS morphology similar to RBBB.

- During ventricular pacing, the ST segments and T waves are usually discordant with the QRS complex, i.e, the major terminal portion of the QRS complex is located on the opposite side of the baseline from the ST segment and T wave.

- The width of the paced QRS complexes in the above EKG varies depending on the degree of fusion between the paced rhythm and the native supraventricular conduction from sinus bradycardia.

Pacemaker codes

The North American Society of Pacing and Electrophysiology and the British Pacing and Electrophysiology Group have developed a code to describe various pacing modes.[1] It usually consists of three to five letters:

- Letter 1: chamber that is paced (A = atria, V = ventricles, D = dual-chamber, 0 = none, i.e, pacemaker is off).

- Letter 2: chamber that is sensed (A = atria, V = ventricles, D = dual-chamber, 0 = none).

- Letter 3: response to a sensed event (T = triggered, I = inhibited, D = dual).

- Letter 4: rate-responsive features; an activity sensor (e.g, an accelerometer in the pulse generator) in single or dual-chamber pacemakers detects bodily movement and increases the pacing rate according to a programmable algorithm (R = rate-responsive pacemaker). Other sensors may use minute ventilation or other physiologic signals to determine the appropriate rate of pacing.

- Letter 5: anti-tachycardia pacing.

VVI Mode - (above example). Ventricle paced, ventricle sensed; pacing inhibited if intrinsic beat sensed.

- A pacemaker in VVI mode denotes that it paces and senses the ventricle and is inhibited by a sensed ventricular event. Also known as ventricle demand mode.

- Used in patients with chronic atrial impairment, e.g, atrial fibrillation or flutter.

- The DDD mode denotes that both chambers are capable of being sensed and paced.

---

1   Bernstein, Alan D., JEAN-CLAUDE Daubert, ROSS D. Fletcher, DAVID L. Hayes, B. E. R. N. D. T. Luderitz, DWIGHT W. Reynolds, MARK H. Schoenfeld, and R. I. C. H. A. R. D. Sutton. "The revised NASPE/BPEG generic code for antibradycardia, adaptive-rate, and multisite pacing." *Pacing and clinical electrophysiology* 25, no. 2 (2002): 260-264.

Commonly Used Pacemaker Modes: The codes[1] are:

- **AAI:** The atria are paced, when the intrinsic atrial rhythm falls below the pacemaker's rate threshold. Used in sinus node dysfunction with intact AV conduction. Also known as atrial demand mode.

- **VVI:** The ventricles are paced, when the intrinsic ventricular rhythm falls below the pacemaker's rate threshold. Similar to AAI mode but involving ventricles instead of the atrium.

- **VDD:** The pacemaker senses atrial and ventricular events, but can only pace the ventricle. This type of pacemaker is used in patients with a reliable sinus node, but with AV conduction abnormalities.

- **DDD:** The pacemaker records both atrial and ventricular rates and can pace either chamber when needed. Most commonly used mode. Atrial pacing occurs if no native atrial activity above pacemaker rate cutoff. Ventricular pacing occurs if no native ventricle activity for set time (programmed AV interval) following atrial activity.

- **DDDR:** As above, but the pacemaker has a sensor that determines the patient's physical activity and adjusts the lower rate of pacing accordingly.

1   Vardas, Panos E., Angelo Auricchio, Jean-Jacques Blanc, Jean-Claude Daubert, Helmut Drexler, Hugo Ector, Maurizio Gasparini et al. "Guidelines for cardiac pacing and cardiac resynchronization therapy." *Europace* 9, no. 10 (2007): 959-998.

This page intentionally left blank.

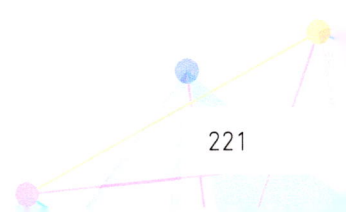

EKG Case 101

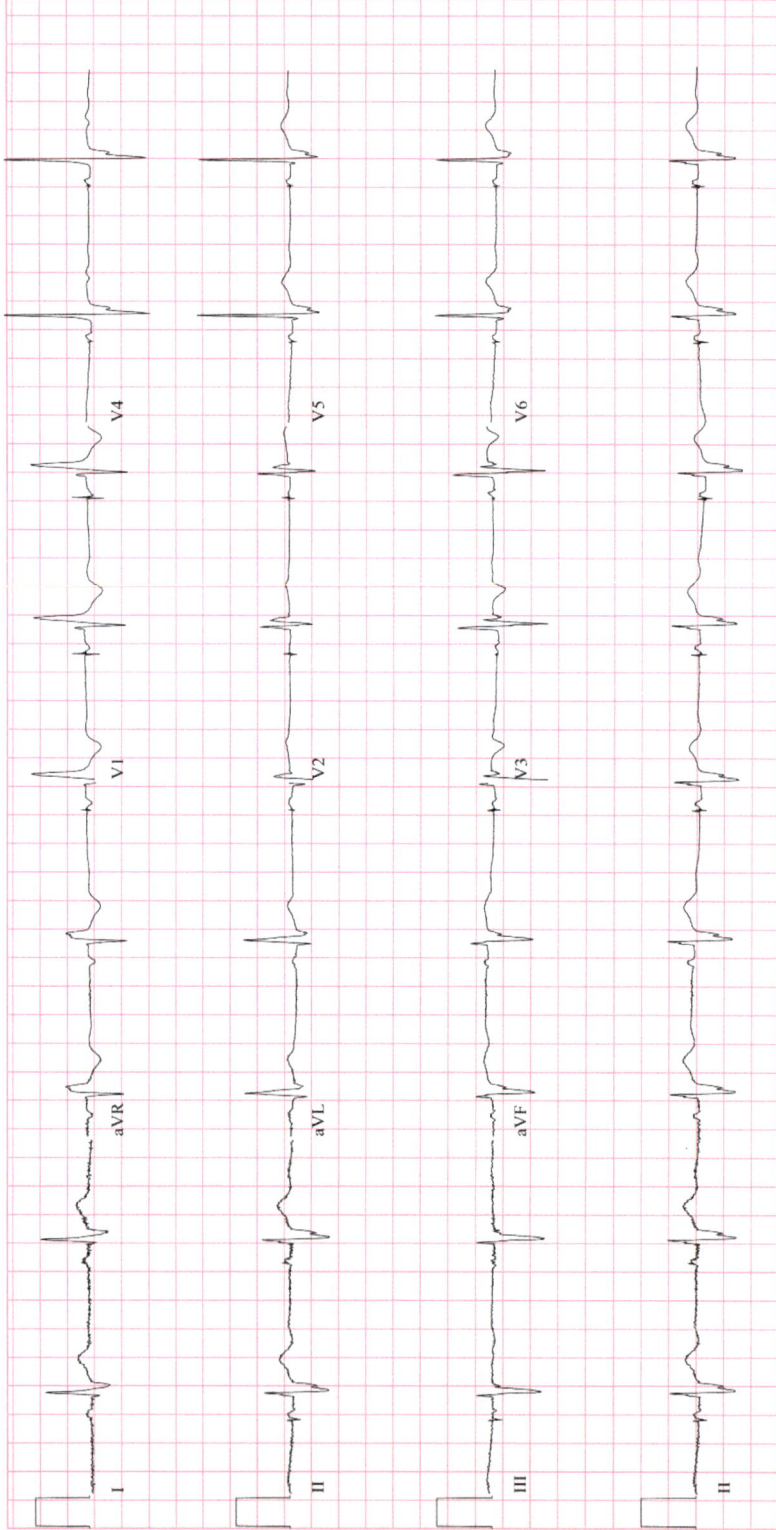

A 28 year male with a history of Down's syndrome, AV septal defect including endocardial cushion defect status post repair presents to office for a routine follow up. An EKG is obtained. What does the EKG show?

DIAGNOSIS: Atrial Paced Rhythm

This EKG shows atrial paced rhythm with intermittent sinus rhythm, fusion, and pseudofusion, left axis deviation (LAFB), and right bundle branch block.

- In above example, the sinus rate is almost equal to the set pacing rate from the pacemaker; thus the 3rd and 4th beats are not paced.

- The second beat shows pseudofusion, i.e, the P wave starts before the pacing spike is delivered but not early enough to inhibit pacing.

- Other beats show varying degrees of fusion (pacing spike to P wave distance is varying). Best seen in the two complexes highlighted below.

- In atrial pacing, pacing spike (highlighted below) precedes the P wave.

- Morphology of the P wave depends on atrial lead placement and may accordingly appear normal, biphasic, or negative.

- PR interval and configuration of the QRS complex are similar to those seen in sinus rhythm, but often there is evidence of first degree AV block on the paced EKG that is not apparent on their baseline tracing. This is because the intraatrial time may be prolonged depending on where the atrial pacing lead is placed.

- The rhythm can be entirely paced or exhibit demand function, i.e, the pacing is only activated when the intrinsic atrial rate falls below a preset rate.

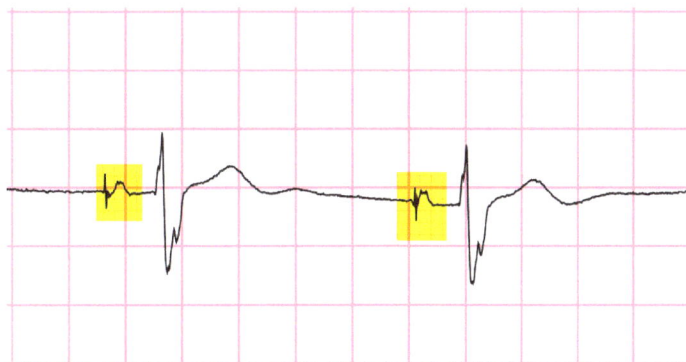

Figure: A single atrial pacemaker spike followed by P wave as seen in atrial pacing rhythm

EKG Case 102

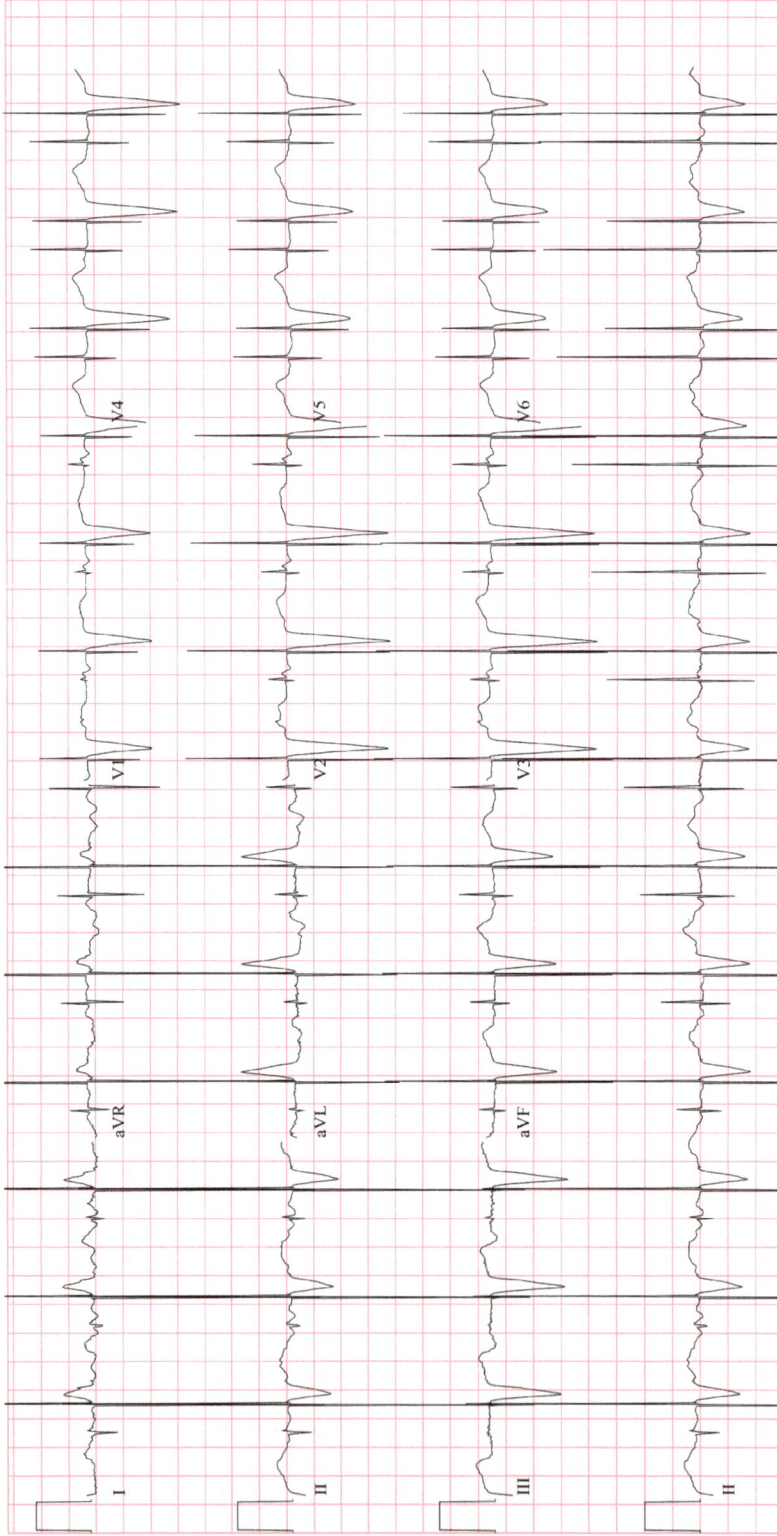

An 86-year-old female with a history of ischemic heart disease, hypertension, and congestive heart failure presents with complaints of fatigue. An EKG is obtained. What does it show?

DIAGNOSIS: Dual Chamber Atrioventricular (AV) Sequential Pacing

- Atrial and ventricular pacing spikes are visible before each P wave and QRS complex.

- There is 100% atrial capture - small P waves are seen following each atrial pacing spike. In demand pacing, if the intrinsic atrial rate is faster than the programmed lower rate of the pacemaker, then no pacing spikes are delivered. The paced P wave morphology depends on the location of the lead within right atrium. The programmed AV interval on the pacemaker (in DDD mode) determines the actual time delay between the atrial and ventricular stimuli.

- There is 100% ventricular capture - a QRS complex follows each ventricular pacing spike. QRS complexes are broad with a LBBB morphology, superior axis, and a negative deflection in V5 and V6, indicating that the pacing electrode is in the inferior right ventricle at the apex.

- Chronic RV pacing may contribute to the development of cardiomyopathy and heart failure, presumably through dyssynchronous activation of the ventricles.

EKG Case 103

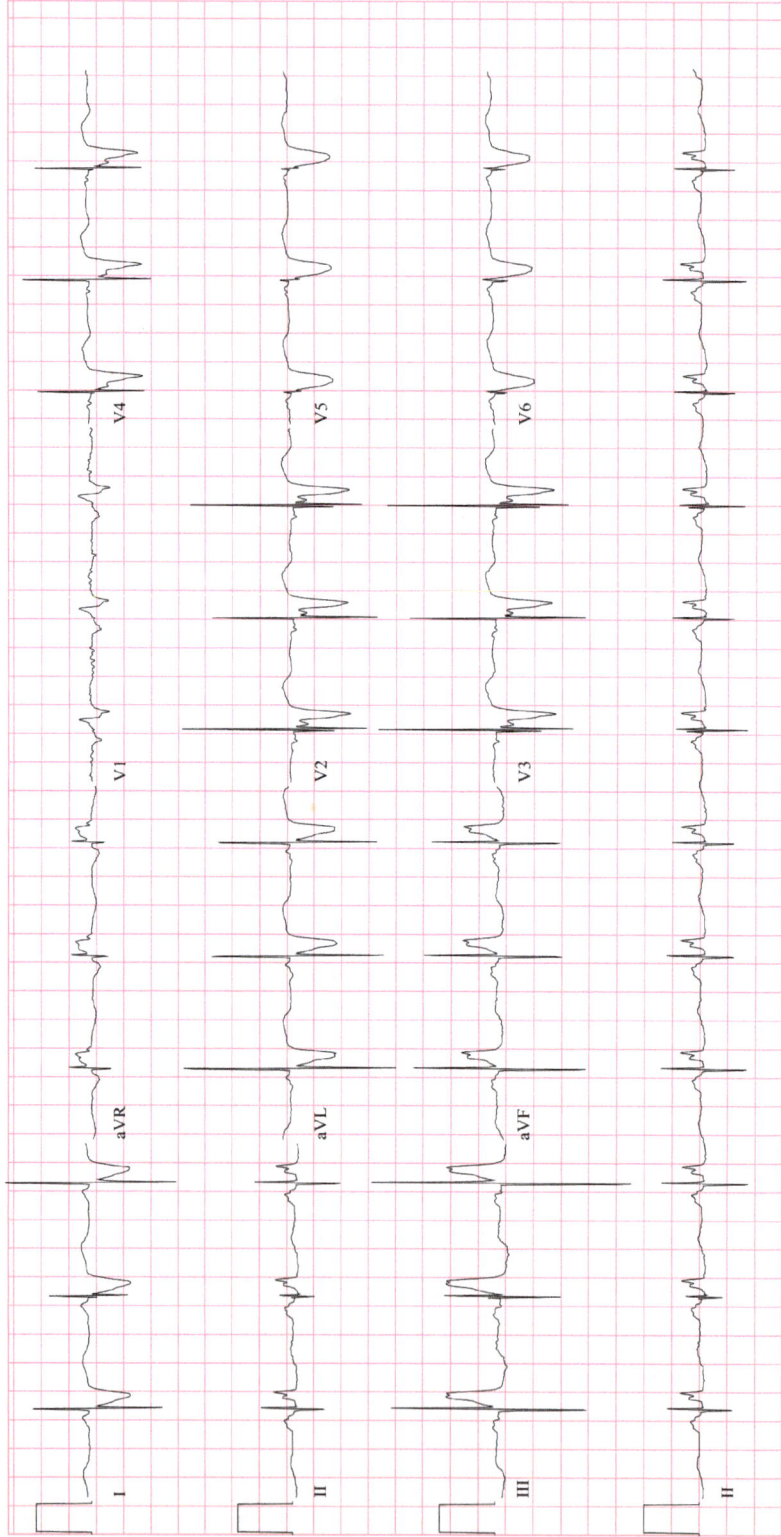

A 65-year-old male with a history of ischemic heart disease, congestive heart failure (NYHA class III), hypertension, and an ejection fraction of 20% presents for a routine checkup. An EKG is obtained. What does it show?

DIAGNOSIS: Biventricular Pacing - Cardiac Resynchronization Therapy

The above EKG shows normal sinus rhythm at 70 bpm with pacemaker spikes preceding QRS complexes. The rhythm is an atrial-sensed, ventricular-paced rhythm. The QRS morphology shows a positive R wave in V1 and a relatively narrower paced complex, consistent with biventricular pacing.

Congestive heart failure (CHF) is a common, debilitating, and usually lethal condition responsible for enormous burden on health care. The association of asynchronous right ventricular contraction with ventricular dysfunction has been recognized for many years. In recent years, the presence of left bundle branch block (LBBB) has been shown to correlate with decreased LV function. LBBB results in asynchronous ventricular contraction with the LV lateral wall, contracting much later than the interventricular septum. In addition, there is an RV-LV asynchrony with RV contracting earlier than LV. Cardiac resynchronization therapy (CRT) attempts to fix this problem by simultaneously pacing both ventricles (biventricular or BiV pacing).

Standard ventricular pacing is from right ventricle and leads to the QRS complex which has left bundle branch morphology. The impulses are generated from the right ventricle and are conducted to the left ventricle. On the EKG, it produces tall and broad R waves in leads I, V5, and V6, with deep QS complex in lead V1.

In BiV pacing, the pacing leads are placed in right atrium, right ventricle, and the coronary sinus branch (which results in stimulation of the left ventricle). Ventricle pacing occurs from both the right ventricular and coronary sinus/left ventricular leads. Biventricular devices allow separate programming of LV and RV stimulation, with the aim of "optimizing" the depolarization vector to overcome the adverse hemodynamic effects associated with ventricular conduction delays. Depending on the timing of pacing between the two leads, the QRS axis and morphology may change significantly. A QS complex in leads V5 - V6 and a tall R wave in lead V1 are strongly suggestive of biventricular pacing. Also, an initial Q wave or a QS complex in lead I is definitive for left or biventricular pacing.

An interesting review article by S. Serge Barold, MD, titled "Usefulness of the 12-lead electrocardiogram in the follow-up of patients with cardiac resynchronization devices" [1] evaluates the EKG morphologies in biventricular pacing in depth.

---

1   Barold, S. Serge, and Bengt Herweg. "Usefulness of the 12-lead electrocardiogram in the follow-up of patients with cardiac resynchronization devices. Part I." *Cardiology journal* 18, no. 5 (2011): 476-486.

EKG Case 104

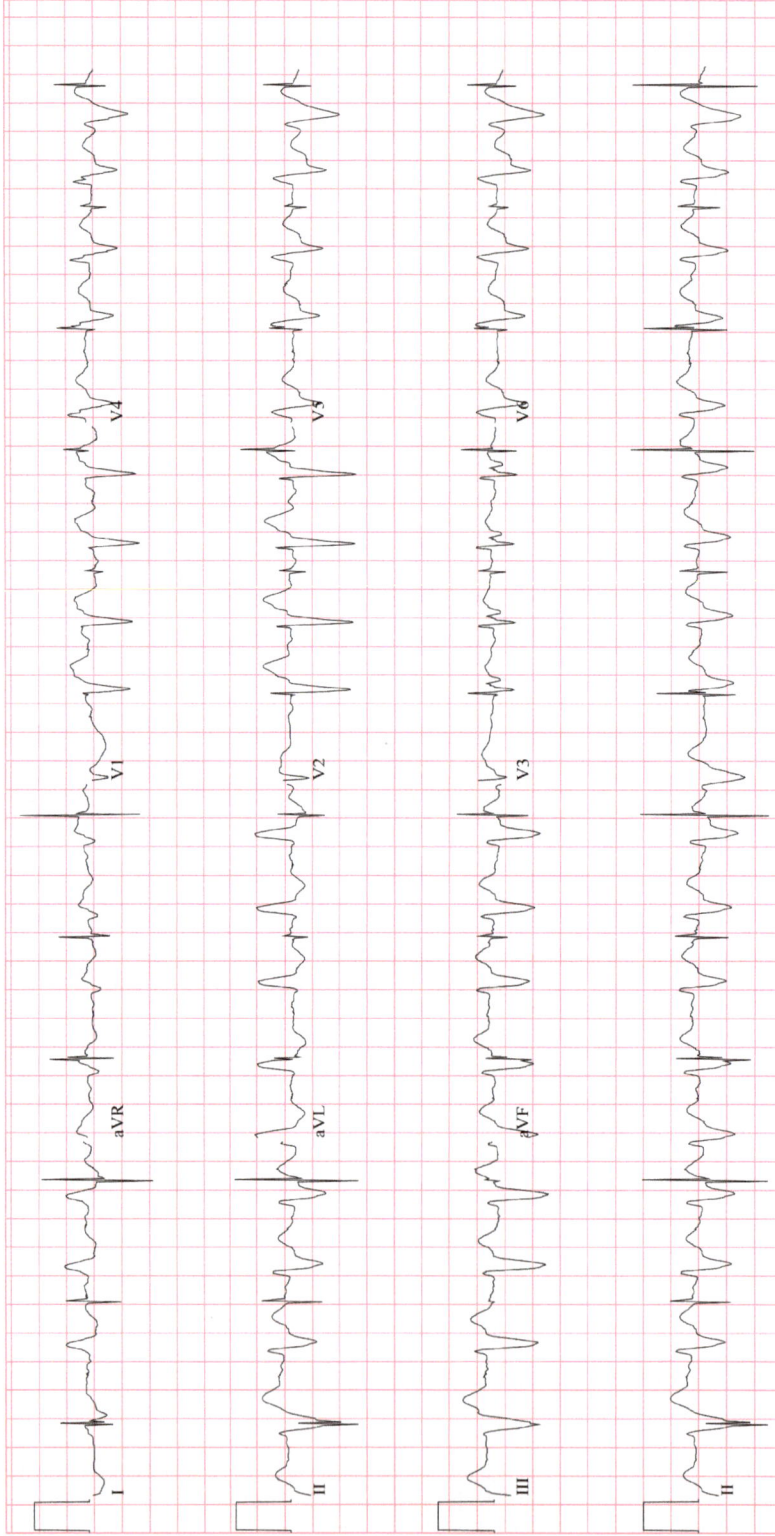

A 75-year-old male with a history of atrial fibrillation and congestive heart failure is brought from a nursing home with shortness of breath. Chest x-ray reveals pulmonary edema and bilateral pleural effusion. An EKG is obtained. What does the EKG show?

DIAGNOSIS: Atrial Fibrillation with Rapid Ventricular Rate and Pacemaker Malfunction; Failure to Sense (Undersensing)

The above EKG shows atrial fibrillation with ventricular response of 120 bpm. The EKG also shows asynchronous pacing spikes completely independent of the intrinsic rhythm going at a rate of about 70 bpm, compatible with failure to sense or undersensing.

- Pacemaker has both a sensing circuit and an output, or pacing circuit. The pacer has to sense whether or not the patient is generating an intrinsic rhythm, in which case pacing in the corresponding chamber is inhibited.

- Undersensing occurs when the pacemaker fails to recognize ("see") intrinsic activity in the chamber of interest. Depending on the refractoriness of the tissue, the pacing spikes that are delivered asynchronously may or may not capture the myocardium.

- This results in asynchronous pacing, where the pacing spikes occur indiscriminately throughout the cardiac cycle.

- Causes of undersensing include, asynchronous mode (pacemaker programmed not to sense intrinsic cardiac signal), intrinsic ventricular activity in blanking period of device, lead position, low QRS voltage, break in connection (poor lead contact), faulty generator, battery failure, etc.

- EKG findings may be minimal, although presence of pacing spikes within QRS complexes is suggestive of undersensing.

- Failure to sense can rarely lead to R-on-T phenomenon, which may result in ventricular fibrillation.

- Undersensing requires identification of the cause and treatment, which often consists of device reprogramming.

EKG Case 105

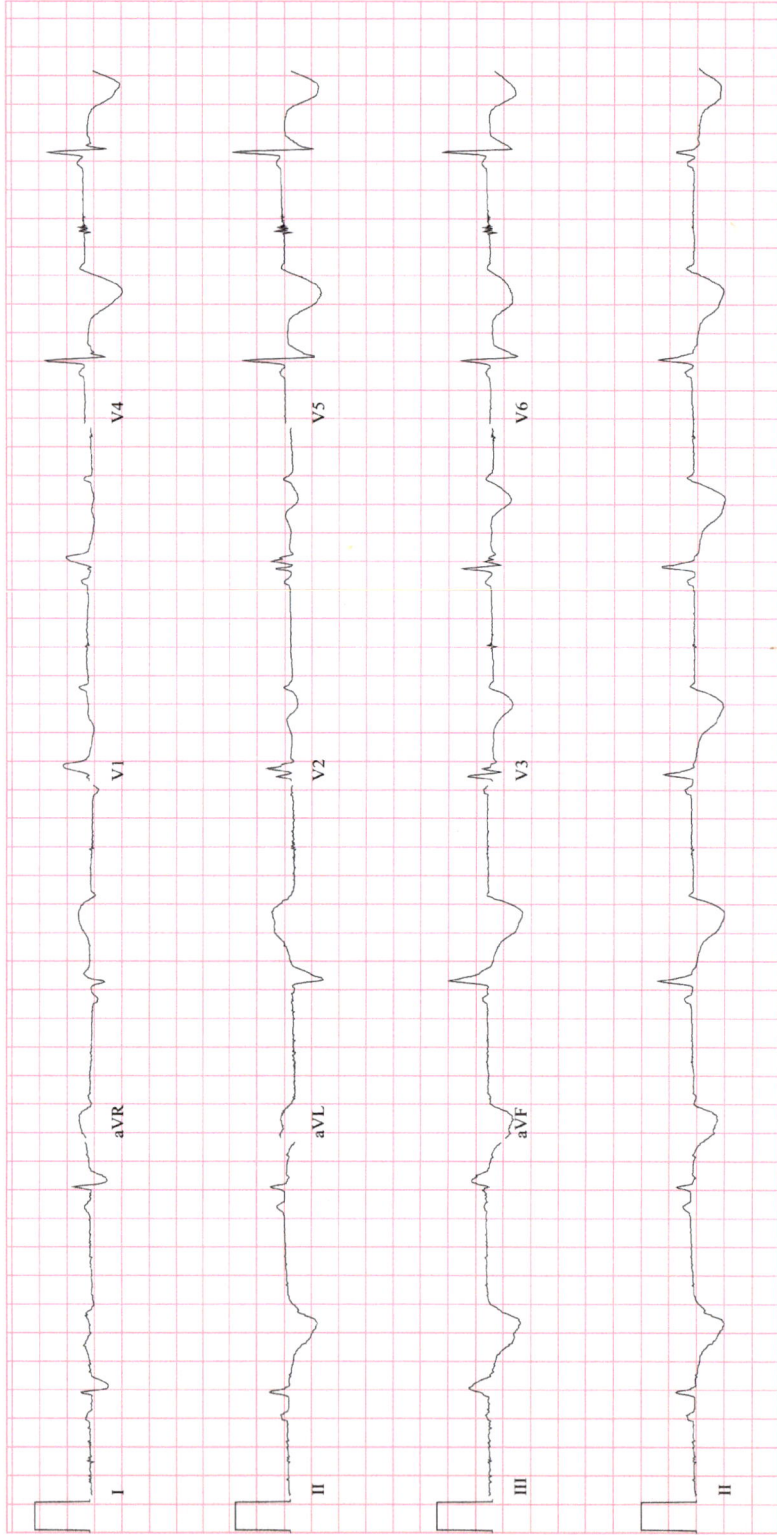

A 82-year-old female is brought to the ER by EMS after a witnessed fall and syncope. On arrival, the patient is obtunded and she is emergently intubated. An EKG is obtained. What does the EKG show and can it explain the syncope?

DIAGNOSIS: Sinus Bradycardia with Complete Heart Block, Long QT, Junctional Escape Rhythm. Pacemaker Malfunction; Failure to Capture

This EKG shows sinus bradycardia with AV dissociation. Underlying rhythm is junctional escape at 35 bpm. Small (bipolar) pacing spikes (highlighted below) are delivered from an implanted pacemaker but do not capture either the atria or the ventricles.

- Failure to capture can be diagnosed when the pacing spikes are not followed immediately by myocardial depolarization as either a P wave (atrium) or QRS complex (ventricle).

- Failure to capture may be intermittent, so that only occasional non-captured pacemaker stimuli are seen.

- It could be persistent, where no capture complexes are seen following any of the pacing spikes. If an intrinsic activity is present (junctional escape above example), the pacemaker stimuli are dissociated from the native P waves and/or QRS complexes. There may be no underlying activity in pacemaker-dependent patients with failure to capture, which could lead to asystole and death.

- Loss of capture may be due to lead dislodgement, perforation, or malposition of a pacing lead, inflammation or fibrosis at the lead/tissue interface, low pacemaker output (below capture threshold), lead failure, or battery depletion.

- If the patient's native heart rate is above the pacemaker lower rate cutoff, no pacemaker spikes are seen and therefore output failure and capture failure cannot be recognized on the EKG.

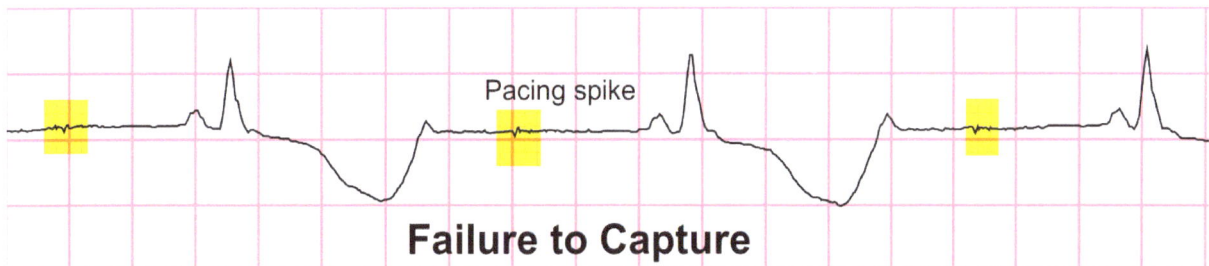

Pacing spike

Failure to Capture

EKG Case 106

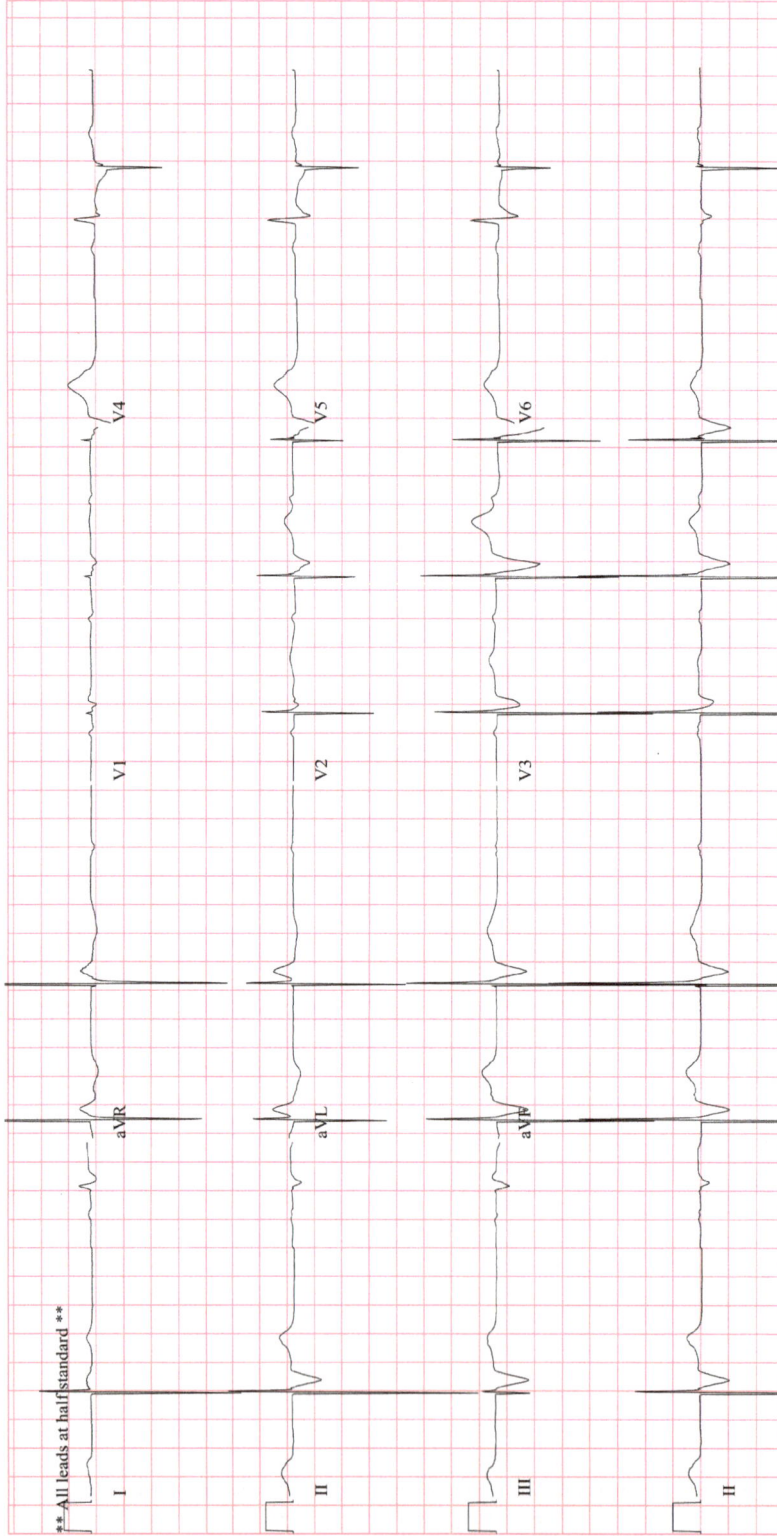

** All leads at half standard **

I   aVR   V1   V4

II   aVL   V2   V5

III   aVF   V3   V6

II

A 75-year-old male presents to the office with intermittent dizziness. Physical examination reveals irregular heart rhythm. An EKG is obtained. What does it show?

DIAGNOSIS: Sinus Rhythm (Atrial Rate 75 bpm), High Grade AV Block, Ventricular Electronic Pacemaker with Intermittent Failure to Pace (Oversensing)

- Failure to pace, also known as oversensing, occurs when the pacemaker does not generate an electrical impulse when it is expected to do so. On an EKG tracing, pacing spikes are missing.

- Oversensing occurs when physiologic (e.g, T wave) or non-physiologic (e.g, noise) electrical signals are inappropriately sensed as native cardiac activity and pacing is consequently inhibited.

- Abnormal signals may not be evident on EKG, but the absence of pacing spike indicates the presence of a signal that was picked up by the pacemaker.

- Oversensing can result from electromagnetic interference, such as from electrocautery or other electrical interference, diaphragmatic myopotentials, and pectoral muscle myopotentials, particularly if unipolar sensing mode (from pacemaker can to the tip of the pacing lead) is programmed. Noise due to lead fracture and far-field signals from pacing in another cardiac chamber (so called "crosstalk") are also causes of oversensing.

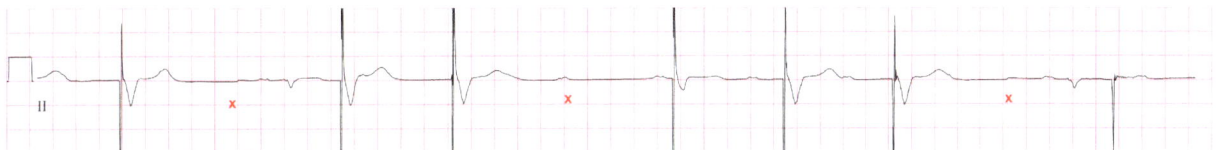

In above example, x marks failure to pace

Notes:

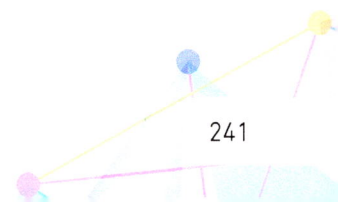

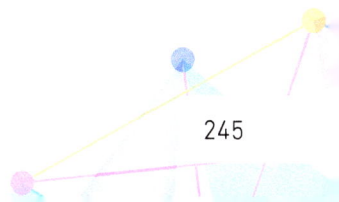